Integrative Treatment of Male Infertility with Chinese Medicine

of related interest

Increasing IVF Success with Acupuncture
An Integrated Approach
Nick Dalton-Brewer
ISBN 978 1 84819 218 8
eISBN 978 0 85701 165 7

Understanding and Treating Hot Flashes in Menopause with Chinese Medicine
Brian Grosam
Foreword by Dr Yubin Lu
ISBN 978 1 78775 538 3
eISBN 978 1 78775 539 0

Acupressure and Acupuncture During Birth
An Integrative Guide for Acupuncturists and Birth Professionals
Claudia Citkovitz
ISBN 978 1 84819 358 1
eISBN 978 0 85701 317 0

Integrative Treatment of
Male Infertility
with Chinese
Medicine

DR OLIVIA POJER

Forewords by Jane Lyttleton and Ashok Agarwal

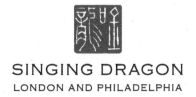

SINGING DRAGON
LONDON AND PHILADELPHIA

First published in Great Britain in 2023 by Singing Dragon, an imprint of Jessica Kingsley Publishers
An imprint of Hodder & Stoughton Ltd
An Hachette Company

2

*The information contained in this book is not intended to replace the services of trained medical
professionals or to be a substitute for medical advice. The complementary therapy described in
this book may not be suitable for everyone to follow. You are advised to consult a doctor before
embarking on any complementary therapy programme and on any matters relating to your
health, and in particular on any matters that may require diagnosis or medical attention.*

A CIP catalogue record for this title is available from the British Library and the Library of Congress

ISBN 978 1 78775 732 5
eISBN 978 1 78775 733 2

Printed and bound in the United States by Integrated Books International

Jessica Kingsley Publishers' policy is to use papers that are natural, renewable and recyclable
products and made from wood grown in sustainable forests. The logging and manufacturing
processes are expected to conform to the environmental regulations of the country of origin.

Jessica Kingsley Publishers
Carmelite House
50 Victoria Embankment
London EC4Y 0DZ

www.singingdragon.com

*Dedicated to my daughter Mirjam,
my very personal miracle of life.*

Contents

Foreword

The state of male fertility in most countries in the world is dire and it continues to deteriorate. Sperm numbers are dwindling, their shapes are not normal and some are swimming in circles. And yet there is surprisingly little discussion about this global fertility problem. At the time of writing, there are no quick easy medical cures for male infertility on offer. So here is a book of its time, and it's not before time! Infertility affects 15% of couples. That (the WHO tells us) means that 96 to 186 million people are affected worldwide. Male infertility contributes to a half of this number. That's a heck of a lot of men!

But what are these men doing about it? Sadly, if my patient population (and that of my colleagues) is anything to go by, not very much. From our perspective as clinicians working in fertility, it is not unusual to note that there is often minimal pro-activity in terms of men seeking out treatment for infertility. Added to these shocking global figures is the fact that male infertility is one of the most common reasons for couples attending an IVF clinic. But IVF clinics don't have any cure for under-performing and poor looking sperm (they do however offer a bypass technique – known as intracytoplasmic sperm injection or ICSI). In the current era of the ICSI fix for all male infertility issues, IVF clinics have reduced their focus on the male partner to not much beyond a quick semen collection in a jar followed by the steady hand of an expert embryologist. It would not be unreasonable to say that men have been left undervalued, undermanaged and undertreated in this field of infertility.

Enter Chinese Medicine and Olivia Pojer, and the book you hold in your hand – which, with its chatty and humorous approach, leaves no stone unturned in its examination of all things male fertility. Let me add that it is not just modern Western Medicine that has neglected men in this field. Historically not much attention was paid to male fertility in Chinese Medicine either (unless of course there were problems with sexual function, and then it got the highest level of attention, a situation not dissimilar to what we might see in modern clinics in the West).

'Nan Ke' (the study of men) is therefore a relatively new speciality in TCM, and in this book, is compellingly informed by a modern Western understanding of anatomy and physiology. We all have a lot to learn about the intricacies of what goes on in those amazing testicular factories churning out millions upon millions of extraordinary cells shaped like, but much more powerful than, torpedoes. While acknowledging it is still a new science, this book covers everything we currently know about sperm genesis, sperm health, semen analysis and what factors affect these – all presented in detail and in easy-to-follow diagrams. And the second half of the book presents what Olivia Pojer calls a 'bag of tricks', listing many acupuncture and herbal treatment options gathered from Chinese Medicine doctors, both historical and modern.

But let's be honest about this – talking (and writing) about treating male infertility is much easier than actually doing it. As alluded to above, it's my experience and the experience of most of my colleagues that it's not easy to get the blokes to come in for treatment… It's not something that just happens in Australia (where I practice TCM); my American and European colleagues have described the same. Those men that do come for treatment for infertility are referred by their female partners – (often presenting reluctantly) and many don't stay the distance. In my last few decades of working in infertility I have, more times than I can count, observed the frustration and despair of my female patients who carry most or all of the burden of improving fertility and trying to conceive, while her male partner does little to change habits that might be compromising fertility – often because the male reproductive specialist they consulted said *No worries mate, your swimmers are great*. I see this as a reflection of a blokey culture and am pleased to say it is changing – but slowly.

A book like this one is an excellent step in this direction of positive change. Hopefully it will not only inform its readers about TCM and other approaches for male infertility but will also give its readers the confidence to reach out to and educate our young male population (the ones who will be fathering our next generation) to let them know that infertility has *nothing* to do with virility, that it is *common*, and that there are some things that can be done – other than IVF/ICSI. For us clinicians this book adds important information on what can be gleaned from the semen analysis lab results – not the least of which is the window on general and future health that such an analysis can indicate.

We have long relied on menstrual cycle details to give us useful insights to whole body systemic health of women, but do not have an equivalent useful insight for men. As we continue to learn more about what the fine details of semen analysis mean, this may help fill some of this gap. A semen analysis that records normal range values for sperm count, morphology and motility usually gets a big tick from the reproductive specialist – and the man leaves the consult relieved and smiling. Nothing wrong with me!

Well wait a moment, that may not be the end of the story. As Olivia Pojer points out, sperm health and male fertility is more than the number, the shape and the purposeful wriggling. What is inside the chromosomes in the invisible-to-the-eye DNA makes a huge difference to embryo quality and establishing a viable pregnancy. How many patients do I see who suffer the pain of a first trimester miscarriage who then add to their grief with self-recrimination? 'I shouldn't have flown, shouldn't have drunk that champagne, shouldn't have lifted heavy shopping' and so on, but none of them say 'my partner shouldn't have been drinking so much, working out and overheating so much, had those back X-rays'.

The author makes a compelling case for a much closer look at DNA integrity in sperm, implicated as it is in IVF failures, miscarriage and the future health of the baby. She explains that the methylation patterns of the DNA and the way it is packaged are important indicators that warrant more investigation before the couple heads straight for ICSI (and couples relying on assisted reproduction should know that embryos formed with IVF do better than embryos formed with ICSI). There are many strategies to be considered in addressing this issue of DNA damage.

This book covers current knowledge on the impact diet and supplements can have, the effect of elevated temperature from clothing, exercise or laptops, the roles of sleep and stress, dental health, sex timing and arousal, the effects of cigarettes, marijuana, caffeine, alcohol and medications and finally hidden infections or other medical conditions affecting the genitals. There's more to think about than any of us have imagined – and certainly a lot more than our male patients might have envisioned!

Back in the TCM clinic, understanding of sperm manufacture and the meaning of the semen analysis (SA) is fascinating but how can we use it for our TCM diagnosis? And for deciding upon what treatment might help? As you may now have gleaned, management of male infertility is complicated. Moreover, the symptom pictures we TCM doctors rely on to inform pattern differentiation don't always apply. In clinical reality a lot of male infertility (as evidenced on the SA) does not necessarily have an obvious accompanying TCM symptom picture and diagnosis. And this is not just because the guys are being reticent and not giving us all the details. They are often young and healthy, with good Tongue and Pulse – and are shocked that their SA has revealed that they are not 100% perfect.

Nevertheless, if we are going to offer a TCM treatment we need to hunt for patterns, even subtle or hidden ones. In modern city life, Liver Qi stagnation is not at all unusual, Kidney Yin deficiency shows itself in some overworked or burnt-out men, but Kidney Jing and Kidney Yang deficiencies are less commonly seen in clinics in the West. While Damp Heat conditions were more common in pre-antibiotic China, jock itch still turns up sometimes here in the West, and the author suggests we may need to start looking more closely at hidden infections like mycoplasma and chlamydia and most likely at the local microbiome as well.

Although we can't always rely on the SA to inform our TCM diagnosis, other medical exams might add useful information. Prostatitis, for example, may indicate damp-heat, varicocele Blood stagnation, erectile disturbance Kidney deficiency or Blood stagnation and hypogonadism Kidney Jing deficiency, and so on. It is the great strength of TCM in its careful attention to subtle details and patterns that allows the administration of the correct and effective treatment. And in our clinics, we find that outcomes from clinical trials can be a useful add-on where there is congruency with our TCM analysis.

There is a saying we find in Chinese Medicine texts, that says 'Women are ten times harder to treat than men'. Maybe once we understand all the information discussed in Olivia Pojer's book, that complexity gradient could be nudged back a little towards the male side.

Jane Lyttleton, BSc (Hons) NZ, MPhil Lond, Dip TCM Aus, Cert Acup/Herbal Medicine China, Adjunct Research Fellow (WSU), Fellow AACMA, Reg AHPRA

Foreword

Infertility is a huge global concern, affecting approximately every 6th couple of reproductive age. Male infertility contributes to up to 50% of couple's childlessness. Still society doesn't focus equally on male infertility, but rather tends to overlook the sperm qualities' importance for conception. As sperm quality has been declining over the last several decades, we need to use every tool we can to improve it for couples' reproductive capacity. Therefore, there is an urgent need not only to explore the opportunities that Chinese herbal Medicine and acupuncture offer to treat male fertility problems, but also to inform clinicians and scientists about the effects of herbal extracts and needles on male reproductive functions.

Combining the knowledge of Western Medicine and evidence-based Chinese Medicine with an integrative approach brings together the best of two worlds, helping men to regain their fertility. Bridging this gap is exactly the author's intention in this book, as Dr Olivia Pojer is wearing the hat of a Western Medical doctor as well as that of a TCM practitioner. This new book provides useful information for professionals dealing with the treatment of male infertility consisting of eight chapters focusing on Western medicine and ten chapters of relevant knowledge of Chinese Medicine.

In this book Dr Pojer addresses Chinese Medicine practitioners who need the basics of Western Medical knowledge on how sperm develops and what is essential vs harmful during the development. As a licensed acupuncturist or herbalist one might benefit from greater insight into specialists' work, e.g. what tests are done by the andrologists and reproductive endocrinologists to diagnose male sub/infertility and what these mean. On the other hand, this publication was also written to encourage medical doctors to network with a fertility acupuncturist trained in treating male factor issues and provide information on what tools could be used from the Integrative Chinese Medicine toolbox.

We do know that there is quite a wide range of reasons for male infertility – and these are not always physical. Lifestyle has become an important factor, which is a domain of Chinese Medicine and easy to be integrated into Western Clinical work.

I enjoyed reading this unique book and hope that this volume will support and enrich your clinical approach in the treatment of male fertility problems.

Dr Ashok Agarwal, Director Andrology Center, Director American Center for Reproductive Medicine,
Professor Case Western Reserve University and Lerner College of Medicine, Cleveland Clinic, USA

Introduction: How to Use This Book

This book is an integrative manual of male fertility treatment with Chinese Medicine.

To be able to treat your fathers-to-be properly in an integrative way, knowledge of the Western Medicine foundations of andrology is essential. As the level of knowledge of readers may vary, with some readers beginning their journey with this book and others wanting to use it as a source of further reading, I have invented Professor Sperm.

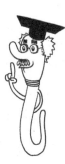

You'll be able to distinguish easily between foundational text, which is essential knowledge you need to achieve, and further content for those who want to dive deeper.

Plain text indicates knowledge you need to gain, whereas every time Professor Sperm appears and a shaded vertical line is included, additional and further knowledge is being passed on. You can skip these sections if you want to focus on basic knowledge or save them for a second read of the book.

This book is all about sperm cells and their function and how to improve their quality. So our main companion is Sam the Sperm, who will guide us through the book and help us understand his species.

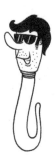

Throughout the book we will meet several of Sam's buddies and supporters. That way, with the help of these little friends, studying is much more fun and our brain memorizes more easily.

So enjoy the book, read it the way that is appropriate for you and your therapeutic situation, gain knowledge in a fun way and stand up for the integrative aspect of treating male fertility patients.

Welcome to Team Sperm!

PART I
Western Medicine

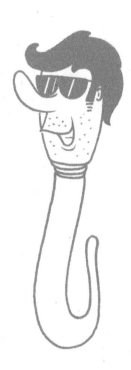

— CHAPTER 1 —

Male Anatomy

ANATOMY AND PHYSIOLOGY OF THE MALE REPRODUCTIVE ORGANS ('THE HARDWARE')

In order to understand how sperm cells are produced, what semen consists of and why that composition is useful, we need to take a journey back to anatomy class. So let me take you through the organs of the male reproductive system and its fascinating physiology to discover how brilliantly our body works to create such a miracle as sperm cells (spermatozoa)...

The components of the male reproductive system include not only the external and internal sexual organs, but also the hypothalamic–pituitary–gonadal (HPG) axis. We will cover them all step by step.

In order to support the study of the male anatomy, the major reproductive organs of the male can be grouped into three categories.

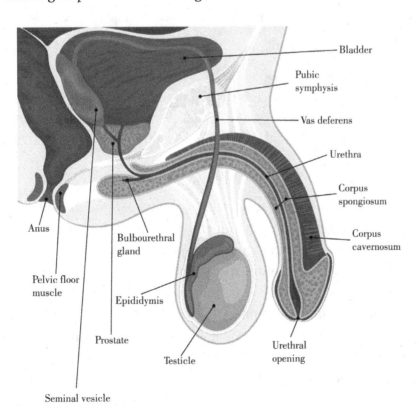

Bladder

Pubic symphysis

Vas deferens

Urethra

Corpus spongiosum

Corpus cavernosum

Anus

Bulbourethral gland

Urethral opening

Pelvic floor muscle

Epididymis

Prostate

Testicle

Seminal vesicle

The first category produces and stores sperm (spermatozoa). Sperm is produced in the testes, which are housed in the temperature-regulating scrotum; immature sperm then travels to the epididymis for development and storage.

The second category consists of the ejaculatory fluid-producing glands which include Cowper's gland (also called the bulbourethral gland), seminal vesicles, prostate and vas deferens.

The third category focuses on copulation and the deposition of the sperm within the female; these include the penis and the urethra.

Let's get a brief overview before diving deeper into how sperm is produced and what semen consists of.

Testes

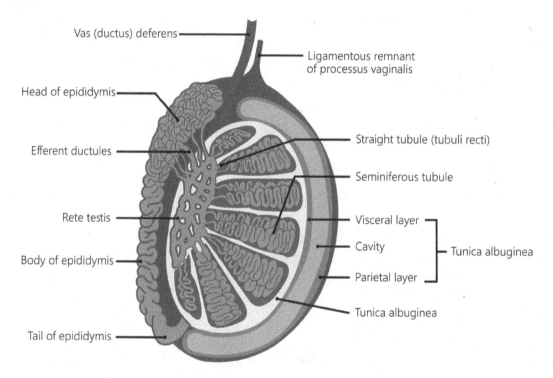

The testes are a pair of oval-shaped structures of about 15–25 ml in volume. (For visual learners, that is something between a quail's egg and a small chicken egg.) They act as a two-in-one organ as they are both exocrine glands producing spermatozoa and endocrine glands producing testosterone. The testes are covered by an outer capsule, called the tunica albuginea. Every testicle is divided by septa into 250 lobuli. Within them there are very fine coiled tubes called seminiferous tubules. If the body wants to store something really long in a very small organ, the trick is to coil it, like a ball of wool. Imagine that this tubal system is 200 metres long! The ends of the seminiferous tubules connect to form the rete testis which directly connects the testicle to its neighbour, the epididymis. The developing sperm travel through the seminiferous tubules (where they are produced) to the rete testis, from there to the efferent ducts, and then to the epididymis where they are stored and receive their functional fine-tuning. They typically do not move in a self-directed way until after ejaculation but are transported by the flow of fluid in the testes and thereafter by contraction of the organs.

The testes don't hang loose but are fixed at the spermatic cord, which is a cord-like structure in males formed by the vas deferens (also called the ductus deferens) and surrounding tissue containing blood vessels and nerves, which runs from the deep inguinal ring down to each testicle.

WANT TO KNOW MORE?

As the testes are the 'sperm factory', which is a very important job, they are hidden in the scrotum.

Each testicle embryologically develops in the abdomen and migrates into the scrotum during its descent, which is testosterone-driven. Descended testes are a sign of maturity of a newborn baby boy; during the first 12 weeks of the life of a newborn, most of the testes show up in the scrotum. The testicles are the only organs in the human body that are located externally.

The scrotum

The scrotum covers and protects the testes and epididymis and helps to regulate the temperature. The process of producing sperm is called spermatogenesis and it works perfectly at temperatures 2–4°C below core body temperature. To maintain this optimal 'production temperature', the scrotum has certain twists.

WANT TO KNOW MORE?

These twists include the very thin scrotal skin, sparse distribution of hair, minimal subcutaneous fat and a great number of sweat glands. On top of that, the scrotum uses the aid of two muscles to help with temperature regulation. The lesser-known one is the dartos muscle which is a very thin layer of smooth muscle fibre right beneath the scrotal skin. When it contracts, heat can be conserved; in a relaxed state, it helps to cool the testes. The more well-known muscle is the cremaster muscle that surrounds each testis and the spermatic cord, and helps with the regulation of temperature by either bringing the testes closer to the body by contracting (if it is too cold outside or during arousal) or by letting them hang further from the body if the testes need to be cooled. If that is not sufficient, the large number of sweat glands of the scrotum help by initiating sweat secretion to actively lose heat.

Epididymis

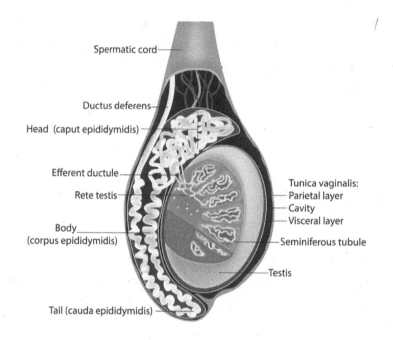

Lying behind and on the testis, the epididymis is directly connected to the testes via the rete testes. Macroscopically, the epididymis is divided into head (caput), body (corpus) and tail (cauda), the head being the one to connect with the upper pole of the testis.

It contains a tubal system, also coiled to be space-efficient, known as the ductus epididymidis, with a total length of 5–6 metres. Here, the sperm cells that were produced in the testis are matured and stored until they are needed.

WANT TO KNOW MORE?

The epididymis produces a secretion which is slightly acid and causes a kind of freezing of the sperm cells to keep them immotile for the time of storage. If the storage gets too full, then the body helps itself to get rid of the older ones via nocturnal emissions which medically is called 'pollution'.

Besides storage, the main function of the epididymis is to ensure the functional maturation of sperm. The morphologic fully developed but functionally immature sperm cells coming from the lumen of the tubuli seminiferi of the testes mature in the tubulus system of the epididymis within their journey. The complete passage through the duct system of the epididymis takes the immotile sperm cells 8–17 days. They achieve motility by having contact with the epithelium of the epididymis and being nourished by its secretions. Finally, the now fully motile sperm is stored in the caudal region, but they typically do not move on their own until they are ejaculated.

Spermatic cord

This cord consists of the ductus deferens, veins (the plexus pampiniformis, well known for potentially causing a varicocele), arteries, nerves and muscles.

Ductus deferens (vas deferens)

The main function of the ductus deferens is the transport of the mature sperm cells with the ejaculate. It is a muscular tube, 40 cm long, that connects the cauda epididymitis with the part of the urethra in the prostate while passing through the inguinal canal.

WANT TO KNOW MORE?

Prior to the entry of the prostate, the ductus enlarges to the ampulla. This ampulla is where the majority of spermatozoa are stored, waiting for ejaculation. Pulsating bumps caused by muscle contractions transport and deliver the sperm cells within seconds during ejaculation. The ampulla, together with the excretory canals of the seminal vesicle, form the ejaculatory ducts that join the urethra.

Seminal vesicles

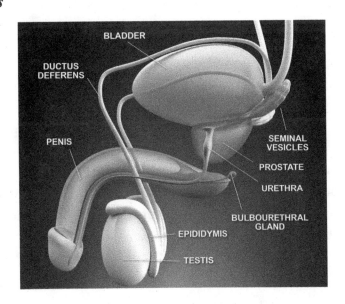

The seminal vesicles produce an alkaline secretion that helps the sperm cells to survive in the acid climate of the vagina. This secretion also nourishes the spermatozoa by providing fructose added to the semen as a provision for the spermatozoa on their strenuous journey to the egg. The secretion of the seminal vesicles accounts for the greatest part of semen composition (approximately 70%).

The seminal vesicle is a twin gland with a length of 5–10 cm, situated behind and attached to the bottom of the bladder, resembling the form of angel wings on the bladder's backside. Its excretory canals merge with the ductus deferens prior to the entry of the prostate to form the 2–3 cm long ejaculatory duct. The seminal vesicle's ability to function strongly depends on androgens. If testosterone is missing, the gland atrophies and stops producing a secretion. The vesicle's secretion is whitish-yellowish in colour and slightly alkaline. It is, as previously mentioned, rich in fructose, which can be used in semen analysis as a marker of whether the seminal vesicles are working properly.

WANT TO KNOW MORE?

These glands produce an important protein called seminogelin, which is the main factor causing the immediate coagulation of the ejaculated semen and thereby inhibiting the overhasty progressive movement of the sperm cells. This makes sense, as it also protects the sperm cells freshly placed in the hostile and acid climate of the vagina within the first 30 minutes after ejaculation, until the seminogelin is antagonized by the prostate-specific antigen (PSA) secreted by the prostate. Brilliant as our body is, the seminal vesicles also add some immune-modulating proteins, namely transforming growth factor (TGF-ß) which is activated by the acid climate of the vagina and plays a very important role in temporarily acquiring an immune tolerance towards male antigens on spermatozoa so that the female immune system is prevented from attacking them immediately.

Prostate

Weighing approximately 25 g and roughly the size of a chestnut, the prostate is the biggest gland of the male reproductive tract and it is situated at the bottom of the urinary bladder, to which it is adhered. At that contact spot on the dorsal aspect, the matched seminal vessels and the ampulla of the ductus deferens meet to form the ejaculatory duct. The urethra runs through the middle of the prostate, and the prostate contributes 15–30% of the average ejaculate with a secretion that has a surface protection function between the ejaculate and the urethra. However, the main function of this secretion is to liquefy the coagulated ejaculate after approximately 30 minutes so that the spermatozoa can move progressively.

WANT TO KNOW MORE?

Most readers might know the PSA (prostate-specific antigen) from being a commonly used tumour marker. Actually, it has a lot to do with activating sperm cells as it antagonizes semigrelin (from the secretion of the seminal vesicles). Semigrelin causes the coagulation of the ejaculate.

Generally the prostate fluid is milky and thin, and contains a high amount of cholesterol, citric acid and acid phosphatase, which together make the secretion slightly acid (pH 6.5). Spermine and the now quite famous spermidine are two components that help stabilize the sperm DNA, but are also responsible for the typical odour of the ejaculate.

Cowper's gland (bulbourethral glands)

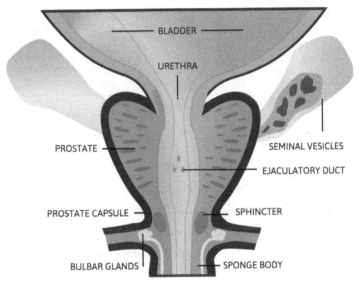

These two glands are the size of a pea and are situated distal to the prostate gland and empty into the bulbus urethrae. When sexually aroused, the glands secrete a fluid that lubricates the urethra prior to ejaculation. This secretion also contains a glycoprotein that inhibits the coagulation mechanism of the ejaculate and hence prevents premature coagulation in the urethra.

The seminal vesicles, the prostate gland and Cowper's gland (bulbourethral gland) are collectively known as the accessory sex glands.

Penis

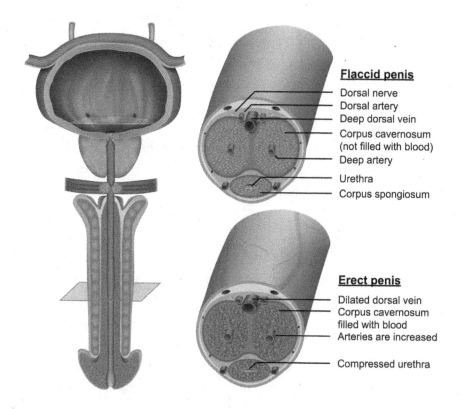

Flaccid penis
- Dorsal nerve
- Dorsal artery
- Deep dorsal vein
- Corpus cavernosum (not filled with blood)
- Deep artery
- Urethra
- Corpus spongiosum

Erect penis
- Dilated dorsal vein
- Corpus cavernosum filled with blood
- Arteries are increased
- Compressed urethra

The penis is a pendulous organ suspended from the front and sides of the pubic arch; the point at which it is fixed to the body is called the root. The male copulation organ mainly consists of three spongy bodies (two corpora cavernosa situated laterally and one corpus spongiosum situated median) with tunica albuginea (connective tissue) wrapped around it, holding them together. The filling of those spongy bodies with blood is the main mechanism of an erection. The urethra runs within the corpus spongiosum and opens at the tip of the glans penis.

WANT TO KNOW MORE?

The process of a normal erection is as follows. First, the smooth muscle chambers in the penis (corpus cavernosa and corpus spongiosa) are in a state of relative tension which restricts blood flow and prevents blood from filling these spongy tissue chambers. Next, in response to sexual arousal, signals from the brain and spinal cord cause the smooth muscles in these chambers to relax. This relaxation allows blood to fill the penile chambers and erection begins.

Biochemically, this process works as follows:

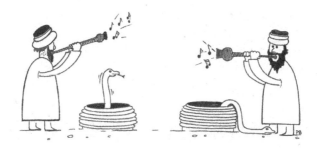

The cascade starts with nerves initiating the release of nitric oxide (NO). The nitric oxide then activates cyclic GMP (cyclic guanosine monophosphate) in the chambers of the smooth muscles, cyclic GMP is needed for the penis to relax. It is this relaxation of the penile smooth muscle chambers (spongy bodies) that allows proper blood flow into them, increasing the blood pressure in the penis. Consequently, the venous return is impeded, trapping the blood in the spongy body of the penis and a complete erection is achieved. For an erection to subside cyclic GMP has to be degraded by an enzyme called PDE5 (phosphodiesterase type 5). The smooth muscles in the chambers cannot stay relaxed without cyclic GMP, the erection decreases as they start to contract and the blood flow to the spongy bodies is squeezed off.[1]

HOW SPERM IS PRODUCED ('THE SOFTWARE')

To learn more about the production of sperm, we need to get back to the inside of the testes.

TESTICLES – A SUMMARY

Remember, testicles are paired, forming a two-in-one organ: an exocrine gland producing spermatozoa (1500 per second or 200 million per day) and an endocrine gland producing testosterone. Testosterone is also necessary for the production of sperm cells.

The share of the work in the testes is 10% testosterone production, 90% sperm production.

Sperm cells are very sensitive to heat during their progress, and therefore the testicles are situated outside the body in the scrotum, where the temperature is approximately 2°C below average body temperature.

Each testis is divided into 250 lobuli, within which are very fine coiled tubes called seminiferous tubules.

Microscopic anatomy of the testis

Functionally, the testis is divided into two compartments:

- The production of the male hormones (androgens, mainly testosterone) takes place in the interstitial compartment.

- The production of the male gametes (spermatogenesis) takes place in the tubular compartment.

And it is the tubular compartment we have to focus on when we want to know more about the production of sperm.

The tubular compartment of the testis

The tubules are lined with a layer of cells (germ cells) that develop into sperm cells (also known as spermatozoa or male gametes) from puberty through to old age.

Histology of the tubular compartment – tubuli seminiferi

Looking at a cross-section of the tubuli, we find three basic structures.

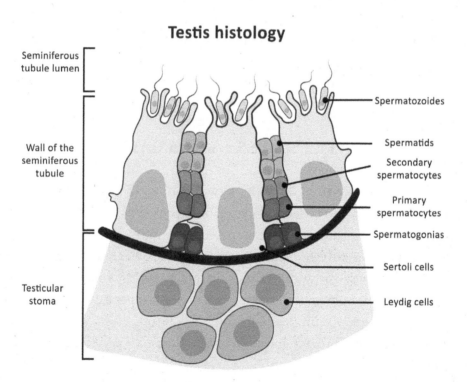

Testis histology

- Germ cells develop into spermatogonia, spermatocytes, spermatids and spermatozoa through the process of spermatogenesis (i.e. the development of sperm). This process goes in the direction from the basal membrane towards the lumen.

- Sertoli cells are the true epithelium of the seminiferous epithelium, critical for the support of germ cell development into spermatozoa.

- Peritubular myoid cells surround the seminiferous tubules to enable the tubuli to contract to move the sperm cells to the epididymis.

GERM CELLS

It all starts with the spermatogonia, which build the basal layer of the tubuli seminiferi's epithelium and represent the gamete's stem cells. They are the foundation of spermatogenesis.

Through multiple intermediate steps (mitosis and meiosis), four spermatozoa arise from one spermatogonia (in reality, there is some drop-out as always in life).

Every hour, approximately one million sperm cells are passed on to the epididymis.

The development from a spermatogonia to a spermatid takes about 64 days. Within this time, the various differentiation forms of sperm can be found. The more abluminal they appear, the more mature they are.

Spermatogenesis

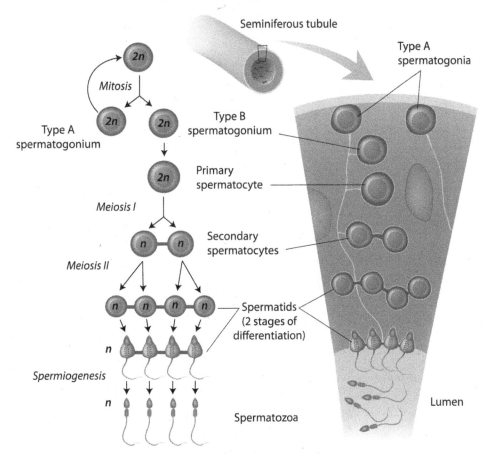

In a nutshell: spermatogenesis starts in the basal compartment of the tubuli seminiferi and ends in the adluminal (apical) compartment. During development, cells are arranged in a highly ordered sequence from the basal membrane to the lumen.

After 64 days of production in the testes, the sperm cells are transported to the epididymis to achieve their functional maturation and their fine-tuning.

WANT TO KNOW MORE?

The most visual change in the development of sperm cells is the formation of tadpole-like spermatozoa out of round spermatids. In humans, there are several different stages involved in the maturation of spermatids to spermatozoa. This step of development is named 'spermiogenesis' (do not confuse this with spermatogenesis which is the development before spermiogenesis). Defects in this phase can cause malformation as well as malfunction of the spermatozoa.

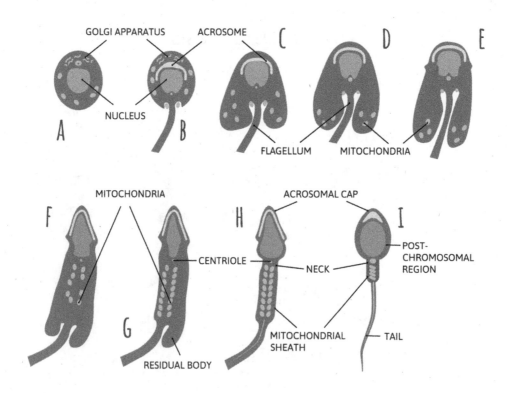

SERTOLI CELLS

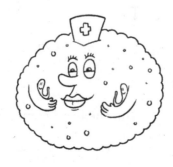

A Sertoli cell (also known as sustentacular cell) is a 'nurse' cell and helps in the process of spermatogenesis, the production of sperm. It is activated by follicle-stimulating hormone (FSH) secreted by the pituitary gland (adenohypophysis).

Sertoli cells are situated at the basal layer of the seminiferous tubule, sitting right above the basement membrane, and are as big as the distance from the basal layer to the lumen. Thus, they are easy to identify as they are the largest cells within the tubules.

One Sertoli cell can only take care and nourish a certain amount of sperm cells in process (just like a nurse).

WANT TO KNOW MORE?

Higher than normal oestrogen levels in the womb might limit the number of sperm a man produces in adulthood by inhibiting the development of Sertoli cells in the forming testicles.

The Sertoli cells are in charge of phagocytosis of the discharged cytoplasm of spermatids that forms during spermiogenesis.

Sertoli cells produce anti-Müllerian hormone (AMH). In males, AMH is involved in embryonic development and contributes to the regression of the Müllerian ducts (which in women form the uterus and the fallopian tubes).

The Sertoli cell secretes two important substances:

• androgen-binding protein (ABP) which binds the testosterone produced in the Leydig cells of the testes and makes it accessible to the gametes. (Note: cortisol – our stress hormone – causes a downregulation of ABP)

• inhibin which regulates the FSH production via a negative feedback cycle.

The occluding junctions of Sertoli cells form the blood–testis barrier, a structure that partitions the interstitial blood compartment of the testis from the adluminal compartment of the seminiferous tubules, which is of massive immunologic relevance. The blood–testis barrier (BTB) is a physical barrier between the blood or lymph vessels and the lumen of seminiferous tubules of the testes. In a nutshell, the tight junctions of Sertori cells make up the BTB and so divide the basal compartment and adluminal compartment.

Spermatogonia are located outside the barrier (they are genetically identical to the somatic cells) and can respond to various factors. Since sexual maturity occurs long after the development of immunocompetence, the differentiating sperm cells can be recognized as 'foreign' and provoke an immune response that will destroy the sperm cells, whereas the spermatogonia cause no immune response. Thus, the BTB protects the developing sperm cells as large molecules (immunoglobulins) cannot penetrate. In other words, the BTB protects highly immunogenic material from leaking out causing autoimmune destruction of the testes (e.g. anti-sperm antibodies – AsAb).

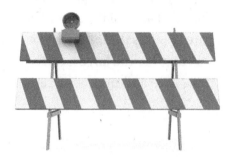

Anything that destroys the BTB will lead to an impairment of meiosis and spermatogenesis.

BTB destroyers include:

- heat

- heavy metals

- pesticides.

BTB can also be damaged by trauma to the testes (e.g. torsion, impact, surgery, vasectomy).

THE INTERSTITIAL COMPARTMENT

In between the tubuli seminiferi, embedded in the connective tissue of the testes, are the Leydig cells.

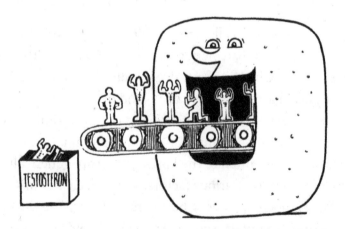

They lie close to each other forming groups. In humans, they account for 10–12% of the volume of the testes. They produce androgens, the male sex hormones – above all, testosterone. This hormone needs the androgen-binding protein (ABP) produced by the Sertoli cells to be administered to the processing sperm.

The whole steroidbiosynthesis is stimulated by luteinizing hormone (LH) and human chorionic gonadotropin (hCG).

WANT TO KNOW MORE?

Just like all cell types that produce steroid hormones, the Leydig cells have lipid drops, a strongly developed endoplasmic reticulum (ER) and mitochondria of the tubule type.

Androgen production of the Leydig cells starts with cholesterol. In the mitochondria of the Leydig cells, cholesterol is converted into pregnenolone.

Interestingly, Leydig cells also have receptors for oestrogen and prolactin. Testosterone can be transformed into oestrogen by an enzyme called aromatase. Such a transformation can cause the growth of breasts in men, for example.

THE HYPOTHALAMIC–PITUITARY–GONADAL (HPG) AXIS ('THE GEARS')

The HPG axis is also part of the male reproductive system, as it stimulates the production of testosterone as well as spermatogenesis. Proper functioning of this three-part system is necessary for male fertility.

Let's have a look into the system as we now know all the gonadal structures involved in it.

Think of the HPG axis by imagining it in terms of a typical company hierarchy. The hypothalamus is the big boss, the pituitary is the supervisor and the testes are the workers.

So the hypothalamus (the boss) releases gonadotropin-releasing hormone (GnRH) to signal to the pituitary to start sending out gonadotropins (LH and FSH) to make the testes work (producing sperm and testosterone).

The testes then give feedback to the pituitary (supervisor) and the hypothalamus (big boss) as soon as they work properly. If they do not work hard enough, the pituitary pushes harder by releasing more LH and FSH to increase the stimulation of the production in the testes. This is called a feedback control cycle. Thus every elevation of the LH and FSH levels in the blood indicates a gonadal problem or failure.

GnRH is secreted in a pulsatile pattern every 1.5 hours and so is LH; FSH release is influenced by inhibin which is produced by the Sertoli cells.

LH acts on the Leydig cells in the testes to stimulate testosterone production through the conversion of cholesterol. When testosterone levels accumulate, it sets a negative feedback effect at the pituitary to suppress the release of LH and at the hypothalamus to suppress GnRH production. Intratesticular testosterone levels are far higher than in the circulation.

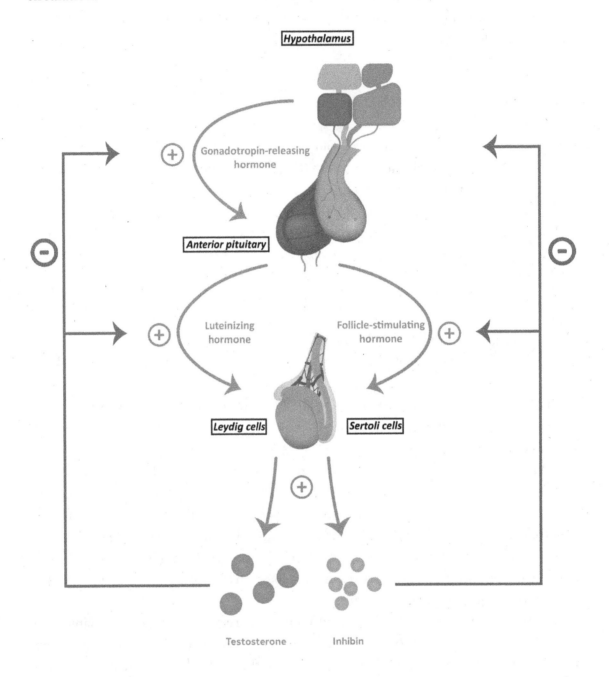

FSH is needed at the onset of puberty when spermatogenesis starts over, as it acts on the Sertoli cells promoting germ cell maturation. Testosterone is necessary to maintain the whole spermatogenesis process. Spermatocytes do not have a testosterone receptor but only ABP receptors. So to allow them access to testosterone, they need the help of the Sertoli cells which do have a testosterone receptor. They can bind testosterone and produce the ABP for the spermatocytes. On top of that, FSH is also needed to convert testosterone in its more active form 5-α dihydrotestosterone (5-α DHT).

CHAPTER 2

The Anatomy and Function of Sperm Cells

THE ANATOMY OF A SPERM CELL

The function of sperm cells is to transport the male genetic information into the egg cell. To do so, those tiny swimmers have to cover quite a distance: from the vagina (where they are deposited) to the ampulla of the fallopian tube (where fertilization takes place), it is 16–24 cm. But it is not only the distance of the journey that needs the sperm cell to have some special features, but also the hostile climate of the female tract and certain physiological barriers that the sperm cells have to overcome. On top of that, they are constantly attacked by female leukocytes and the whole female immune system.

To fulfil its mission to fertilize the egg, a sperm cell needs to be capable of certain functions that are associated with special morphologic structures. In order to understand how a sperm works, we need to know about its anatomy.

Spermatozoa (sperm)

A sperm cell of normal morphology consists of head and tail and has a length of roughly 45–50 µm. The head is the most important part of a sperm cell as it contains the male nucleus with all the male genetic information – in short, DNA packed in 23 chromosomes.

To provide deposition of the genetic material in the head, the sperm cell needs to be able to move towards the egg cell. The tail can be divided into neck, midpiece, principal piece and endpiece, all fulfilling slightly different jobs in terms of motility.

Let's look at this in detail.

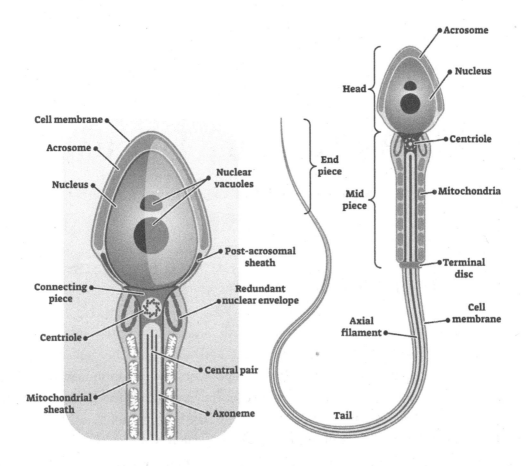

HEAD

The head is oval in shape and at only 4.3–5.2 μm in length it is the smallest cell of the body. It mainly consists of a compact nucleus with chromatic substance. The nucleus contains the paternal genetic material, the DNA, stored in 23 chromosomes (a haploid set of chromosomes), 22 autosomes and one sex chromosome (X or Y) that determines the future sex of the baby.

WANT TO KNOW MORE?

A single sperm contains capacity for 35 megabytes of data. On this basis, the average ejaculation contains 1500 terabytes or 1.5 petabytes of data (or the capacity for 10 billion Facebook photos).

Right above the nucleus lies a cap-like structure called the acrosome, which secretes a bunch of hydrolytic enzymes (e.g. hyaluronidase, acrosin) that are needed to be able to penetrate the egg. This functionally important step for fertilization is called the acrosome reaction. We'll come back to its exact explanation later in this chapter.

The head and its morphology have a predictive value in terms of fertilization ability.

WANT TO KNOW MORE?

A proper morphology according to the Kruger strict criteria (which are the criteria for a sperm's morphology that a sperm test relates to) indicates that a morphologically normal-shaped head should be symmetrically oval and smooth with a tapering apex as well as a broad base. The normal head has a length of 3–5 µm, width of 2–3 µm and a width/length ratio of 3/5–2/3. The acrosome has to cover 40–70% (approximately two-thirds) of the head and no big vacuoles should be seen, as it is assumed that those contain a high percentage of damaged DNA.

NECK (OR CONNECTING PIECE)
The neck connects the sperm head and the flagellum. It is the smallest part (0.5 µm in length) and among other things it contains the centrosome.

WANT TO KNOW MORE?

This centrosome consists of a proximal and a distal centriole (cylinders) and the pericentriolar material. The centrosome and centrioles play an important role in the first mitotic division in humans as they provide the spindle and aster. Human oocytes do not possess any centrioles, so in fact the material of that connecting piece, the centrosome, initiates the first cleavage division of the fertilized egg. Studies have demonstrated that injection of the sperm tail alone can induce aster formation.[1]

MIDDLE PIECE
This is the powerhouse of the sperm cell as it consists of tightly packed mitochondria supplying energy in the form of adenosine triphosphate (ATP) for the tail movement in the presence of magnesium.

WANT TO KNOW MORE?

It has 10–14 spirals of mitochondria (helical pattern) around the axonema. The mitochondrial structure in the sperm is the same as in other types of cells but more stable. This mitochondrial stability is necessary to provide resistance to osmotic changes as well as resistance to compression and stretching during flagellar beating.

PRINCIPAL PIECE OF THE TAIL
This is the longest part (ten times longer than the sperm head). It flagellates, which propels the sperm cell (at about 1–3 mm per minute in humans) by whipping in an elliptical cone.

This movement pattern is similar to the lash of a whip. This motility is essential in fulfilling the mission of deposition of paternal genetic material in the oocyte. Only a well-formed tail ensures a progressive motility towards the egg and a certain speed to avoid phagocytosis by the immune cells of the female tract.

WANT TO KNOW MORE?

In the centre of the flagellum (tail), excluding the end piece, one can find a structure called an axonema. It stretches across the full length of the tail, like a spine, and is the motor of the sperm tail. It has two central microtubules surrounded by nine pairs of microtubules, to form the classical 9+2 pattern. The structural component of these microtubules is tubulin, and those microtubules have 'arms' made of dynein which play an important role in tail movement as they transform the chemical energy of ATP into kinetic energy. That leads to a bending of the flagellum and so initiates the characteristic lash of a whip pattern of tail movement. The axonema is surrounded by outer dense fibres as a protector for the axonema against shear forces during ejaculation (flagella without outer dense fibres break and hence lack motility), moreover, they help in facilitating sperm movement, just as spine and paravertebral muscles work together. For the outer dense fibres to work properly, zinc needs to be incorporated during spermatogenesis. Hence, zinc is important for proper sperm movement.

THE FUNCTIONING OF A SPERM CELL

Remember that sperm cells are produced in the testes, are then passed on to the epididymis to get their fine-tuning in terms of maturation and are stored there. They look mature and they can move, but a sperm cell still needs to take two further steps to be able to fertilize an egg at all.

Capacitation
The first step is called capacitation. Without this, no fertilization would be possible as all the following steps depend on a sperm being capacitated. This penultimate maturation process starts when the spermatozoa enter the female genital tract, where cervical mucus and secretion from the uterus help by activating this biochemical occurrence.

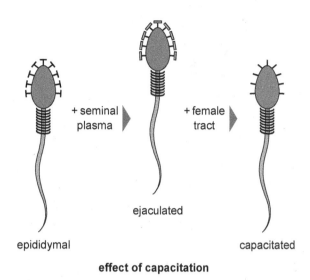

ejaculated

epididymal   capacitated

effect of capacitation

In short, capacitation has two effects: destabilization of the acrosomal sperm head membrane which allows it to penetrate the outer layer of the egg, and chemical changes in the tail, to allow greater motility in the sperm (by the increase of Ca^2+ levels within the sperm cell).[2]

WANT TO KNOW MORE?

Capacitation is a time-dependent phenomenon which prepares the sperm to undergo the acrosome reaction. It must occur at exactly the right time, not too early and not too late, to ensure fertilization ability. To guarantee the right timing, certain decapacitation factors are secreted by the epididymis, seminal vesicles and prostate into the seminal plasma, such as fertilization-promoting peptide (FPP), cholesterol or spermine to prevent early capacitation. Later these are removed in the uterus and tubes.

Sperm transport through the female genital tract happens quite fast (in as little as 15–30 minutes, but usually approximately 45–90 minutes) whereas capacitation may take between three and 24 hours. Capacitation is not completed until after spermatozoa have entered the cumulus layer of the oocyte.[3] The uterus aids in the steps of capacitation by secreting albumin, lipoproteins and proteolytic and glycosidasic enzymes such as heparin.

Besides significant molecular changes in every compartment of the sperm cell (head, tail, membrane, cytosol, cytoskeleton), capacitation also causes the elimination of epididymal decapacitation factor such as spermine that prevents premature capacitation. Capacitation also leads to the reorganization of the membrane's lipids (especially cholesterol) and proteins which results in a more fluid membrane with an increased permeability to Ca^2+. That influx of Ca^2+ produces increased intracellular cAMP levels and, hence, an increase in motility. This elevation of Ca^2+ levels within the sperm cell induces a phenomenon called hyperactivation.

Hyperactivation

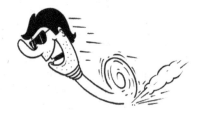

Hyperactivation coincides with the onset of capacitation and at the same time is a consequence of it. It is initiated by progesterone, which is secreted by the cumulus cells of the outer layer of the egg. The chemotactic stimulus of the attractant progesterone induces an influx of Ca^2+ into the sperm tail, changing the swimming pattern of the sperm. Hyperactivated sperm tails do not show progressive movement but circling movement due to asymmetrical flagellar beating. Hyperactivation seems to give the sperm cell the final power at the end of a marathon. They swim faster (2–3 times) and their tail movements become more forceful and erratic. The sperm's head gets a lateral displacement. Those two changes allow spermatozoa to dig into the cumulus layer surrounding the ovum.

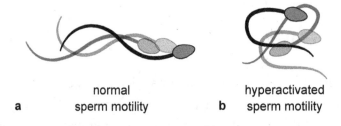

a   normal sperm motility   b   hyperactivated sperm motility

WHAT IS HYPERACTIVATION FOR?

Prior to fertilization, sperm become entrapped within the finger-like projections of the microvilli of the oviduct. In order for the sperm to fertilize the oocyte, hyperactive motility is needed, allowing the sperm to escape the microvilli and reach the oocyte for fertilization.[4]

WANT TO KNOW MORE?

The influx of calcium ions into the tails while progesterone is present has been researched a lot recently. We now know that the flagellum of the sperm is studded with ion channels formed by proteins called CatSper. These channels are selective, allowing only calcium ions to pass. The opening of CatSper channels is responsible for the influx of calcium; hence, CatSper plays a key role in mediating hyperactive motility.[5]

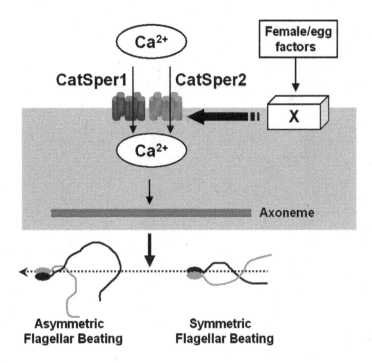

Acrosome reaction

The precondition of the acrosome reaction is sperm's capacitation. The elevated intra-cellular calcium levels of hyperactivation induce acrosome reaction; at the same time, low-dose reactive oxygen species (ROS) initiate the irreversible acrosome reaction. (It is important to know that a certain amount of ROS is not harmful but necessary!) Natural stimulants for the acrosome reaction include follicular fluid and progesterone (produced by cumulus cells).

The acrosome reaction is an exocytotic event in which the acrosome (the cap of the sperm's head) fuses with the overlying plasma membrane. The multiple fusions between the outer acrosomal membrane and the plasma membrane result in the release of hydrolytic enzymes (e.g. acrosin and hyaluronidase) and exposure of new membrane domains.[6]

These enzymes are responsible for the digestion of the zona pellucida, allowing the sperm cell to enter the perivitelline space that surrounds the egg membrane. Only acrosome-reacted spermatozoa can break through the zona pellucida. The special tail movement as a result of hyperactivation helps to dig a channel in the zona.

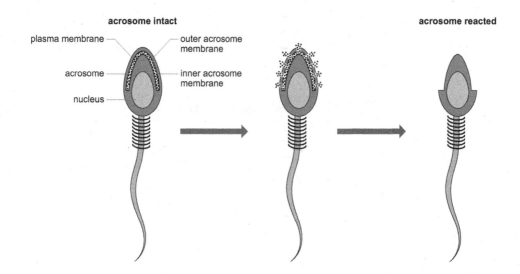

WANT TO KNOW MORE?

The acrosome has an inner membrane and an outer membrane. The acrosomal enzymes are in between these two acrosomal membranes. All the membranes are wrapped by the plasma membrane. At the beginning of the acrosomal reaction, the outer acrosomal membrane fuses with the plasma membrane. This leads to the building of vesicles with, for example, acrosin as lytic content, followed by the perforation of the acrosome which finally peels off. The former inner acrosomal membrane becomes the new frontier membrane. Within this process the acrosomal content, consisting of a bunch of enzymes, such as hyaluronidase, acrosin, collagenase and phospholipid A, is set free. Those hydrolytic vesicles are set free during the passage through the zona pellucida and digest it to allow a breakthrough. Only acrosome-reacted spermatozoa are able to bind to the oolemma, the membrane of the ovum. That is because on the surface of the former inner acrosomal membrane a protein is expressed which is essential for binding to the oolemma. This sperm-specific protein Izumo, named for a Japanese shrine dedicated to marriage, is essential for sperm–egg plasma membrane binding and fusion.[7] The acrosome reaction is also a time-dependent phenomenon; it cannot take place prematurely or too late.

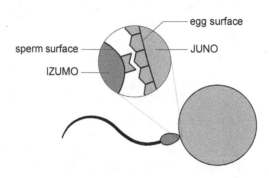

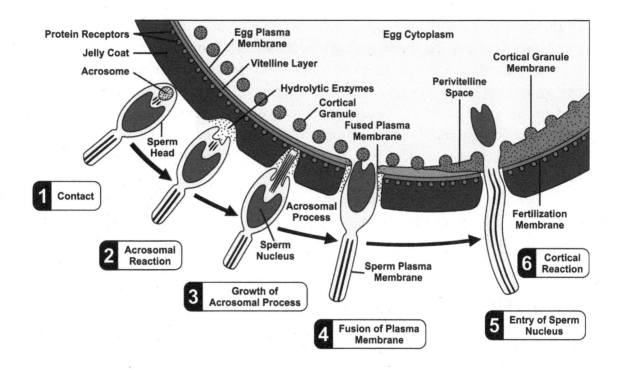

EJACULATION

Ejaculation is a reflex that is initiated and coordinated by various hormonal factors as well as by a complex neuronal system of autonomous and somatic nerves (central and spinal).

The most important players are the parasympathetic and the sympathetic system which normally play against each other as antagonists. In ejaculation, those two systems synchronize to make it happen.

Ejaculation needs the availability of two main steps.

The starting point is a psychological, visual and/or acoustical stimulus which leads to parasympathetic impulses. These induce the release of acetylcholine which causes a dilatation of the pudendal artery. This increases bloodflow to the spongy bodies of the penis but prevents the venous effusion, leading to a swelling of the penis – the erection. Parasympathetic impulses also lead to secretion of the Cowper's glands to moisten the urethra for the future ejaculate.

The next step is called emission, which takes place after a certain threshold is reached and is controlled by the sympathetic nervous system. Via stimulus of certain nerves, adrenalin is set free, which leads to contractions of the muscles around the ductus ejaculatorius, the ductus deferens itself and the cauda of the epididymis. Those contractions finally cause spermatozoa to be pulled out in the urethra.

During the ejaculation itself, parasympathetic fibres initiate – due to increasing pressure of the urethra filled with semen – contractions of the bulbocavernosus muscle (3–10 rhythmic contractions) to force expulsion of the seminal fluid with the spermatozoa out of the urethra. Due to the rhythmic contractions of the pelvic floor muscles, the secretions of the various glands composing semen are partly mixed together during ejaculation. Simultaneously, ascending nerval impulses impart a strong mental-sexual arousal, the feeling of an orgasm. Thereby, a powerful activation of the sympathetic system is responsible for all the typical physical signs and symptoms of immediately before and during orgasm: an increased tonus of the skeletal muscles, increased sweat secretion, tachycardia, hyperventilation and mydriasis (dilation of the pupils).

At the end of the orgasm, noradrenalin is set free, causing a constriction of the corpus cavernosum of the penis, thus leading to the process of subsiding from the state of swelling and arousal (detumescence).

COMPOSITION OF SEMEN

Ejaculate is the commonly used word for seminal fluid (semen). The volume of the ejaculate of a human male usually is more than 1.5 ml (according to the WHO 2010 threshold) and is composed of spermatozoa (sperm cells) and a fluid called seminal plasma, which includes the secretions of the accessory glands (Cowper's glands, seminal vesicles and prostate).

> Sperm cells + secretions of the accessory glands = semen

WANT TO KNOW MORE?

Semen is not an even mixture of its components; in fact, the different secretions are expelled in four fractions during ejaculation.

Right before ejaculation occurs, the secretion of the Cowper's glands is expelled to lubricate the urethra and inhibit premature coagulation of the semen within the urethra. This precursor is followed by the first real fraction of the ejaculate, consisting mainly of acid prostate secretion. The second fraction includes secretions of the testes and the epididymis (here come the sperm cells!) and the main amount of the alkaline secretion of the seminal vesicles. This second fraction also contains the rest of the prostate secretions. The last and third fraction consists of the leftover secretion of the seminal vesicles and hardly contains any sperm cells.

It is very important to keep in mind that gametes (sperm cells) only account for 5% of the semen; the vast majority is secretion of the accessory glands.

Composition of semen

	% of total	Description or mechanism for delivery/purpose
Spermatozoa	2–5	Formed in testes, stored in epididymis and vasa differentia
Seminal fluid	60–75	Alkaline fluid, primarily responsible for nutritional support through amino acids, enzymes, fructose; also suppresses possible immune response by female
Prostate fluid	25–30	Acid phosphatase, citric acid, proteolytic enzymes and zinc
Bulbourethral glands	1–5	Galactose, mucous

Source: Rebecca Lane, 'Urinalysis and Body Fluids CRg' (https://slideplayer.com)

Why is this composition of semen essential for the fertilization process? What role do its components play?

In a nutshell, the seminal plasma is responsible for maintaining osmolarity and the ionic balance as well as for transportation and nutrition of the sperm cells. In addition, it has a protective function for the spermatozoa in terms of preventing damage due to shear forces (during high-speed expulsion) as well as protecting them from inflammatory and oxidative damage. It also prevents premature capacitation or acrosome reaction and prepares the endometrium for the future implantation of the embryo.

Its main components are:

- Sperm cells – the players – carry the genetic material to be placed in the ovum.

- Cowper's glands neutralize the milieu of the urethra and lubricate it, and hinder the semen from premature coagulation within the urethra by secretion of a certain protein.

- Prostate fluid is a slightly acid secretion that seems to have a surface protective function between urethra and ejaculate to prevent damage from shear forces. The prostate secretes the tumour marker known as PSA (prostate-specific antigen) which is originally useful for the liquefication of the coagulated ejaculate and therefore plays an important role in mobilization of the spermatozoa. Prostate fluid is rich in zinc, which is essential for coagulation and liquefication of semen – in fact, the prostate is the organ of the body richest in zinc; therefore, zinc threshold in seminal plasma has a certain diagnostic value in measuring prostate function. Citric acid is also secreted by the prostate. It helps to maintain the pH balance, and reduced thresholds can indicate a silent prostatitis or dysfunction of the gland.

- Seminal vesicles produce an alkaline secretion to neutralize the acid climate in the vagina. Their main function is nutritional support (fructose) for the sperm cells – incidentally, fructose content impairs with age. As only the seminal vesicles supply fructose to the semen, the fructose content can be used to measure the gland's function. It also secretes the enzyme semenogelin that is responsible for the coagulation of the semen immediately after ejaculation to prevent unnecessary movement and hence energy loss of sperm cells. Additionally, the secretion of the seminal vesicles has bacteriostatic and immune-modulating abilities.

WANT TO KNOW MORE?

Further contents:

- So-called round cells which are spermatids from spermatogenesis – their content in semen could be up to 10% even in fertile men.

- Leukocytes are a steady content of semen too, so up to 1 million/ml is normal; if above, this is called leukocytospermia which is the case in up to 35% of infertile men. Leukocytes play an important role in oxidative stress as they produce reactive oxygen species (ROS) that can – if too much – damage sperm cells and their DNA.

- Growth factor-ß, cytokines and prostaglandins from prostate and seminal vesicles imitate the cascade of inflammation to a certain level, which is necessary to prepare the female endometrium for the upcoming implantation.

- Glucose, sorbitol, inositol, ribose, fucose, n-acetyl-neuraminic acid as carbohydrates, which, in addition to fructose, nourish the sperm cells on their journey. Also, citric acid to maintain pH balance.

- Amino acids glycine, glutamic acid, arginine, serine, alanine and asparagine acid as well as ornithine and carnitine (carnitine can be used as a marker of the function of the epididymis as it is produced from it).

- Immunglobules, mainly IgG.

- Electrolytes such as potassium and loads of zinc (the electrolytic situation within the semen is very similar to blood serum except the level of potassium is far higher in semen).

- Spermine as antioxidant and main decapacitation factor (that means prevention of premature capacitation). This substance is responsible for the typical odour of semen.

- Hormones such as testosterone, estradiol, DHEA, cortisol, prolactin and FSH.

Due to the rhythmic contractions of the smooth muscles of the pelvic floor, those ejaculatory fractions are partly mixed up in the expelled semen, but even directly after ejaculation the different fractions are not equally distributed in the semen. The even distribution of semen's components takes place after liquefication of the initially coagulated semen, so after about 15–60 minutes post-ejaculation.

The cellular component (the sperm cells) and the lipid vesicles of the prostate secretion are responsible for the milky-white appearance of the ejaculate. Any other colour would indicate the presence of other cells.

Appearance of semen

Opaque normal, grey, white, light yellow	Normal
Shades of yellow	Correlate with flavin concentration Deep yellow could also indicate contamination with urine
Deep yellow	Associated with certain drugs
Brown or red	May contain blood
Highly turbid	Usually contains leukocytes indicating infection or inflammation

Source: Rebecca Lane, 'Urinalysis and Body Fluids CRg' (https://slideplayer.com)

THE JOURNEY OF A SPERM CELL – A SUMMARY

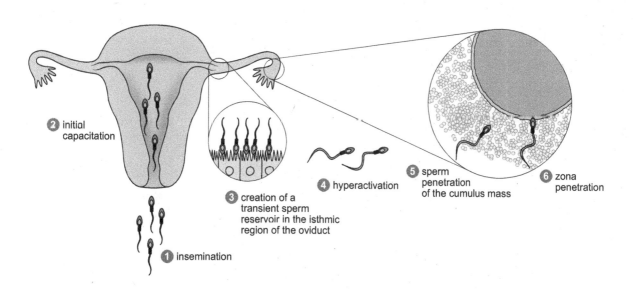

- Spermatozoa can survive up to seven days in the female genital tract, but the perfect fertilization day is the first day of entering the female body.

- When spermatogenesis is finished, the spermatozoa are stored in the epididymis; when ejaculating, they are pushed out via the urethra.

- Approximately 300 million sperm cells enter the female vagina during intercourse. Only a small percentage gets to the fallopian tube and reaches the egg there.

- A higher percentage never get to the fallopian tube; they have other jobs to do in addition to fertilizing the egg.

- On their way to the egg that 'waits' in the fallopian tube, the spermatozoa are directed by chemotaxis (fragrances, attractants from progesterone and other substances) as well as the pH value and difference in temperature.

- Due to the many obstacles on their way, only 300 sperm cells reach the egg and only one fertilizes the egg.

— CHAPTER 3 —

Oxidative Stress and Its Role in Male Infertility

Male infertility is a pathology that has many causes; in most cases, there will be several co-factors that together turn the wheel from fertile to infertile – co-factors such as physiological, environmental, epigenetic and genetic issues. What they all have in common is that on the molecular level they have an impact on male fertility via the imbalance of generating reactive oxygen species (ROS) and male antioxidant capacity. That imbalance causes oxidative stress (OS) and negatively affects several components of the male reproductive functioning.

But what are these mysterious ROS?

ROS are a normal by-product of producing energy in the mitochondria. Precisely, ROS are the oxygen metabolism derivatives generated as a result of physiological cellular metabolism.

At normal physiological levels, ROS participate and therefore are essential in intracellular signalling cascades to ensure proper reproductive functions such as capacitation, hyperactivation of sperm and acrosome reaction.[1] ROS are essential to trigger the maturation and fertilization potential of sperm, so we actually do need a certain amount of reactive oxygen species. The problem arises when too much ROS is produced, far more than needed, and which is more than the antioxidant capacity of the semen can balance and neutralize. That imbalance between ROS and antioxidant levels has deleterious effects on sperm cells because spermatozoa are very vulnerable to oxidative stress as they lack proper cell repair mechanisms and have inadequate antioxidant capacities themselves.[2]

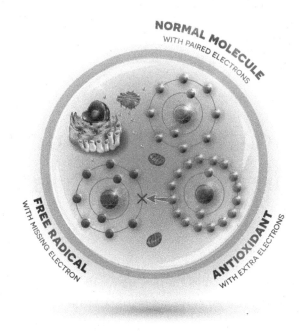

WANT TO KNOW MORE?

Antioxidants are mainly in the seminal plasma, as spermatozoa lose their cytoplasmic content, which includes antioxidants, during spermatogenesis when the cell turns from a round cell into the spermatozoa shape.

The number-one ROS molecule is superoxide anion (O_2-) radical. This most famous one can then be transformed to peroxyl radical (ROO–), hydroxyl radical (OH) or hydrogen peroxide (H_2O_2). We could call them 'the ROS gang'.

Spermatozoa generates ROS via two mechanisms:

- in sperm plasma membrane

- in sperm mitochondria – and as we've already learned, spermatozoa have loads of mitochondria in their middle piece!

But what are the sources of ROS in the male reproductive tract? We need to divide between endogenous and exogenous sources.

Let's start with the endogenous sources. Those are:

- **Leukocytes:** There are physiologically a lot of leukocytes (peroxidase-positive ones) and macrophages in the specimen. They originate from the accessory glands (prostate and seminal vesicles). If their number gets over 10^6, the pathology is called leukocytospermia, which is a sperm-disrupting disorder. Leukocytes are the number-one source of ROS production, as any infection or inflammation triggers these cells to produce 100 times more ROS than the normal production rate as a defence mechanism. This generation of ROS is one of the prime mechanisms of leukocytes-induced immune defence with leukocytes being quite potent OS-inducing cells.[3]

- **Immature sperm cells:** In normal development of sperm cells through spermiogenesis, the cytoplasm is extruded. This can be seen as mature spermatozoa have their tadpole-like shape (no cytoplasm), whereas developing sperm cells are round (contain cytoplasm). These immature sperm cells should not be found in large numbers in the ejaculate. They are called immature teratospermic (= teratozoospermic) sperms. Teratospermic means that they have a different morphology to normal spermatozoa. They not only look abnormal, but they also produce an abnormally high amount of ROS compared with morphologically normal sperm.

- **Infections, inflammatory conditions and autoimmune issues:** Genitourinary tract infections such as prostatitis, even if it is chronic but caused by bacteria, can commonly produce acute inflammatory responses by promoting leukocyte influx into the male reproductive tract and ultimately triggering ROS production. But it is not only bacterial infection that can cause oxidative damage to spermatozoa; viruses can too. Herpes simplex DNA has been found in semen of 4–50% of infertile men.[4] Also systemic infections can cause OS in the male genital system, such as HIV or hepatitis B and C, all of which cause elevated seminal oxidative stress via an increase of leukocyte numbers. Chronic abacterial prostatitis is an inflammatory condition that seems to trigger adverse autoimmune responses to seminal or prostate antigens, leading to an elevation in pro-inflammatory mediators and ROS-generating leukocytes.[5]

- **Varicocele and cryptorchism:** Varicocele is a condition with an abnormal dilation of the venous plexus pampiniformis around the spermatic cord. This pathology might be found in fertile men too, but it is found in approximately 40% of infertile men and is therefore thought to be the leading cause of male infertility. Why is this? The dilation of that venous plexus leads to testicular hyperthermia and, as we know, the testicles like it cool to be able to produce properly. Varicocele can also lead to hypoxia. Both hypoxia and hyperthermia result in OS-induced testicular dysfunction. This ROS generation also causes a lack of sperm DNA integrity associated with the grade of the varicocele. Cryptorchism, another common cause of male infertility, impairs spermatogenesis. Even if surgically treated in the early days of life, spermatogonia of these boys will continue to possess increased sperm ROS generation and DNA fragmentation.[6]

- **Diabetes and hyperhomocysteinemia:** Diabetes has a negative impact on spermatogenesis and thus leads to OS-induced sperm DNA fragmentation. Hyperhomocysteinemia occurs via suboptimal homocysteine re-methylation to methionine. The responsible enzyme for that transformation is the well-known MTHFR (methyl tetrahydrofolate reductase). This process cannot take place properly for one of two reasons: either due to a dietary folate deficiency or because of a defect in the MTHFR gene. The latter is commonly reported in infertile men, rendering these men at elevated risk for homocysteine-induced OS.

Exogenous sources:

- **Radiation:** Mobile phone radiation increases ROS production in the seminal plasma and therefore has a negative impact on sperm quality, on three parameters: motility, count and vitality. It also induces DNA damage. Radiofrequency waves affect male fertility via the temperature-regulating pathway, but also via nonthermal mechanisms. We do know that radiation elevates temperature, which isn't good at all for the testes as sperm factories. Even if temperature increases by just 1°C, proper spermatogenesis is already affected. Radiation can also induce OS which disrupts germ cell proliferation and cause DNA fragmentation as well as epigenetic modifications.[7]

- **Smoking and alcohol:** Smoking destroys the balance of ROS production and antioxidant capacity as it elevates the concentration of leukocytes in the seminal plasma by almost 50%, which leads to an increase of ROS by more than 100%. Furthermore, smoking elevates cadmium and lead concentrations in blood and semen, which also increases ROS generation and damages sperm motility. Germ cell apoptosis and DNA damage are commonly seen in infertile smokers.

- **Toxins:** Industrialization has led to the generation of a mass of environmental toxins and so-called endocrine disruptors which we will discuss in a later chapter. These can enter the body and cause massive ROS production in the testicles, and hence impair morphology and sperm function. They can also cause ROS-induced germ cell apoptosis.

What are the mechanisms of ROS-mediated male-factor infertility?

- Sperm DNA fragmentation.

- Apoptosis of spermatozoa.

- Lipid peroxidation.

Bear in mind that ROS (at a physiological level) plays an essential role in certain steps in sperm development, such as maturation, capacitation, hyperactivation and acrosome reaction!

How to test for elevated ROS?

ROS-induced sperm damage is a major contributing male reproductive pathology (almost 30–80% of idiopathic male infertility). However, ROS assessment is difficult due to high costs, screening inconveniences and lack of an accepted specific analysis method. Nevertheless, more than 30 different ROS measurement assays have emerged recently that can predict the level of OS in infertile men.[8]

HINTS IN NORMAL SEMEN ANALYSIS TO ASSUME HIGH ROS

- **Asthenozoospermia** (= asthenospermia, sperm motility deficiency) is a major OS marker as high ROS leads to impaired sperm motility.

- **Hyperviscosity of the seminal plasma** may indicate elevated ROS levels (due to high malondialdehyde (MDA) levels as a marker of a high level of peroxidative damage to spermatozoa).

- **Round cells** could indicate leukocytospermia, if present to an abnormal high level, as we know leukocytes are a common source of ROS.

- **Teratospermia** (abnormal morphology) is presumed to indicate OS.

SPECIAL TESTING METHODS

- Total antioxidant capacity (TAC). The antioxidant capacity of the seminal plasma can be tested.

- Lipid peroxidase markers. Spermatozoa often carries accumulated lipid peroxides. Its metabolites such as MDA can be used as OS indicators.[9]

- Seminal oxidation-reduction potential (ORP). This helps to infer the association between oxidants and antioxidants and thereby suggests the level of OS.[10]

- Direct laboratory assessments of OS. Seminal ROS can be directly measured. Luminol, for example, measures both intracellular and extracellular ROS.[11]

WANT TO KNOW MORE?

The sixth edition of the *WHO Laboratory Manual for the Examination and Processing of Human Semen* recognizes the increasing clinical relevance of seminal OS by dedicating a section to the methods assigned for ROS testing. Possibly due to the limited availability of such testing, this assessment has been incorporated in the 'Advanced Examination' section, suggesting that this should still be considered a research tool. However, given the large number of recent papers on the reproductive impact of OS and the clinical utility of

ROS testing, along with the description of Male Oxidative Stress Infertility (MOSI) as a clinical entity, one may consider ROS testing as part of the extended semen examination in clinical practice.[12]

How to treat elevated ROS causing male infertility

Besides Chinese Medicine, which is what this book is about, Western Medicine also has some important recommendations which are not so far away from the general Asian approach.

LIFESTYLE CHANGES

- Cease substance abuse, alcohol intake, smoking.

- Improve diet.

- Minimize exposure to endocrine and reproductive disruptors as much as possible. Specifically, try to avoid pollutants, heavy metals and other toxins as they greatly account for OS development.

- Observe scrotal temperature, knowing that an elevation of it can impair spermatogenesis. Therefore, where possible, avoid hot baths, driving for long periods, seat heating, rigorous exercise, sitting for long periods as heat stress can also create OS.

VITAMIN AND ANTIOXIDANT SUPPLEMENTATION

- Antioxidant supplementation may eradicate excess ROS or decrease its production. Preventive antioxidants such as transferrin and lactoferrin prevent OS by restricting ROS generation, and scavenging antioxidants such as vitamins C and E combat OS by mitigating excess ROS. There are some antioxidants that are well researched and shown have an effect on OS-induced male infertility such as vitamins C and E, N-acetyl-cysteine, selenium and zinc.[13]

SURGERY

- Varicocele repair decreases seminal ROS, preventing further oxidative damage. It not only improves several sperm parameters, but it also improves pregnancy rates.[14] This can be proved by measuring antioxidant levels as well as inflammatory and OS markers such as MDA, H_2O_2 and nitric oxide (NO) pre- and post-surgery.[15]

CHAPTER 4

Enhancing Sperm Quality with Nutraceuticals

DR KALI MACISAAC

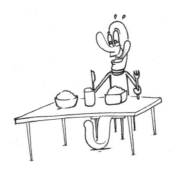

You now have sound knowledge of the complex and delicate processes that govern spermatogenesis and understand that these processes can be easily disrupted by alterations to the hormonal, nutritional or transport systems within the male reproductive system. My goal is to familiarize you with how to support optimal sperm production in the presence of these potentially damaging factors. For this, we need to consider not only whether the patient is nutritionally replete enough to produce high-quality sperm, but also the degree of attack their sperm cells are under. This section will highlight nutraceuticals that impact each of these targets.

Developing spermatozoa are incredibly sensitive to their environment – recall that they are the smallest cells in the human body, containing half of the genetic material necessary to create life within a headpiece protected by a single plasma membrane. For the optimal production of high-quality sperm, we need to ensure that the patient is nutritionally replete in the building blocks required by the body to manufacture sperm. While a patient's diet is foundational for this process, oral or intravenous nutrients can more quickly assist a patient in recovering from a nutrient deficiency and will flood the cellular environment with targeted nutrition. Here is where elements like specific fats play a key role, along with nutrients such as zinc and the B complex vitamins.

When it comes to damage of spermatocytes, the literature has demonstrated that male infertility results from three major harmful influences: seminal oxidative stress, sperm DNA damage and apoptosis.[1] These three influences are, in fact, linked to one another – excessive seminal reactive oxygen species (ROS) lead to several types of DNA damage (chromosome deletion, chromatin cross-linking, DNA strand breaks and base oxidation) and they also mediate apoptosis through the mechanism of inducing single- and double-stranded DNA breaks responsible for cellular death.[2] In order to combat the three major damaging influences, we must focus our efforts on balancing seminal ROS levels. It has been well demonstrated that oxidative stress is a major cause of male infertility, as a large proportion of infertile men have elevated levels of seminal ROS. We now know that 80% of men diagnosed with idiopathic infertility (idiopathic = no known cause) have high levels of oxidative stress in their semen samples.[3] Supplementation with antioxidants has been shown to be a cost-effective way to improve sperm quality and pregnancy rates, both for spontaneous pregnancies and through assisted reproductive technology (ART).[4] Supplementation with antioxidants such as Coenzyme Q_{10} and vitamins C and E must be considered together with a high-antioxidant diet rich in brightly coloured vegetables and fruits.

In our modern world, it is unfortunately impossible to avoid everything that can potentially damage sperm. Thus, even in the face of impeccable diet and lifestyle, sperm quality is often less than optimal. The quality of the cellular environment during spermatogenesis is key – whether necessary nutrients are present and the degree to which harmful agents are controlled determine if the developing spermatocytes reach their fertile potential. It's our job as functional practitioners to equip our patients with a plan to clean up their diet and lifestyle as much as possible, decreasing the toxic load and increasing nutritional status, and implement a supplement regime that amplifies these efforts. While diet and lifestyle adjustment is always the first priority when it comes to improving sperm quality, a well-planned oral nutraceutical protocol containing vitamins, minerals, essential fats and antioxidants is an essential component of your well-rounded treatment plan because most of our patients want to have been pregnant yesterday. That said, we must keep in mind that producing new sperm takes between 60 and 90 days. Every change you help your patient make will impact their sperm quality after at least three months of continuous effort. In the literature, most interventions show weak responses after three months, and more significant change after six months (i.e. two cycles of sperm production). It's good to remind our patients ahead of time that this is what we expect to see – any changes they make today will impact their sperm quality in 3–6 months.

Fortunately, brand new sperm are being produced all the time, Recall that, unlike women, who are born with virtually all of their oocytes for a lifetime, men constantly generate new sperm. This is good news for those who wish to optimize sperm quality, as subtle tweaks to the cellular environment often pay out massive dividends for one's fertile potential.

This chapter will address nutraceuticals that should be considered when aiming to improve sperm quality, which is one of the simplest and most cost-effective interventions for male-factor infertility.

NOTES ON BUILDING A SUPPLEMENT PROTOCOL

Before we begin, let me first say that I would never recommend every supplement on this list to a single patient. While you may want to (because they all sound beneficial), always keep in mind the power of a high-dose nutrient – having a patient take all of them at once might actually become problematic. You're likely familiar with the axiom from Traditional Chinese Medicine (TCM) that 'too much is too much, and too little is too little'. When we're talking about supplements, this becomes incredibly important. Antioxidants, for example, are a necessity in your oral supplement protocol for sperm quality; they will help to shift the seminal ROS levels, reducing the amount of physical and genetic damage the sperm cells are up against. But small amounts of ROS are actually necessary for many physical processes when it comes to fertility and conception. If we wipe out 100% of the ROS, we may be doing more harm than good. A great place to start when building a protocol is to test your patient's nutritional status and antioxidant levels. While a seminal ROS meter exists, it isn't a staple of every functional medicine practice (at least not yet!). Luckily, we can run tests for our patients that indicate intracellular concentrations of vitamins, minerals and antioxidants, along with parameters such as essential fatty acid ratios. The results of tests like these are invaluable as you decide which nutrients to add to your patient's regime. If time and finances don't allow for testing, build a protocol starting with the nutrients that fit your patient's picture best – choose zinc if you see a testosterone deficiency and a fish oil if they present with inflammation and a diet low in essential fatty acids. Use your professional judgement to hand-select the nutrients you think will be most beneficial based on how the research shows them to benefit sperm quality. This chapter will help you select!

A second consideration with your protocol is being mindful of the quality of the products you recommend to patients. There are so many different options when it comes to nutritional supplements these days that it can be difficult to keep up with new brands and formulations. At the time of writing, I do my best to recommend what to look for in a particular supplement, based on what's available to us. Things change quickly in the supplement industry, and what's available in North America is quite different from what you'll find in Europe, for example, but if you know the key things to look for (dosage and form, encapsulation method), it should help to simplify things. The quality of a supplement is extremely important. If you're not using therapeutic doses (because a 'cheaper' supplement may not contain enough of an active ingredient), your patients won't see results. And if you're reaching for supplements that contain too many fillers, you're risking an unpleasant set of side effects. We want the sperm quality to improve and we don't want to give your patients digestive problems! I'll try to help you avoid those pitfalls.

A NOTE ON SUPPLEMENT FILLERS AND INGREDIENTS TO AVOID

In general, try to avoid the following in the supplements you recommend (contact the manufacturer if it's unclear whether they allow the addition of these ingredients): artificial colours, artificial flavours, chemical preservatives, high-fructose corn syrup, hydrogenated oils, sulphites, BPA or other plasticizers, stearic acid or magnesium stearate, irradiated ingredients, and gluten/egg/dairy/nut-derived ingredients if your patients have sensitivities.[5]

Last, while this is a chapter focused on nutraceuticals, I'll also mention food sources of the various nutrients we'll discuss. I think it's important to know where these nutrients come from and to encourage our patients to seek them in both dietary and supplemental forms. Always keep in mind that patients can't simply out-supplement a poor diet (believe me, if you don't tell them this, they'll try!). There's no easy way around it: the foods our patients eat form the foundation of their protocol, and nutritional supplements should literally 'supplement' that. They're incredibly powerful and useful, but won't be nearly as effective as they could be if you're fighting against a poor diet and sedentary lifestyle. I'm sure you've seen this clinically as often as I have, and it's so disappointing when a patient isn't seeing the results you both want for them. Focus on foods with your patients first, and consider the following nutrients in supplement form as additions to this.

Throughout this chapter, we'll be discussing how a particular nutrient is known, or suspected, to enhance sperm quality. While there is a growing body of evidence for the utility of supplements to improve male fertility, research is often contradictory. However, knowing the mechanism of why a nutraceutical may be beneficial can help to guide your consideration of it. Most of the literature focuses on how a nutrient can alter the classic semen analysis parameters. You'll often find reference to changes in count, concentration, motility, morphology, volume, viscosity and total motile count with a given supplement protocol. Occasionally, you'll find research conducted on nutrients and sperm DNA fragmentation or the effects of nutrients on the ability of sperm to undergo capacitation. While not all of our patients will be regularly running a DNA fragmentation test, knowing that a nutrient can reduce fragmentation tells us a bit about how it works and why it may benefit the ability of your patients to conceive and create healthy babies. In some cases, a nutrient will not show significant effects on the semen analysis parameters, but will influence fragmentation, efficiency of the acrosome reaction or pregnancy rates. Have this discussion with your patients ahead of time so that they aren't disappointed if their semen analysis results don't change significantly. In fact, even if their semen analysis results look stellar, there could be room for improvement. We know that genetic and epigenetic information from spermatocytes form the blueprint for the health of their child and at least two subsequent generations. The choices we help our patients make prior to conception impact their fertility and their family's health overall. In the end, the goal is a pregnancy and a healthy family!

If a patient manufactures sperm, regardless of what it says on their semen analysis, you can communicate that they should be actively interested in making changes that impact their sperm quality. Addressing diet, lifestyle, toxic exposures and emotional health and relationships prior to conception is my best advice for success with fertility and improved health for their children and future generations.

A NOTE ON SEMEN ANALYSIS PARAMETERS VS DNA FRAGMENTATION

In a 2018 study by Kaarouch and colleagues,[6] a group of couples with a male partner over the age of 41 (called the advanced paternal age group = APA) had nearly indistinguishable semen analysis results compared with younger men (younger than 41). Count, motility and morphology were not significantly different – you couldn't tell a patient's age by his results. However, the degree of DNA damage assessed by DNA fragmentation was significantly higher in the APA group than in the younger men (they had higher DNA fragmentation, chromatin decondensation and sperm aneuploidy rates). They also found significantly more cancelled embryo transfers (29% vs 10%), lower clinical pregnancy rate (17% vs 32%) and a higher miscarriage rate (60% vs 42%) in the APA group when compared with the couples with a younger male partner. Luckily, combination antioxidant formulas have been shown to improve sperm DNA fragmentation.[7]

SUPPLEMENTS TO SUPPORT SPERM HEALTH

Semen contains trace amounts of every single nutrient in the human body – and higher concentrations of nutrients that humans are commonly deficient in (including zinc, potassium and magnesium). The following vitamins, minerals, essential fats and antioxidants all play a role in the proper formation and protection of sperm.

Zinc

I consider zinc to be one of the most important trace minerals when it comes to male hormonal and sperm health. It is one of the best-studied minerals for male fertility, and it has a multitude of proven benefits. Research has correlated zinc levels in seminal plasma with sperm count and normal morphology in male test subjects.[8] Fertile men have been shown to have higher seminal plasma zinc levels when compared with their infertile peers, and smokers tend to have a diminished zinc status compared with non-smokers.[9] Zinc is known to play a crucial role in sperm capacitation, affecting a sperm's ability to fertilize an oocyte.[10] And studies have shown that zinc supplementation benefits those trying to conceive naturally as well as through ART.[11]

As zinc cannot easily be stored in the human body, adequate dietary or supplemental intake is necessary to ensure a constant supply to growing sperm cells. Zinc is found abundantly in many foods (listed below), but its absorption may be hindered by issues in the digestive tract. I frequently find suboptimal zinc levels when testing patients in my office. When a deficiency is present, dietary shifts may not be enough and supplemental zinc must be added either orally or through nutritional IV therapy.

Dietary sources: Oysters and crab, organ meats, muscle meats (beef, pork, chicken), eggs, soy beans, pine nuts, cashews, yogurt, sunflower seeds, pumpkin seeds, pecans, Brazil nuts, chickpeas.[12] Note that animal proteins and eggs contain zinc that is significantly more bioavailable than plant sources, due to the phytate activity of plant foods.

Supplemental sources: Consider zinc picolinate (preferred for ease of absorption), 25–50 mg per day depending on the patient's needs. Suggest a zinc supplement containing copper if you plan to use these doses long-term, as supplementing with zinc in high doses may create a copper deficiency. As it causes nausea on an empty stomach, always recommend zinc with food, and push it to lunch or dinner if a patient is particularly sensitive.

Selenium

The main action of selenium in the male reproductive tract is that of its role as an antioxidant. Selenium plays a major role in glutathione activity and, ultimately, the protection of sperm cells against oxidative stress.

A NOTE ON GLUTATHIONE

There are five major glutathione peroxidase enzymes that require selenium for proper functioning, and one of them (called GPx4) plays a crucial role in protecting immature sperm from damage due to oxidative stress. Animal test subjects that lack the SEPP1 gene, responsible for selenium supply to the testes, are infertile due to defective GPx4 formation and impaired sperm maturation.[13]

Data on selenium supplementation for human fertility is mixed, but this may be because clinical trials continue to use different dosing strategies when it comes to this antioxidant.

One trial of selenium supplementation showed no impact on sperm parameters or hormone levels when 300 mcg (µg) per day was used for nearly a year,[14] but two others (using 100 mcg for three months and 200 mcg per day for six months, respectively) showed improved motility and chance of conception, and improved count and morphology.[15]

Interestingly, when N-acetylcysteine (NAC) has been studied along with selenium, participants have also benefitted from some hormonal effects – increased testosterone, LH and inhibin B, and decreased FSH[16] – so they may work well in concert. More on NAC a little later.

I always encourage patients to focus on selenium-containing foods and will add supplementation (typically along with NAC) if we find a deficiency in testing.

Dietary sources: Brazil nuts (far and away the richest dietary source – I recommend 2–3 Brazil nuts per day for most male fertility patients), organ meats, seafood, muscle meats, rice, sunflower seeds.[17]

Supplemental sources: Consider a selenomethionine supplement, 100–200 mcg per day. Exercise caution with selenium supplements in patients with type 2 diabetes as it may impact glycaemic control.

Coenzyme Q-10 (CoQ10)

If you have done any research on supplements to support fertility, chances are you've come across the research on coenzyme Q10 (CoQ10). Why? CoQ10 supports mitochondria in their ability to manufacture cellular energy (ATP), something the egg, sperm and early embryo all use to survive. Every single cell in the human body contains CoQ10, in amounts that reflect the energy demands of the individual tissue type. In fact, the body uses so much ATP that it's estimated that we recycle our own body weight in the molecule every single day. I'm sure you can imagine that an early growing embryo, undergoing cell division at a rapid rate, is no exception. It takes a lot of ATP to make a baby!

CoQ10 supplementation is particularly important for older fertility patients (both male and female), as endogenous CoQ10 production peaks in the mid-20s and declines steadily thereafter.[18]

A NOTE ON THE MITOCHONDRIA AND COQ10

Our mitochondria serve multiple cellular functions. While we classically think of them as the cellular powerhouses that produce ATP, mitochondria also regulate calcium signalling, thermogenesis and apoptosis, and produce ROS. In the spermatocyte, a functional mitochondrial membrane potential is required for many processes, including motility, hyperactivation, capacitation, the acrosome reaction and maintenance of DNA integrity.

It has been shown that men with abnormal semen parameters have increased mitochondrial DNA (mtDNA) copy number and decreased mtDNA integrity.[19]

CoQ10 serves two main functions within the mitochondria: it plays a central role in oxidative phosphorylation and the production of ATP, and it serves directly as an antioxidant to combat ROS-mediated damage.

Both excessive ROS production and ageing of our mitochondria are at least partially responsible for the decline in both male and female fertility over time – not only do older cells make less ATP, but older mitochondria also generate more reactive oxygen species that damage DNA.

Studies of CoQ10 and sperm health that last six months or longer have shown improvements in sperm count, motility and morphology,[20] and an increase in acrosome-reacted sperm in the ejaculate.[21] This translates to better-looking sperm that are more likely to be able to fertilize an oocyte. Because it takes at least two weeks for CoQ10 levels to stabilize in the body after the onset of supplementation, it should be taken for at least two cycles of sperm production (six months+) in order to expect to see a change in sperm quality.

Aside from length of time to supplement, other important considerations for CoQ10 are the dose and the form. Endogenous synthesis and dietary intake typically provide enough CoQ10 to avoid deficiency in young healthy individuals, but as humans age, we find a decline in cellular CoQ10 concentrations. While some foods contain CoQ10 and should be incorporated into the diet of our male fertility patients, quantities sufficient to impact sperm quality must be derived from CoQ10 supplements (dietary intake is typically ~5 mg per day).

In supplement form, you'll find there are two versions of CoQ10: ubiquinol and ubiquinone. Because your patients will definitely ask you about it, it's worth knowing the difference between the two and specifically which one you'll choose to recommend in supplement form.

A NOTE ON ABSORBABILITY, PRODUCT QUALITY AND UBIQUINOL VS UBIQUINONE

Ubiquinols are a class of fat-soluble molecules that have anywhere from one to 12 isoprene units. The ubiquinol found in humans, ubidecaquinone or CoQ10, has a tail of ten isoprene units (hence CoQ'10'). It exists in three different redox states: ubiquinol (fully reduced), ubiquinone (fully oxidized) and ubisemiquinone radical in between (see figure opposite), and can be found in supplements in either the ubiquinol or ubiquinone form, with various emulsification and encapsulation techniques used by different manufacturers to affect absorbability.

ubiquinol
CoQ10H2

ubiquinone
CoQ10

ubisemiquinol
CoQ10H•

The difference in effectiveness between the various forms of CoQ10 in supplements (ubiquinol vs ubiquinone, oil carrier vs powder tablet, different encapsulation techniques) comes down to these manufacturing techniques that influence absorbability. CoQ10 is a large, fat-soluble molecule, difficult for us to absorb through the intestinal tract. While both ubiquinol and ubiquinone supplements have been shown to raise serum CoQ10 levels, the long-standing 'general opinion' has been that ubiquinol supplements are superior to ubiquinone, as the fully reduced ubiquinol form is the one with the antioxidant capacity, and because the initial absorption of ubiquinol in the intestinal tract was thought to be superior to that of ubiquinone. However, the body constantly inter-converts between ubiquinone and ubiquinol to continue the antioxidant action of CoQ10, and the body transports CoQ10 in both forms. It has been demonstrated that the ubiquinol form is transported in serum (bound to LDL (low-density lipoprotein) and VLDL (very-low-density lipoprotein) cholesterol), regardless of the original dietary form of the molecule that was ingested.[22] We also know that all CoQ10 is oxidized to the ubiquinone form during stomach-to-intestinal transport, for ultimate absorption in the duodenum.[23] It is reduced to ubiquinol in the enterocyte, exists as ubiquinol in circulation, and in the mitochondria, ubiquinone is used in ATP production. So you can see, the body is constantly inter-converting between the two forms during the different stages of absorption and transit. Supplement companies capitalize on the misunderstanding of how CoQ10 is absorbed, transported and used to market their products' superiority.

Most CoQ10 on the market today is synthesized via a fermentation process by the Kaneka company in Japan. The type of CoQ10 made from this process is the trans form (vs the cis form) of the molecule that is bioidentical to that which we make in our bodies, but in its raw form it comes as a polymorphic crystal that cannot be absorbed by humans. It is then up to the supplement manufacturer to dissociate these crystals into individual CoQ10 molecules, and their product must keep the CoQ10 dissociated and stable throughout its shelf life.

I'm sure you're beginning to see that ubiquinol vs ubiquinone isn't the whole story. It really comes down to the encapsulation process: how the crystals are dissociated and how they are emulsified and packaged determines how effectively a CoQ10 supplement will raise serum CoQ10.

Therefore, you can't simply look at a supplement label, see that it's in the reduced ubiquinol form and know that it's superior to the ubiquinone sitting next to it on the shelf at the store. Nor can anyone who prescribes supplemental CoQ10 say with any authority that one form is, across the board, superior to the other. The encapsulation of ubiquinone, if done properly, can result in a product that raises serum CoQ10 as much or even more than a competitive ubiquinol. In fact, failure to subject CoQ10 to de-crystallization can hinder absorbability of the product by up to 75%![24] That's a major difference.

For reference, the absorption rate of different CoQ10 preparations is as follows:

- powder form (in a capsule or hard-pressed tablet): <1%

- oil-based softgel: 2–4%

- colloidal emulsification softgel: 10–12%.[25]

This means that if you ingest 250 mg of CoQ10 from a colloidal emulsification softgel, you're absorbing the equivalent amount of CoQ10 to what would be reached by 750–1000 mg of a comparable oil-based softgel.

My best advice? Call up the supplement company you're interested in and ask them about their CoQ10. If they are aware of the importance of how it's processed and encapsulated, you can trust that their product will be effective. Be sure that, at a minimum, it's in an oil carrier softgel (e.g. rice bran oil, olive oil) and has undergone de-crystallization. Ideally, they will have used an emulsification technique to improve absorption further.

Dietary sources: Humans make CoQ10 out of precursor amino acids (tyrosine, phenylalanine) and co-factors (vitamins B5 and B6), but consume it mainly from meat, poultry and fish. Other good sources are high-quality oils and nuts and seeds. Small amounts of CoQ10 are found in some vegetables and fruits such as broccoli, cauliflower, oranges and strawberries. However, the amount of CoQ10 one can consume in food would never reach the therapeutic levels necessary to change sperm quality.

Supplemental sources: Research demonstrates benefit from 200–600 mg of CoQ10 per day, and most of the literature to date uses a softgel ubiquinone (although newer research is being conducted on ubiquinol and also shows positive benefits to sperm health). There are two forms of CoQ10 that you'll find at your natural supplement store (ubiquinol and ubiquinone), and several ways that the absorption of CoQ10 can be enhanced by a supplement company. See the box above for an explanation of the difference.

You can choose to supplement your patients with either form, in my opinion, but you should know how the raw materials have been processed and encapsulated to know what dose to use. I'll often recommend 250–400 mg of a highly absorbable emulsified ubiquinol or ubiquinone, and 600–800 mg of a softgel ubiquinol or ubiquinone that has not been engineered for better absorbability. I don't recommend powder formulations. Lastly, always spread out the dose. Research shows that intestinal absorption can easily reach saturation, and taking 200 mg three times a day will result in higher serum CoQ10 levels than taking 600 mg all at once.

N-acetylcysteine (NAC)

NAC is a powerful antioxidant that is used in many conditions involving high levels of oxidative stress. It directly scavenges free radicals and also leads to elevated levels of glutathione (the body's master antioxidant). Interestingly, NAC is also a mucolytic agent – this means that it helps to thin mucous secretions. I consider NAC in patients who have highly viscous semen, those in whom I've found low levels of glutathione and in cases where I want to support detoxification as glutathione is a crucial component of phase two detoxification within the liver.

Although research on NAC for male fertility is lacking, one study showed that NAC added to selenium had beneficial effects on sperm count and morphology, and increased testosterone, LH and inhibin B while decreasing FSH levels.[26] Clinically, I have found beneficial effects with the use of NAC for male fertility, especially in the cases mentioned above.

Dietary sources: Foods such as pork, beef, and poultry contain cystine, but in order to ingest the oxidized version cysteine, you'll need to supplement with NAC to benefit from this nutrient.

Supplemental sources: I use anywhere between 600 mg and 1800 mg per day of NAC, depending on the patient, in divided doses. As it can cause digestive upset for some, it's advisable to start with the lower dose and always take it with food.

Alpha-lipoic acid

Alpha-lipoic acid (ALA) is another antioxidant that you may want to consider using to improve sperm health if the main concerns are sperm count or progressive motility (ability of sperm to swim in a forward motion).

ALA, also known as thioctic acid, is a naturally occurring organosulfur compound that is synthesized by both plants and humans. In humans, it is bonded to proteins that function as essential mitochondrial multi-enzyme complexes involved in energy (ATP) and amino acid metabolism. Several of the citric acid cycle steps require ALA to function.

As an antioxidant, ALA can be found in the oxidized or the reduced form, and because it has an asymmetric carbon molecule, it can also exist in either 'S' or 'R' enantiomer forms. The 'R' form of ALA is biologically identical to that manufactured and used by humans; although you can find R-ALA and a racemic mixed S+R-ALA version in supplemental form, research has shown that R-ALA has slightly better absorbability.

Although data on ALA for male fertility is limited, one 12-week trial showed an improvement in sperm count, concentration and progressive motility in subjects who took 600 mg of ALA daily.[27] Semen volume and morphology were not impacted by the intervention, but the researchers showed a significant improvement in total antioxidant capacity of the semen.

Dietary sources: The body manufacturers ALA endogenously. It is also found abundantly in foods bound to an amino acid called lysine (lipoyllysine), but intake of lipoic acid in this form has not shown to produce a detectable increase in free lipoic acid in human plasma or cells. However, foods high in lipoyllysine include organ meats, spinach and broccoli, which are beneficial foods to encourage patients to consume for reasons including and beyond their lipoyllysine content.

Supplemental sources: Consider 600 mg r-ALA daily, taken between meals to enhance absorption. Do keep in mind that ALA is a strong detoxifying agent – use caution in patients with high heavy metal or other environmental toxic loads as you may start moving more than you plan to.

Vitamins C and E

I often consider these two antioxidants together, as clinical trials often put them together when studying their effects on male fertility. What's interesting about these two nutrients is that most trials looking at their effects on the standard sperm parameters (count, motility and morphology) show minimal to no impact, but they have been shown to increase pregnancy rates along with a couple of other alternative sperm health indicators. Therefore, while a semen analysis report may not drastically improve, the patient may be able to get his partner pregnant after using a combination of vitamins C and E (the ultimate pay-off!).

One clinical trial showed an improvement in results of the zona binding test after three months of vitamin E supplementation,[28] and another showed improvement in sperm DNA fragmentation after two months of vitamins C and E given together.[29] The most important indicator of fertility, pregnancy rate, has shown to improve after 3–6 months of vitamin E supplementation both in conjunction with clomiphene (a pharmaceutical anti-oestrogen) and without.[30]

Dietary sources, vitamin C: Kiwis, grapefruits, oranges, strawberries, red bell peppers, broccoli, Brussels sprouts.[31]

Dietary sources, vitamin E: Oils (best sources: grapeseed, olive), sunflower seeds, almonds, hazelnuts, pecans, tomato sauce, dried apricots, avocado.[32]

Supplemental sources: I typically recommend a multivitamin formula that contains both vitamins C and E. Consider vitamin C (ascorbic acid, liposomal version if there are digestive sensitivities) 500–1000 mg daily, and vitamin E 200–400 mg daily.

Vitamin D

Vitamin D (also known as cholecalciferol) is synthesized from a cholesterol precursor in the skin upon stimulation with UVB light. In humans, about 80–90% of our vitamin D is generated this way, with the remaining being derived from food and supplementation.

The role of vitamin D in male fertility has been debated by doctors in the field since we first learned that vitamin D receptors are found in the testes and spermatozoa, and research to date shows mixed results on the effects of supplementation. We know for sure that a deficiency of vitamin D negatively impacts semen and hormone function in both animals and humans,[33] but researchers have had a harder time proving that supplementing with vitamin D creates a benefit. The theories that exist are that vitamin D may support male fertility via hormone production (support of testosterone generation), calcium regulation and a possible influence on sperm count, motility and morphology. But for every study that shows a positive influence of vitamin D on these parameters, another shows no change. This is likely to be because studies use different dosing strategies and don't always take an individualized approach to treatment, testing levels and titrating vitamin D doses specific to each patient.

That said, if what we know for sure is that vitamin D deficiency is associated with poorer semen and hormone function, it's a good idea to test your patient's vitamin D status to see if supplementation may be of benefit. While the research at this point can't suggest an optimal range of vitamin D for male fertility, I like to see values in the upper 25th percentile of the 'normal' range on a 25-OH vitamin D lab test.

Dietary sources: The inactive form of vitamin D (called D2) is partially derived from food sources such as animal protein, dairy products and mushrooms, but the biologically active version (D3) is primarily produced in the skin from sunlight exposure. If results of the 25-OH blood test show deficiency, levels should be increased via supplementation and safe sun exposure.

Supplemental sources: I prescribe anywhere from 2000–10,000 IU vitamin D3 per day, depending on the patient's 25-OH test results, and sometimes give vitamin D3 injections in the case of poor absorption or incredibly low serum levels. Vitamin D is fat-soluble – a supplement should either contain a carrier oil (e.g. coconut oil) or be taken with a meal containing a significant amount of fat in order for it to be efficacious. It is also a smart idea to use an oral supplement containing vitamin K2 in addition to the D3, as these two nutrients work in concert. Supplementing with high amounts of vitamin D3 without K2 can create a relative deficiency in K2 over time, hindering D3's biological activity.

B vitamins

The B complex vitamins have hundreds of biological functions in the human body. For nearly all male fertility patients, I recommend a multivitamin formula that contains a mixture of the B vitamins, as many of them work in concert to support processes such as DNA synthesis, mitochondrial function and amino acid and fatty acid metabolism. We also incorporate the B complex vitamins into our intravenous therapies aimed at enhancing both male and female fertility. Two particular B vitamins – B9 (folate) and B12 (cobalamin) – have been shown to significantly impact sperm quality and physiology.

Often recommended for women who are trying to conceive, folate (vitamin B9) has shown some benefit for sperm quality. Folate levels have been shown to impact sperm quality by influencing DNA integrity and the epigenome.[34]

There are several different types of folate that can be given supplementally. Folic acid, the synthetic version of the vitamin, folate, which is the version found in foods, folinic acid, an intermediary, and methylfolate (also known as 5-methyltetrahydrofolate or 5-MTHF), the biologically active version. While most research suggests supplemental folic acid, most functional practitioners prefer to use either folate or methylfolate as they are easier for the body to use, and unmetabolized folic acid can cause problems in some patients. If you test genomic panels including MTHFR and MTRR status in your patients, it can help to guide your supplementation suggestions. If not, choose either folate or methylfolate, and change the form if your patient has trouble tolerating it.

Most of the research done to date on vitamin B12 and sperm quality has shown improvements in sperm count, in addition to some literature that has shown that fertile men have higher seminal B12 levels than their infertile peers. The doses used in clinical trials have varied, but studies using as little as 1000 mcg/day and as much as 6000 mcg/day of methylcobalamin have shown benefit.[35] Like folate, vitamin B12 can be supplemented in four different forms – cyanocobalamin, hydroxocobalamin, adenosylcobalamin and methylcobalamin – depending on the molecule that the cobalamin is attached to. While some patients tolerate one version over the others, the biologically active forms adenosyl- and methylcobalamin are preferred.

A NOTE ON THE FOLATE AND VITAMIN B12 FORMS

Although beyond the scope of this chapter, it is interesting to note that the methylation ability of your patients can predict which form of folate or B12 they will both benefit from and tolerate best. In general, I recommend supplementing with anything other than folic acid and cyanocobalamin. Folic acid needs to undergo conversion to gain the ability to be biologically active in methylation processes, requiring the action of various enzymes in order to be activated. Cyanocobalamin is a cheap version of B12 that is complexed with a cyanide molecule, and while it's incredibly stable in this form, it's not easily absorbed or directly useable in the system. Methylcobalamin and adenosylcobalamin are the active forms of B12, and methylcobalamin is by far the easiest to find in supplements. Testing your patient's genetic profile, looking at gene SNPs (single nucleotide polymorphisms) such as MTHFR, MTR, MTRR, TCN2 and others, will provide you with the best guidance on the form of B vitamins to supplement.

Other B vitamins – including B5 and B6 – are cofactor nutrients in a number of enzymatic pathways involving hormone regulation and the steps of spermatogenesis. Riboflavin (B2) is a critically important nutrient involved in methylation and mitochondrial and immune function. For these reasons, in most cases it's smart to supplement your patients with a B vitamin complex as opposed to the individual Bs.

Dietary sources: Folate is found in highest concentrations in dark-green leafy vegetables, fruits and nuts. Synthetic folic acid is added to fortified cereals and other baked goods, but must be converted to biologically active 5-MTHF in the body before it is useful. I prefer patients to consume naturally derived folate or supplements containing active methyl-folate. Vitamin B12 is rich in animal foods such as meat, fish and dairy products. Other B vitamins, such as B5 and B6, are also found predominantly in muscle and organ meats but mushrooms, avocados, nuts and seeds are good vegetarian sources. When patients are recommended to follow a 'fertility promoting diet', rich in non-starchy vegetables, a combination of animal and vegetarian proteins, whole grains or starchy vegetables and healthy fats, they will likely consume an array of B-vitamin rich foods. It is still ideal to supplement on top of dietary intake, as research shows that often patients need more of the Bs than they're getting in their diet.

Supplemental sources: Consider folate or 5-MTHF, 250–500 mg/day, vitamin B12 (hydroxo-, adenosyl- or methylcobalamin) 1000–6000 mcg/day, or a B complex vitamin containing active folate and B12.

Omega 3 fatty acids

Fats are what make up the cell membranes in every cell in the human body including (you guessed it!) sperm cells. The type and quality of the fats available to build cellular membranes impact the health and function of sperm. In particular, the group called poly-unsaturated fatty acids (PUFAs), which includes omega 3 and omega 6 fats, are responsible for the fluidity and function of cell membranes. Diet plays a primary role in the ratio of omega 6:omega 3 available, and while it has been suggested that the optimal human ratio is 1:1, in many industrialized countries the ratio falls somewhere between 25:1 to 40:1. Researchers have shown these higher ratios to be hazardous to sperm health,[36] and several studies have demonstrated that fertile men have higher levels of omega 3 in their blood and spermatozoa.[37] Further, supplementation with omega 3 fats (EPA and DHA, sourced from high-quality fish oil) in two separate trials showed improvements in count/motility/morphology and sperm DNA fragmentation index.[38] The omega 3 oils EPA and DHA have a mild to moderate anti-inflammatory effect as well.

Considering that most men I treat have high omega 6:omega 3 ratios from years of following a standard North American diet, I almost universally suggest an omega 3 supplement for sperm health. Be very careful which one you choose – many on the market are either incredibly low dose (making them a waste of money) or low quality (making them not only ineffective but potentially harmful). Be sure to select a fish oil with an appropriate dose of both EPA and DHA that comes from a manufacturer with strict standards for oil stabilization and testing of various toxicants such as heavy metals.

Dietary sources: Fish and seafood. Encourage consumption of higher welfare/sustainable fish and seafood varieties, and be sure to avoid fish that are high in mercury and other environmental contaminants. A good place to find out which seafood varieties are both healthiest and sustainable in your area is www.seachoice.org.

Supplemental sources: Consider a high-quality fish oil supplement containing at least 1000 mg EPA and 500 mg DHA daily. Higher doses may be necessary in the case of concomitant inflammatory conditions.

Carnitines

L-carnitine is synthesized in the body from the amino acid precursor lysine. It is considered a 'conditionally essential' nutrient – meaning that although the body can produce it, in certain scenarios (e.g. high stress) the body may not be capable of producing enough and begins to require it through food or supplementation. There are two different versions of carnitine that have been studied in regard to sperm quality – l-acetyl carnitine (LAC) and l-carnitine (LC). While they both benefit mitochondrial function by shuttling fatty acids into the mitochondria for conversion to ATP, LAC has further benefits via its antioxidant activity; it protects mitochondria from metabolic toxins, stabilizes cell membranes and has anti-apoptotic effects.[39] One of the first research studies on carnitines and sperm quality, published in 1984, showed that men with higher concentrations of l-carnitine in their semen had higher sperm counts and higher percentages of motile sperm.[40] Both LC and LAC have been found to benefit sperm motility, which makes sense considering carnitines support mitochondrial activity.[41] Some studies have shown beneficial effects also on sperm count and morphology, but given the body of evidence and my clinical experience, I tend to reach for the carnitines when I'm trying to improve sperm motility.

Dietary sources: Meat, poultry, fish, dairy products, avocado, wheat, asparagus.[42]

Supplemental sources: Some of the difference in activity between LC and LAC lies in their respective abilities to penetrate different tissues. They both assist in mitochondrial ATP production, but while LC is active only in the peripheral tissues, LAC can cross the blood–brain barrier and influence energy production there. LAC has also shown antioxidant effects, and while LC is often less expensive, it may also be less well absorbed. One research paper compared the two versions for sperm quality effects and found that both were beneficial for sperm motility. Doses at 3 g of either LC or LAC or 2 g of LC + 1 g of LAC have shown benefit.

L-arginine

L-arginine is a semi-essential amino acid, meaning we produce it endogenously, but certain situations can require us to obtain it from dietary sources. It functions in the production of a number of biologically important molecules including urea, polyamines, proline, glutamate, creatine, nitric oxide (NO) and agmatine. There are several mechanisms by which l-arginine can enhance sperm quality. First, it can cross the blood–brain barrier and stimulate growth hormone production, necessary for instigating spermatogenesis. Second, it serves as a precursor to spermine, an alkaloid necessary for sperm production. Third, its roles in cellular and protein building contribute to proper sperm formation. And fourth, as it enhances NO production, it also supports blood flow and erectile function.

Research dating back to the 1970s has shown that 4–8 g per day of l-arginine can boost both sperm count and semen volume in oligospermic men.[43] When test subjects are fed an arginine-restricted diet, spermatogenesis is significantly reduced after just a few days in those who previously had normal function. In the 1990s, research further proved that l-arginine can significantly influence sperm motility[44] and pregnancy rates in men with low sperm counts.[45]

In order for your patient to see noticeable results, l-arginine should be supplemented for a minimum of three months; for some, it will take up to six months (two cycles of sperm production) to see a noticeable difference in sperm count. Because nitric oxide is produced and metabolized quickly, you may want to consider a sustained-release product in a base of methylcellulose. This will help to maintain tissue arginine levels for a 24-hour period. If you are just prescribing l-arginine for erectile function, a quick release formula may be best.

A cautionary note on l-arginine: if your patients get cold sores or have frequent herpes outbreaks, l-arginine will likely exacerbate them. Always ask your patients about this before prescribing it.

Dietary sources: Meat, poultry, fish, dairy products, eggs and grains, nuts, pumpkin seeds.[46]

Supplemental sources: Use a slow-release l-arginine to support sperm count and motility, 1000 mg per day in divided doses.

Pycnogenol

Pycnogenol is the trade name for an extract from French maritime pine bark that is a source of several antioxidants. It is used in a number of high oxidative stress conditions, and a few small trials have shown benefit to sperm quality. While most of the research on Pycnogenol has been done on combination formulas containing a mixture of some or all of l-arginine, taurine, roburins, l-citrulline, and Pycnogenol, one trial of 200 mg daily Pycnogenol alone for 90 days showed improvements to sperm morphology and mannose receptor binding.[47] Combination formula studies have shown improvements to erectile function, orgasmic function, sperm concentration, morphology and percentage of motile sperm; in fact, a cross-over design trial showed that when men stopped supplementing with the l-arginine and Pycnogenol formula, their sperm quality returned to previous functionality/infertile status.[48] These results suggest that Pycnogenol improves sperm functionality and enhances natural male fertility when taken for a minimum of three months.

Dietary sources: None.

Supplemental sources: Doses in the trials vary from 60 mg to 200 mg daily. If using Pycnogenol as an add-on to l-arginine and other antioxidants, start with a lower dose. If using Pycnogenol alone, a 200 mg daily dose would be appropriate.

Myo-inositol

The inositols are a family of compounds that are all stereoisomers of each other – meaning they are all basically the same molecule arranged in different spatial patterns, giving them slightly different activities in different tissues. Myo-inositol has long been used as a supplement to improve female fertility, especially in women with polycystic ovary syndrome (PCOS) because of its ability to improve insulin resistance, balance excessive androgens and improve oocyte quality. Interestingly, myo-inositol has also shown some promise for sperm functionality. In men, myo-inositol is produced by Sertoli cells in response to FSH release, and is involved in processes that regulate motility, capacitation and the acrosome reaction of sperm.

A NOTE ON HOW INOSITOLS AFFECT MOTILITY

In a really interesting initial research paper, spermatozoa from patients with oligospermia, asthenospermia and/or teratospermia (OAT) was found to be covered in an 'amorphous fibrous material' not seen in healthy controls. The fibrous material both increased seminal fluid viscosity and reduced sperm motility, not surprisingly. It was also observed that the cristae forming the mitochondria in these sperm were damaged. After incubation with inositol, researchers observed that the fibrous material disappeared – improving viscosity of semen and motility of sperm – and the damage to mitochondrial cristae diminished.[49]

The positive effect of myo-inositol on sperm motility has been confirmed by more recent research investigating the effects of myo-inositol on male fertility. Further studies have shown that while myo-inositol seems to 'stimulate' motility of sperm of men with OAT, it also plays a protective role in men with normal sperm. It was then suggested that myo-inositol be used in vitro during ART procedures (both for intrauterine insemination (IUI) and in vitro fertilization (IVF)) to enhance the activity of sperm. Physicians who have tested this hypothesis have seen some promising results: the oocyte fertilization rate during intracytoplasmic sperm injection (ICSI) procedures where the sperm have been incubated in myo-inositol was significantly improved, and the number of grade A embryos on day 3 was higher in a myo-inositol test group versus placebo.[50]

In addition to the research showing improvements to sperm motility, a randomized controlled trial (RCT) showed no adverse reactions to myo-inositol in a group of 194 men diagnosed with idiopathic male infertility after supplementing with 2 g myo-inositol and 200 mcg folic acid twice daily for three months. Encouraging results were seen: significant improvements in acrosome-reacted spermatozoa, sperm concentration, total count and progressive motility compared with placebo. Hormones reacted as well – researchers observed normalization of LH, FSH and inhibin B levels.[51]

Dietary sources: Fruits, vegetables, beans, grains and nuts. Notably, fresh vegetables and fruits contain significantly more myo-inositol than frozen or canned varieties.[52]

Supplemental sources: Consider 2 g myo-inositol twice daily. I use myo-inositol in a powder form, as it has a subtly sweet flavour that is well tolerated and easy to take. Some patients experience digestive upset (diarrhoea) if this dose is taken straight away – we often tell patients to start slow and increase their dose over a couple of weeks to help the bowels adjust.

Probiotics and prebiotics

Although a recent development, scientists are beginning to discover the important roles of both the gynaecological and seminal microbiomes in various aspects of fertility. We are starting to see that the steps of fertilization, embryo transport through the fallopian tubes, implantation, early development and the maintenance of a healthy pregnancy (as well as others) are mediated, at least in part, by the microbiome. Not only our conception rates, but the type of sperm that are selected (or rejected) in the female system are driven by the seminal microbiome.[53] If we change the microbiome, we can change sperm quality and a couple's fertility.

The seminal microbiome certainly has lower bacteria concentrations than the vaginal microbiome, but the makeup of this microbiome has shown to be different in infertile men compared with fertile men. Testing in IVF clinics has shown that low-quality semen has high concentrations of *Anaerococcus*, *Prevotella* and *Pseudomonas* species. Healthy *Lactobacillus* strains are heavily concentrated in both the healthy female vaginal microbiome and in a healthy seminal microbiome – they are commensal and also protective for other potentially infectious organisms. It is important to encourage healthy *Lactobacillus* levels in semen. *Lactobacilli* not only preserve sperm motility and viability (in vitro) but also prevent membrane damage induced by ROS.[54]

While there certainly hasn't been enough research done to say that particular strains of probiotics will definitely benefit male fertility for every individual, considering the microbiome of your patient is important in your consideration of their clinical case. Although, at the time of writing, a test for the seminal microbiome isn't currently available for clinicians, you can identify potential microbiome concerns by a careful evaluation of the semen analysis (SA) and sperm parameters. High agglutination results on an SA are often found in the presence of infectious bacteria, and we find this correlated with elevated DNA fragmentation and sperm antibodies. If the female partner has any gynaecological infections (especially hidden ones such as asymptomatic mycoplasma), it is important to consider treating both partners and rebalancing both microbiomes. In some cases, this is a missing link in a couple's fertility journey.

Dietary considerations: Encourage a diet high in fibre (high-fibre vegetables in particular, apples and pears), moderate amounts of fermented foods (kimchi, sauerkraut), resistant starch (cooked and cooled potatoes or rice) and some vegetarian meals to promote pH balance and growth of healthy bacteria.

Supplemental considerations: In the case of infectious microbes, treat the infection with herbs or with antibiotics as indicated and follow up with oral (and/or topical) probiotic preparations high in *Lactobacillus* strains. For prebiotics, my favourites are inulin, PHGG (partially hydrolyzed guar gum, aka Sunfiber), FOS (fructooligosaccaharides) and GOS (galactooligosaccharides). You can often find these within probiotic supplements themselves, but supplementing with them in addition to probiotics and a high-fibre diet is sometimes necessary.

Turmeric and sperm: yes or no?

One last supplement we should address (because your patients will ask about it all the time!) is the use of turmeric in the context of sperm quality. A quick internet search will reveal fears that the use of supplemental curcumin (the active antioxidant derived from turmeric) could be detrimental to sperm health and male fertility. In reality, these fears are likely overblown, and when curcumin is indicated as an antioxidant in a particular case, I use it without concern (but with a good discussion with the patient ahead of time, warning of this internet myth). A powerful anti-inflammatory agent, I'll reach for curcumin when there are other inflammatory concerns or blood sugar dysregulation, and use it with good success to balance the cellular environment and ultimately improve fertility. That said, you should know why the fear exists and decide with your patient if it's right for them.

The fear of curcumin stems from older research that investigated it as a possible contraceptive agent. When sperm were incubated in petri dishes with high concentrations of curcumin, researchers found negative impacts on sperm motility and capacitation/acrosome reaction[55] – so much so that sperm are completely immobilized in an environment where curcumin concentrations are very high. Further research showed that intravaginal administration of curcumin significantly blocked sperm function – something we'd never do clinically, but it was an interesting contraceptive idea at the time.[56]

However, other research on supplemental curcumin shows positive results for sperm quality. What seems the likely case in the context of curcumin and sperm is 'the dose makes the poison'. A study released in March 2020 showed improvements to sperm motility at moderate concentrations of curcumin, but decreases in motility at higher concentrations.[57] Turmeric is thus another example where 'too much is too much, and too little is too little'. I have found that when curcumin is used therapeutically in the right context and at the right dose, the patient and their semen analysis results benefit.

SUMMARY

There are several different approaches to supplementation, and the route you choose will depend on the patient in front of you, with consideration taken for their diet, lifestyle, environmental exposure and emotional health. Some patients may need only one or two specific nutrients to make a difference, in combination with some foundational dietary and lifestyle changes. In many instances, I recommend a pack-a-day supplement that contains several of the above nutrients in an easy-to-take once-daily vitamin pack. This is for convenience, as asking my patients to do one thing per day is much more likely to produce compliance than asking them to take several different supplements throughout the day. That said, when it comes to certain nutrients such as CoQ10, dividing doses becomes important.

In cases where I want to supplement more specifically one aspect of sperm quality, I'll often rotate through nutrients, specifically the antioxidants, using a bottle of one before swapping for another. The reason for this approach is that I never want to overwhelm the body with all of the antioxidants at once! In truth, a small amount of oxidative stress is necessary for many healthy bodily processes – regarding fertility, for example, there needs to be a bit of oxidative stress allowed around the time of fertilization or else the sperm can't penetrate the zona pellucida of the egg. Miss this crucial step, and while you may be helping your patient produce healthy sperm, they may not succeed with a pregnancy.

I urge everyone trying to create a pregnancy and a healthy baby to take a good look at their diet, lifestyle, environmental toxic exposures and emotional health/relationships when the time comes to prepare for conception. A well-structured supplement protocol is a worthy addition to lifestyle adjustments, considering the major impact they have on fertility and the health of our future generations.

— CHAPTER 5 —

Epigenetics

Epignetics is one of the youngest fields of research when it comes to reasons for male infertility. The term is a confusing one – hardly anyone knows what exactly is meant by epigenetics. As it has huge importance in our understanding of and finding treatment options for male infertility, especially in unexplained male infertility, where sperm tests are normal and no further pathology can be found with routine testing, we're going to look at epigenetics more closely in this chapter.

WHAT IS EPIGENETICS?

The term was first coined by C.H. Waddington in 1942 based on the idea of an 18th-century French naturalist Jean Baptiste Lamarck, who created the term 'soft inheritance'. He outlined a pathway for evolution that involved passing along traits that were gained from simply living and surviving. In a nutshell: environment can influence genetics.[1]

Helpful in understanding the term is to know that the prefix 'epi' comes from the Greek meaning 'on top of' or 'in addition to'. So epigenetics implies features that are in addition to genetics. It is everything that is related to gene expression but is not coded in genes.

The thing about the queen bee

The best example for understanding what exactly is meant by the term is the queen bee. All bees (workers, queens) have the same genome; what makes the difference is what is fed to the bees. Future queens are fed with royal jelly. That diet has compounds that will change the expression of enzymes involved in the methylation (activation or silencing) of key genes responsible for brain development and morphogenesis of the bee.[2]

In other words, epigenetics is a way for a cell to control the genes that need to be expressed for the proper functioning of that cell. Epigenetics is a kind of gene control item, responsible for what is expressed and what is silenced in terms of genes. That has an importance for gene functioning and new phenotypes.

THE ROLE OF EPIGENETICS IN MALE FERTILITY

Concerning male fertility, epigenetics describes all types of information on the molecular level that are transmitted from the spermatozoa to the embryo. To guarantee proper embryo development, certain epigenetic regulatory mechanisms are required:

- DNA methlation/genomic imprinting

- histone modifications

- chromatin remodelling

- role of RNA transcripts and telomere length.

The sins of the father

As spermatozoa are not just a DNA cargo, the roots of inheritance may extend beyond the genome, but the mechanisms remain a puzzle! (V. Hughes)

Aberrant epigenetic reprogramming in male germ cells can lead to sperm abnormalities and/or embryonic or foetal development. Some epigenetic regulations are linked to environmental factors, which may explain infertility in the context of exposure to some environmental toxins (e.g. smoking, alcohol, endocrine disrupters, diet, pollution).[3]

To put it all together, especially for couples suffering from unexplained male infertility, but also male-factor infertility in general, advice and recommendations concerning obesity, alcohol consumption and smoking may help to reduce infertility-related epigenetic errors in sperm and moreover help in understanding and treating male fertility problems.

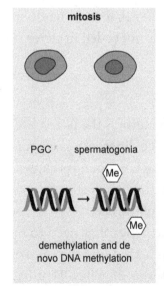
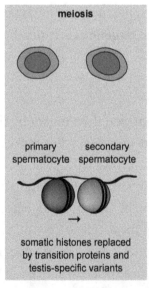
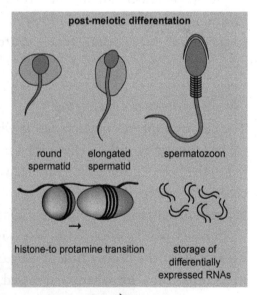

WANT TO KNOW MORE?

All these mechanisms are far beyond our common knowledge, so if you want to dig deeper let's go through them step by step starting with a short summary on genetic concepts for a better understanding of epigenetic terminology.

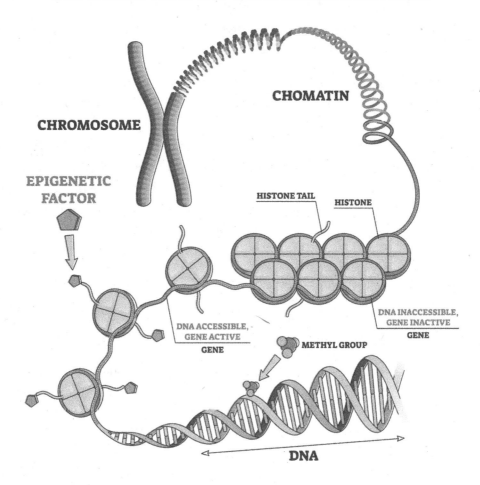

Somatic cells have 23 pairs of nuclear chromosomes; however, germ cells (oocytes and spermatozoa) contain only 23 chromosomes (not paired). The human genome also includes mitochondrial chromosomes that originate from the cytoplasm of the fertilized ovum, and are thus inherited maternally. Nuclear chromosomes (the common ones, not the mitochondrial ones) are composed of chromatin. Chromatin is a complex of unbroken long double-stranded helical DNA that carries genes and proteins and that is wrapped around proteins (histones). This DNA+histone complex is called nucleosomes. Each DNA single strand is formed from nucleotids, which include a composition of the nitrogenous bases adenin (A), cytosine (C), thymine (T) and guanine (G), desoxyribose and phosphate. Hydrogen bridges interconnect base pairs (A–T) and (C–G) to form a DNA helix. Our genome consists of 6–7 billion of these base pairs. Approximately 140 DNA base pairs are associated with the histone complex as its centre and wrapped around it. In between two of these DNA complexes (nucleosomes), there is always a short 'spacing segment' of DNA. Genes can best be described as DNA sequences that encode different functions including protein synthesis after transcription of messenger-RNA (mRNA), a functional RNA synthesis. There are about 40 million genes in our body. Genes can be coding (if so, they are called exons) or non-coding regions (introns). Introns are transcribed to RNA in the nucleus, but they do not end up as a protein end product. The locus defines the exact position of a gene on a chromosome. Generally, each gene has two copies, one from the mother and one from the father. These copies are called 'alleles'.[4]

DNA methylation: The greatest amount of research has been done on this regulatory tool of epigenetics, so we know a lot about it. DNA methylation means that a methyl group (CH_3) is added to the DNA strand, typically to a carbon atom of a cytosine ring. To be exact, it is added to the fifth position of cytosine in a CpG dinucleotide by DNA methyltransferases. Cytosine is the only base that can be methylated. Methylated cytosine is called the 'fifth base' of DNA. It fixes genes to the 'off' position, meaning that the gene is inactivated. In that way, DNA methylation regulates gene expression. In sperm cells, promoters of developmental genes are highly hypomethylated.

Hypermethylation: gene silencing

Hypomethylation: gene expression

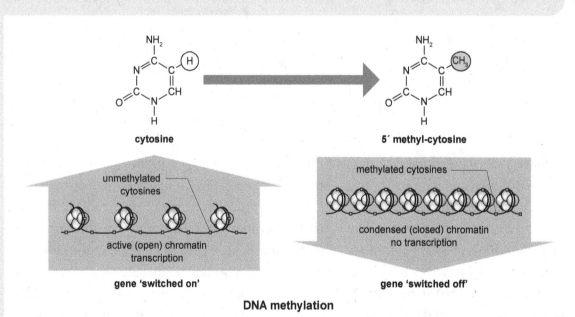

DNA methylation

Aberrant DNA methylation in sperm cells is associated with male infertility and has been found as abnormalities in semen parameters, as several recent studies show. Even in unexplained male infertility, when no pathologies in semen analysis can be found, DNA methylation errors are evident in sperm cells, causing male-factor infertility. Sperm DNA methylation may therefore be used to predict fertility and is potentially predictive of embryo quality during IVF.[5]

To put DNA methylation errors in a more practical context, smoking has a strong correlation with CpG methylation, which has an impact on sperm count, morphology and motility. Smoking is strongly associated with changes in sperm DNA methylation patterns. Alcohol has also been shown to have a negative impact on proper DNA methylation at regulatory regions. Even paternal diet seems to have an influence on proper DNA methylation processes in sperm. Recent studies pointed out the effect of paternal age, when DNA methylation defects are concerned. Interestingly, DNA methylation defects that occurred in older fathers were found to be located in regulatory or promoter regions that govern neurological, psychiatric and behavioural disorders such as autism, and mood disorders including schizophrenia. To enable proper methylation, men need certain dietary components that may serve to regulate the availability of methyl donors for the subsequent methylation process. Those are methionine, folate, choline, betaine, vitamins B2, B6 and B12 and, of course, the proper functioning of MTHFR, a key enzyme of the folate metabolism.

To prevent the passing on of DNA methylation aberrations, there are two major reprogramming events that involve genome-wide erasure and re-establishment of DNA methylation patterns during mammalian development. The first occurs in primordial male germ cells on day 6.5–13.5 and the second following fertilization in the pre-implanted embryo (male pronuclei are actively and rapidly demethylated in the zygote, whereas the maternal genome is passively demethylated in a replication-dependent manner until cleavage).[6]

Genomic imprinting: This means that although genes are inherited as two copies (diallelic) – one maternal and one paternal – only one copy will be expressed. Which of the two is being expressed depends on whether it is paternally imprinted in sperm or maternally imprinted in the oocyte. For a gene to be imprinted, it needs to be hypermethylated. Then it is switched 'off' and not being expressed.

Paternal imprinting means that an allele inherited from the father is not expressed in the offspring. It is silenced by hypermethylation. Maternal imprinting, on the other hand, means that an allele inherited from the mother is not being expressed in the offspring as it is frozen by hypermethylation. This methylation pattern occurs in the somatic cells throughout their lifetime.

Chromatin remodelling: DNA is usually wrapped around proteins called histones to facilitate packaging into chromosomes and into the nucleolus. So chromatin consists of DNA and histones. In a step that is unique to sperm, throughout spermiogenesis (where motile spermatozoa develop from round spermatids) these histones are being replaced by other arginine-rich proteins called protamines. These far tighter packages of DNA create a doughnut shape (toroid), which allows no further transcriptions from the DNA – in other words, no nuclear activity. Within this 'histone-to-protamine transition' 90–95% of the histones are replaced by protamines. However, there should be no more than 10% of remaining histones, as an increased histone-to-protamine ratio can be found in infertile men, so obviously harms fertility. For many years, researchers thought that the remaining 5–10% of histones were a mistake of nature. Nowadays, we do know that these retained male histones are essential for the early embryo development; interestingly, they are located at promoter genes for that purpose. They bring the 'already open' paternal genes that are essential for embryo development into the zygote. They also transfer the paternal epigenetic signals into the oocyte. The sperm's protamines begin to be replaced by maternal histones right after fertilization (protamine-to-histone transition) and only the small amount of paternal histones remain and show the paternal epigenetic marks.

Once again, what is this exchange of proteins for?

Histone-to-protamine transition is unique to sperm, is needed for nuclear compaction, protects the sperm DNA and precludes transcriptional activity. Defaults in protamination as well as increased histones retention results in subfertility.[7]

In a practical context, oestrogen in the environment (soy, plastics, hormones such as the contraceptive pill) has a huge impact on that epigenetic modification as oestrogen receptor agonists cause increased histone retention, protamine deficiences and other histone modification issues.[8]

There are two types of protamines, P1 and P2, and their ratio has to be around 1:1, otherwise fertility is impaired.

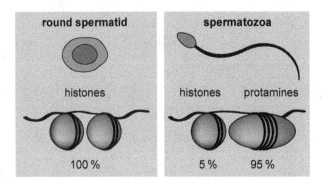

Histone modifications: Histones are subjected to post-translational modifications on their histone tails including phosphorylation, methylation, acetylation and ubiquitination on different residues. Each of these modifications works alone or in concert to influence activation or inhibition of gene transcription.[9] For example, acetylation always takes place on a lysine base and causes gene activation, whereas methylation (either on lysine or arginine) can cause a gene activation or gene silencing depending on site specificity and the number of methyl groups added. Histone modifications in general can alter gene expression and are known to underlie biological processes such as transcriptional activation, chromosome packaging and repair of DNA damage. This process provides another modifiable layer of gene regulation with the potential of heritability.[10] Histone modifications represent epigenetic signals that are transferred into the oocyte. Defects in histone modification are seen in azoospermia, oligospermia and teratospermia, so the proper functioning of that process has an impact on male fertility as well.

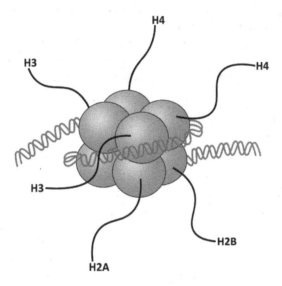

Non-coding RNA: Because of its extreme compaction, the sperm nucleus has long been thought to be inert. In fact, the spermatozoon contains many specific RNAs that could be useful to embryo development by modifying gene expression upon fertilization.[11] A non-coding RNA (nc-RNA) is a functional RNA that is transcribed from DNA but not translated into protein.[12] Nc-RNAs are expressed in male reproductive cells and play a pivotal role in male spermatogenesis. Currently, interest in the functional role of nc-RNA in male infertility has been increasing due to their enormous role in spermatogenesis.[13] Abnormal parameters in semen analysis are reported to be due to abnormal nc-RNA expression, and the abnormal expression of nc-RNAs can also affect the sperm capacitation. Finally, sperm RNA seems to play a role in embryo development as sperm RNAs are carried into the oozyte and therefore translated. Long nc-RNAs are so important for spermatogenesis that they can even be used as a biomarker for sperm quality.[14] Precisely, the comparison of microarray profiles between fertile and infertile men showed up- and down-expression of several transcripts. A 2015 study even suggested that analyzing elements of sperm RNA could be used as an individual predictor of effective fertility treatments.[15]

In contrast to environmentally induced DNA methylation alterations which can be corrected by reprogramming the sperm methylation errors, sperm RNAs and their modifications are maintained transgenerationally. In a 2014 study on that topic, sperm RNAs from mice that were exposed to mentally stressful conditions were injected into normal zygotes, proving that behavioural conditions that were observed in the father could be recapitulated in the offspring. The same applied to metabolism. Studies showed that mice who were fed a high-fat diet also contained sperm RNAs that, when injected in to normal zygotes, would produce offspring with similar paternal metabolic disorders.[16]

Epigenetics and ART: If epigenetic modifications are a key factor in the maturation of sperm cells, alterations in the epigenetic patterns of infertile men may provide a reasonable explanation for complications associated with ART, including low birth weight, premature births, congenital abnormalities, an increased perinatal mortality rate and pregnancy complications.[17]

We do know that the development of ARTs leads to epigenetic changes that may alter the normal gene imprinting processes. Although controversial, a rise of imprinting diseases in children conceived with ART has been reported, particularly Beckwith–Wiedemann syndrome and Silver–Russell syndrome.[18]

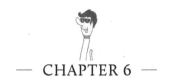

— CHAPTER 6 —

Causes of Male Infertility

Please note that any kind of medical examination mentioned in this chapter needs to be per-formed by a medical doctor; however, it is important to know about these tests and how and why they are done.

Part 1: Common anatomic/organic causes

VARICOCELE

Up to 43% of the general adult male population, and 7% and 10–25% of prepubertal and postpubertal males respectively, have a varicocele.[1] Interestingly, 35% of men with primary and up to 80% with secondary infertility have varicose veins.[2] In healthy veins inside the scrotum, one-way valves move the blood from the testicles to the scrotum, and then send it back to the heart. Sometimes the blood does not move through the veins as it should and begins to pool in the venous plexus, known as the plexus pampiniformis, causing it to enlarge. A varicocele develops slowly over time, and therefore the prevalence of varicoceles increases over time – it is estimated that a 10% rise in incidence occurs for each decade of life.[3] There are no established risk factors for developing a varicocele, and the exact cause is unclear. Varicocele formation is therefore likely to be multifactorial.

An inverse relationship between the occurrence of varicoceles and body mass index as well as intense physical activity over the years seem likely.[4] Varicoceles generally form during puberty and are more commonly found on the left side of the scrotum. The anatomy of the right and left side of the scrotum is not the same, causing a higher incidence of left-side varicoceles.

WANT TO KNOW MORE?

Whereas the right internal spermatic vein inserts into the vena cava inferior directly at an acute angle, the left one inserts at a right angle. So, the left spermatic vein might suffer from compression of the left renal vein and the increase of the hydrostatic pressure of the left spermatic vein may be transferred to the left plexus pampiniformis. Varicoceles can exist on both sides with recent findings showing that bilateral palpable varicoceles are found in more than 50% of cases.[5]

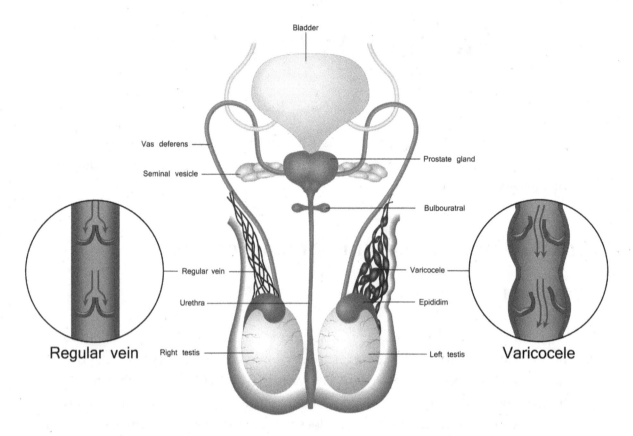

Why does a varicocele affect male fertility?

Proposed mechanisms include hypoxia and stasis (impaired drainage or pooling of blood around the testicles), testicular venous hypertension, elevated testicular temperature, an increase in spermatic vein catecholamine leading to testicular underperfusion and increased oxidative stress. This can lead to germ cell apoptosis and subsequent oligospermia (= oligozoospermia), hypoxia on the Leydig cells and thus reduced levels of androgens as well as ROS-induced DNA integrity problems. One of the main problems with varicoceles appears to be that they cause disruption of the blood–testicular barrier and cause an autoimmune status.

WANT TO KNOW MORE?

A novel hypothesis shows that in varicoceles, via several biochemical reactions, the intracellular pH decreases, causing more ROS damage of sperm, resulting in diminished sperm motility. It is known that the optimum pH for ROS scavenging by the enzymatic antioxidant systems ranges from neutral to slightly alkaline; their activity is depressed in low pH. It has been observed that antioxidant enzyme activity is significantly impaired in infertile men with varicocele and it can further cause sperm motility issues.[6]

Treatment recommendations

- Varicocele treatment is indicated for men with clinically palpable varicoceles and abnormal semen parameters.

- Open microsurgical inguinal or subinguinal techniques are considered the best treatment modalities because they result in a higher natural pregnancy rate as well as higher success rates in ART as concluded in a 2017 recent review.[7]

- Also the chances of retrieving testicular sperm for ICSI are optimized in non-obstructive azoospermic men with treated clinical varicocele.

- Varicocelectomy treatment can be offered to men with clinical varicocele and hypogonadism as a means to improve androgen production and potentially avoid testosterone replacement therapy.

- Lifestyle changes can benefit reproductive health (e.g. losing weight, easing physical activities).[8]

HYPOGONADISM

Hypogonadism means diminished functional activity of the gonads, which may result in diminished production of sex hormones. The official definition of male hypogonadism is a disorder associated with decreased functional activity of the testes, with decreased production of androgens and/or impaired sperm production.[9] The prevalence of hypogonadism increases with age and the major causes are central obesity, comorbidities (e.g. diabetes) and overall poor health.

It is essential to know that infertile men who want to father a child must not be treated with testosterone as this hinders proper spermatogenesis via the feedback mechanism.

There are two types of hypogonadism. According to the origin of the underlying problem, male hypogonadism can be classified as primary, if a consequence of testicular dysfunction, or secondary, if due to a pituitary or hypothalamic dysfunction.

Primary hypogonadism means that the cause of the underproduction of male sex hormones (mainly testosterone) is in the testes. Because the higher-ranking hormone producers – the pituitary and hypothalamus – are working properly and produce even more of their gonadotropic hormones to compensate for the failure of the testes, this type of hypogonadism is called a hypergonadotropic hypogonadism.

In secondary hypogonadism, the cause of a lack of sex hormones is the malfunction of the pituitary gland or the hypothalamus. As neither of those 'big boss' hormone producers (and consequently the testes) produces the right amount of hormones, this type of hypogonadism is called hypogonadotropic hypogonadism.

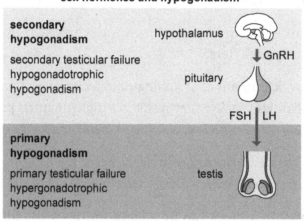

Typical lab test results for the two types of hypogonadism are:

PRIMARY HYPOGONADISM

- Location of problem: testis
- Hormones: serum testosterone ↓, FSH and LH ↑

SECONDARY HYPOGONADISM

- Location of problem: pituitary gland or hypothalamus
- Hormones: serum testosterone ↓, FSH and LH ↓

Causes of primary hypogonadism[10]

- **Congenital:** Chromosomal defects such as Klinefelter syndrome, trisomy 21 (Down syndrome), Noonan syndrome, congenital anorchia, androgen receptor/enzyme defects.

- **Acquired:** Testicular trauma/torsion, varicocele, surgical removal, chemotherapy, testicular irradiation, environmental toxins, drug-induced.

- **Systemic diseases/conditions with pituitary/hypothalamic impact:** Infections such as mumps orchitis, diabetes, renal failure, alcoholic liver disease, cirrhosis, autoimmune damage, Cushing syndrome, malignancies, HIV, ageing.

Those in the 'Acquired' category are the easiest for us to check on:

DRUGS ARE THE NUMBER-ONE REASON FOR HYPOGONADISM

- Leydig cell production of testosterone ↓

Drugs such as: corticosteroids, ethanol, ketoconazole

- Androgen receptor blockers

Drugs such as: spironolactone, flutamide, cimetidine

Causes of secondary hypogonadism[11]

- **Congenital:** Haemochromatosis, Kallmann's syndrome, idiopathic hypogonado-trophic hypogonadism (IHH), Prader–Willi syndrome.

- **Acquired:** Pituitary disorders causing hyperprolactinemia (prolactinoma, pituitary adenoma , hypothalamic tumour), medications (e.g. anabolic steroid abuse, oestrogens, opiates, glucocoricoids), obesity, ageing.

- **Systemic diseases/conditions with pituitary/hypothalamic impact:** For example, in HIV/AIDS, inflammatory diseases (sarcoidosis, histiocytosis tuberculosis), metabolic diseases.

Hypogonadism and risk factors

Low testosterone levels in men frequently coexist with:

- type 2 diabetes mellitus

- erectile dysfunction

- abdominal obesity and obesity in general

- other cardiovascular risk factors.

So could it be a component of the metabolic syndrome?

WANT TO KNOW MORE?

Kallmann syndrome (KS) is a genetic disease associated with hypogonadotropic hypogonadism and smell disorders, including anosmia and hyposmia. The disease can occur in both males and females, but it is more common in men. The prevalence of KS is 1 in 8000 males. The disease has a genetic origin. Based on the type of mutation, it can be autosomal-dominant, autosomal-recessive or linked to X-chromosome inheritance.

People with KS lack the surge of GnRH because GnRH-secreting neurons fail to migrate to the hypothalamus. As a consequence of the hypogonadotropic hypogonadism caused by KS, affected people have an incomplete development of the reproductive system, along with a lack of sexual development and fertility issues such as oligospermia or azoospermia.[12]

CHROMOSOMAL ANOMALIES/GENETIC ABNORMALITIES

Approximately 2–8% of infertile men have an underlying genetic abnormality; in men with azoospermia, this percentage rises to 15%.[13] Two quite common etiologies of genetic causes are karyotypic abnormalities and Y-chromosome microdeletion. Let's start with the chromosomal anomalies.

Klinefelter syndrome (47, XXY)

Klinefelter syndrome affects around 1 in every 660 males; they are born with an extra X-chromosome causing a congenital primary hypogonadism. Klinefelter syndrome does not usually cause any obvious symptoms early in childhood, and even the later symptoms may be difficult to spot. Many boys and men do not realize they have it. Klinefelter syndrome is not directly inherited – the additional X-chromosome occurs as a result of either the mother's egg or the father's sperm having the extra X-chromosome (there is an equal chance of this happening in either), so after conception the chromosome pattern is XXY rather than XY.[14]

Signs and symptoms may include low sperm count or no sperm, small testicles and penis, low sex drive, normal to low testosterone, FSH increase greater than LH, modest elevation of estradiol, taller than average height, weak bones, decreased facial and body hair, less muscular compared with other men, enlarged breast tissue, increased belly fat.[15]

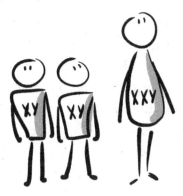

Klinefelter and infertility: Between 95% and 99% of XXY men are infertile because they do not produce enough sperm to fertilize an egg naturally; however, sperm are found in more than 50% of men with Klinefelter syndrome.[16] Advances in ART have made it possible for some men with Klinefelter syndrome to conceive. Aromatase inhibitors and surgical sperm extraction have shown success for XXY males. There is also current debate about testosterone treatment of adolescent Klinefelter patients or even children, but not yet enough data to support that.[17]

Noonan syndrome

Noonan syndrome (NS) is a genetic disorder causing primary hypogonadism. The incidence is one in 1000–2500 live births for the severe phenotype, but mild cases may be as common as one in 100 live births. There is no known disposition by race or sex. A number of genetic mutations can result in NS (chromosome 12, spontaneous mutation or autosomal-dominant inherited). Adolescent males with NS typically experience delayed puberty. They go through puberty starting at age 13 or 14 and have a reduced pubertal growth spurt that leads to shortened stature. Most males with NS have undescended testes (cryptorchidism), which may contribute to infertility later in life. Most affected individuals have characteristic facial features that evolve with age: a broad, webbed neck; increased bleeding tendency; high incidence of congenital heart disease; failure to thrive; short stature; feeding difficulties; sternal deformity; renal malformation; pubertal delay; cryptorchidism; developmental or behaviour problems; vision problems; hearing loss; lymphoedema.[18]

Y-chromosome microdeletions

These occur in approximately 10% of men with azoospermia or oligospermia. On the long arm of the Y-chromosome there is a very special region, the so-called AZF region (AZF stands for azoospermia factor). The AZF area contains three subregions which are named AZFa, AZFb and AZFc. Microdeletions of these three subregions lead to slightly different phenotypes of sub- or infertility. The best of these three microdeletions would be the AZFc microdeletion. It is the most common, found in 5–7% of oligospermatic men. With the AZFc microdeletion, there is a chance – even in men with azoospermia in a sperm test – of retrieving testicular sperm via micro-TESE sperm extraction (a micro-invasive technique described in Chapter 8). Reported success rates range from 35% to 72% to find sperm cells, whereas with AZFa microdeletions the chances of finding sperm cells for ART are very low. AZFa microdeletions lead to the well-named 'Sertoli cell-only syndrome', whereas AZFb microdeletion causes an arrest of spermatogenesis.

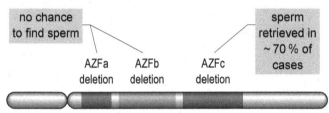

Y-chromosome microdeletion screening

| no chance to find sperm | | | | sperm retrieved in ~70% of cases |

AZFa deletion   AZFb deletion   AZFc deletion

CRYPTORCHISM

A sign of maturity of a male newborn is that the testes should have descended from their former location in the abdomen down via the inguinal canal into the scrotum. This process of 'descensus testis', the travel of the testicles into the scrotal sac, is triggered by testosterone. The location of the testicles outside the body is absolutely necessary to keep the gonads cooler than the usual body temperature. Any remaining of the testicles along that descensus pathway or even in the abdomen is called cryptorchism. It is a well-known cause of sub- or infertility due to a heat issue that has a negative impact on spermatogenesis. In fact, the severity of the cryptorchism effect on fertility is directly proportional to the severity of the cryptorchism itself, with bilateral cryptorchism having poorer effects than unilateral, and with higher testes having worse function than lower testes.[19] The surgical correction of the malposition of the testicles is called orchidopexy. It should be performed as soon as possible, preferably within the first year of the boy's life; when done so, orchidopexy has shown to improve fertility remarkably.

RADIATION

Ionizing radiation can have an immense impact on male fertility. Studies show that sperm counts declined when testes were irradiated and that decline was dose-dependent, as was the time to recovery (e.g. six months recovery time of sperm counts when radiated with 20 cGy while up to 24 months with 600cGy and even no recovery in very high dosages). Decline of sperm count takes place according to the timeline of spermatogenesis, and therefore has its nadir 64 days after the start of radiation. Fractionated radiation, where the dosage is delivered over the course of many days (as in radiotherapy to treat testicular cancer, for example) has been shown to be more damaging than single-dose radiation. One report shows that fractionated radiation with a total dosage of 200 cGy may cause permanent azoospermia.[20]

ORCHITIS

Inflammation or infection of any kind may cause indirect damage of the testes. The most common such infection is the mumps virus. This children's disease not only causes parotitis, but in some cases also causes an infection of the testes. This mumps orchitis is characterized by inflammation and swelling, which is limited by the wrapping of the testicle, the tunica albuginea. Since the 'trapped' swelling puts more pressure on the structure of the testes, this consequently leads to atrophy. It is estimated that approximately 1.5% of postpubertal males with mumps become infertile as a result of that infection, which can show up as low seminal sperm concentrations and poor sperm quality in a semen analysis. Orchitis may even lead to intratesticular obstruction, which is the case in 15% of obstructive azoospermia. However, it is rare in developed countries due to vaccination.

OBSTRUCTION

Any obstruction may be at the level of:

- epididymis

- vas deferens

- ampulla of the vas

- ejaculatory duct.

Obstructive azoospermia (OA) is a common cause of male infertility, and it is defined as the absence of spermatozoa in the ejaculate despite normal spermatogenesis. OA is a common urologic disorder and accounts for between 6.1% and 13.6% of patients who present for fertility evaluation.[21] An absence of fructose in the semen analysis supports the diagnosis, as fructose is present in the secretions from the seminal vesicles.

It can result from:

- **Infection (8–46%):** Epididymitis is a common genitourinary condition, and an infectious etiology should always be considered in men with the diagnosis of obstructive azoospermia. Gonorrhoea, chlamydia, trichomoniasis, brucellosis, BCG, ureaplasma, mycoplasma, coliform bacteria, adenovirus and enterovirus have all been reported as causes of epididymitis. Regardless of the etiology, epididymitis can cause an intense inflammatory reaction, leading to secondary scarring and obstruction of the epididymis. The incidence of post-infectious epididymal obstruction is thought to be low in developed countries due to prompt treatment, but it may account for a disproportionately large percentage of OA in the developing world. Microsurgical reconstruction is a viable option for post-infectious epididymal obstruction.[22]

- **Congenital anomalies:** Conditions where the vas deferens is absent such as congenital bilateral absence of vas deferens (CBAVD). This disease is closely related to cystic fibrosis (CF); not every male with CF presents with it, but most men with CBAVD have the CFTR mutation, which is responsible for cystic fibrosis.[23]

- **Iatrogenic injury (including vasectomy):** Vasal injury has been attributed to a variety of inguinal, scrotal and pelvic surgeries, including hernial surgery, hydrocelectomy, orchidopexy, appendectomy and renal transplant. Trauma is a rare cause of vasal obstruction. Surgical reconstruction is possible in many cases of iatrogenic injury to the vas in the scrotum or inguinal canal. Vasectomy is the most common cause of obstructive azoospermia. Vasal reconstruction is the preferred method for the restoration of fertility after a vasectomy, and due to the popularity of vasectomy and frequency of divorce, the demand for this procedure will continue to grow. The success of surgery to restore fertility is proportional to the age of the male and the time since the vasectomy. Research shows patency rates of approximately 70–95%, but fertilization rates of only 40–55%. This is on the one hand due to the fertile state of the female partner but on the other hand due to impaired motility of the sperm cells as seen in post-operative semen analysis.[24] On top of that, we do know that the probability of anti-sperm antibodies is quite high in any traumatized blood–testis barrier.

Ejaculatory duct obstruction (EDO) is a rare cause of OA. It should be suspected when the patient has low-volume, acidic semen that contains no sperm. An absence of fructose in the semen supports the diagnosis, as fructose is present in the secretions from the seminal vesicles. Occasionally, pain at the time of ejaculation is reported. Traditional treatment consists of transurethral resection of the ejaculatory ducts (TURED). Yurdakul and colleagues retrospectively reviewed the outcomes of 12 azoospermic men with EDO who underwent TURED. Sperm appeared in the ejaculate of 11 of 12 patients.[25]

Part 2: Environmental Causes

In this second part of the chapter, we will be digging deep to search for the influence of environmental and lifestyle factors throughout a man's life and try to figure out the impact they have on the reproductive capacity of a man. Numerous environmental or lifestyle factors can affect testicular development and function during both foetal life and adulthood. Exposure to these factors via the mother during pregnancy can affect the differentiation and/or endocrine functions of the foetal testes, resulting in a reduced synthesis of androgens by Leydig cells and/or reduction in the final number of Sertoli cells. This can lead to an irreversible reduction in sperm count and sperm-fertilizing capacities in adulthood. In adult men, the effects of environmental or lifestyle factors can affect spermatogenesis and/or the production and action of androgens. However, the impact is likely to be reversible because a new cycle of spermatogenesis takes place approximately every 74 days.[26]

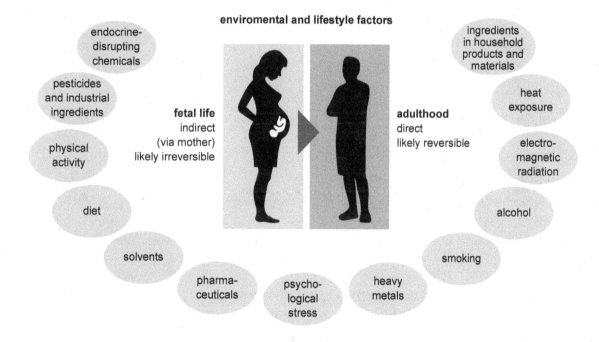

HORMONAL FACTORS

Androgen excess

Through the hypothalamic–pituitary–gonadal (HPG) axis, testosterone facilitates a negative feedback inhibition on the hypothalamic secretion of GnRH. This is not a direct feedback mechanism but an indirect one, transforming testosterone to oestrogen via aromatization. In that way, excess circulation of testosterone can suppress the HPG axis by supressing gonadotropin secretion and thus lead to impaired spermatogenesis.

There are several reasons why too much testosterone could circulate in the male. Alarmingly, one main cause is the illicit use of anabolic steroids. A huge retrospective analysis of over 6000 young men showed that in one-third of the patients with manifest hypogonadism, the reason for it is previous abuse of anabolic steroids. Furthermore, one-fifth of males who were treated for hypogonadism reported former anabolics abuse.[27]

After removing the exogenous source of testosterone, return of spermatogenesis usually occurs within four months but might take up to three years in some cases.[28]

Therapeutic administration of testosterone can also lead to testosterone excess, thus having a detrimental effect on spermatogenesis. That is why it is not recommended to use testosterone therapy to improve spermatogenesis in any cause of hypogonadism. However, one in four urologists prescribe external testosterone to men with the desire to father a child as an attempt to enhance spermatogenesis. This is why I keep pointing out the ambiguity of that therapy in this book; the four-eyes principle is intended to protect men from harm that is otherwise caused by ignorant colleagues.[29] In terms of an adequate treatment, numerous alternative strategies have been studied and proven efficacious, including hCG, FSH and clomiphene citrate.[30]

Of course, androgen excess can be due to endogenous androgen production such as in congenital adrenal hyperplasia and functional tumours.

Oestrogens and oestrogen exposure

Oestrogens are produced in the testis along with testosterone, yet the main source of oestrogen in men is the conversion of testosterone to oestrogen via the enzyme aromatase. This aromatization takes place in the adipose tissue, making obesity one of the main causes of oestrogen excess causing impaired spermatogenesis. Besides the endogenous production of oestrogens, a main source is oestrogen exposure. There are two types of oestrogen exposure:

- **Oestrogens from contraceptives** (e.g. oral contraceptive pill) or hormone replacement therapy make their way into our body orally.

- **Xenoestrogens** are artificially produced substances that have an oestrogen-like effect on our body cells. Those are the silent enemies of male fertility. Xenoestrogens belong to a group of chemicals called endocrine disrupting chemicals (EDCs).

WANT TO KNOW MORE?

The group of molecules identified as endocrine disruptors is highly heterogeneous. A non-exhaustive list includes:

- industrial solvents/lubricants such as polychlorinated biphenyls (PCBs), polybrominated biphenyls (PBBs), dioxins

- perfluorinated compounds (PCFs), such as perfluorinated alkyl acids (PFAA)

- phenols such as bisphenol A (BPA)

- plasticizers such as phthalates

- pesticides and fungicides such as dichlorodiphenyltrichloroethane (DDT)

- pharmaceutical agents such as diethylstilbestrol (DES)

- UV filters and parabens.[31]

These environmental insults in the form of oestrogens have been shown to cause responsive changes in the neuroendocrine system of the mature male with effects notable in reproductive function and spermatogenesis. Xenoestrogens have been found to adversely affect the male reproductive system in the following ways:

- They are able to inhibit FSH secretion by the foetal pituitary gland and thus mess up the proper functioning of the HPG axis, leading to a decreased number of Sertoli cells.

- They also inhibit the formation of Leydig cells and impair their proper function, thus causing decreased testosterone production and decreased gamete differentiation as a result.

- Moreover, they even inhibit androgen receptors within foetal testes.

- Additionally, via the conversion of xenoestrogens to quinones, which are a source of ROS, oxidative stress or damaged DNA can be induced.[32]

Where to find xenoestrogens? Better ask how to avoid them! They are in plastic bottles, cans, wrapping film, suncream, deodorants, preserving agents in food, pesticides, industrial waste, solvents, washing agents and cleaning agents. Bisphenol A (BPA), one of the most common xenoestrogens, was found in the blood of 90% of Americans.[33]

Those artificial hormones also bind to human oestrogen receptors (of reproductive tissue, body fat, hypothalamus and pituitary) just as the normal oestrogen does.

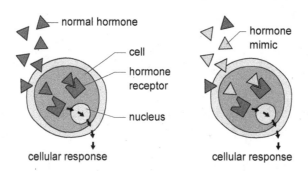

Studies on mice have shown that these artificial hormones lead to progressive degeneration of testicular tissue and can lead to dysfunction of the reproductive system in both sexes.

Another group of xenoestrogens comes from commercially available dairy products, meat and eggs. Commercial farmers often use food additives (for cows or chickens) to increase the milk or egg production. Therefore, such commercially produced eggs, dairy and meat are a main source of xenoestrogens.[34]

A study of 21 infertile men with a poor sperm test found out that their ejaculate contained far more PCBs (polychlorinated biphenyls) and PEs (polyethylene) (both xenoestrogens) than the ejaculate of 32 fertile men in the control group. On top of that, the amount of progressively motile spermatozoa went down the higher the concentration of xenoestrogens was.[35]

Another detailed review also found that exposure to PCBs and polychlorinated compounds in adulthood appears to be negatively linked to sperm motility and sperm morphology, respectively.[36]

A very recent study shows that maternal serum bisphenol A (BPA) concentration at 10–17 weeks of gestation was positively associated with congenital or postnatally acquired cryptorchidism, and n-propyl paraben concentration was associated with shorter adrenogenital distance (AGD) from birth to 24 months of age – the shorter distance causes the testicles to heat up too much.[37]

Phytoestrogens

Soya: There was an inverse association between soya food intake and sperm concentration proven by a study done in 2008. Increased intake of soya- and isoflavone-containing food (e.g. tofu, soya milk) reduced the total amount of sperm by 41 million/ml compared with men without soya intake. Soya food and soya isoflavone intake were unrelated to sperm motility, sperm morphology or ejaculate volume.[38]

Antiandrogens

Some experts claim that a more serious problem than xenoestrogens is antiandrogens (e.g. phthalates). They can be found in everyday products such as plastic, cosmetics, hairspray, shampoo and soap. They seem to be responsible for a high percentage of abnormalities in the sex development (e.g. minor anogenital distance, smaller scrotum and penis, higher chance of cryptorchism).[39] Other male reproductive traits have been shown to be related to EDC exposure in foetal life including genital malformations such as cryptorchidism and hypospadias.[40]

Generational problems (epigenetics): Some agents (insecticides and fungicides) cause infertility in the offspring of pregnant women who come in contact with those agents. This inability gets passed on, even if there is no direct contact with such agents (genetic damage).[41]

PATERNAL AGE

Not only female fertility, but also male fertility declines with age. That is important to know, since higher paternal age and eventually associated fertility decline is a common problem in men with second, often younger partners. Moreover, paternal age is generally increasing.

Several morphological changes that occur in testis histology and changes that occur in semen parameters with advanced age suggest evidence of deteriorating testicular function. The number of Leydig cells, Sertoli cells and germ cells decreases with age. Semen analyses show a noticeable decrease in semen volume, sperm motility and sperm morphology as men get older.[42] For example, in terms of semen parameters, volume of semen decreases by 0.03 ml per year, total motility by 0.7% per year and progressive motility by 3.1% per year.[43]

As paternal age increases, it presents no absolute barrier to conception, but it does present greater risks and complications. What causes far more trouble than a negative impact on sperm parameter is that there is an increased amount of DNA strand breaks in spermatozoa of older men. That DNA fragmentation leads to a higher percentage of early miscarriages.[44]

Advanced paternal age also increases the relative risk of offspring developing conditions such as neurocognitive defects, some forms of cancers and syndromes related to aneuploidies. Physicians and their patients need to be better informed of the risks and problems associated with advanced paternal age.[45]

Summarizing a few studies done on the impact of paternal age, I can say that the higher the age of the father the more increased the risk of low birth weight, premature birth and a low Apgar score.[46] The chance of conceiving within a year for a couple with the man being older that 35 years was 50% lower than with a man being under 25 years old, even when adjusted to maternal age.[47] Interestingly, these younger men interestingly tended to father a boy compared to those aged 25–34 years.

What age is advanced paternal age?

While the age of 40 years was used as a threshold more often than any other age, the number of studies was not so great as to imply an overwhelming consensus.

Why are there more pathologies in offspring from older fathers?

About 30 spermatogonial cell divisions occur before puberty. After puberty, spermatogonial stem cells divide every 16 days (approximately 23 times per year). If the average age of male puberty is 15, sperm produced by a 70-year-old male have formed after around 1300 mitotic divisions. DNA replication preceded each cell division, and mutations often arise as a result of uncorrected errors in DNA replication. Owing to the large number of cell divisions that occur during spermatogenesis, we can speculate that advanced paternal age can contribute to an increased number of mutations.[48] Recent studies have begun to uncover a potential epigenetic link between the ageing paternal genome and health outcomes in offspring. Age-dependent alterations, such as DNA methylation, have been observed in mammalian somatic and germline cells. Additionally, it has been suggested that genomic imprinting influences placental growth, morphology and nutrient transfer, which in part explains the paternal influence on birth outcomes.[49]

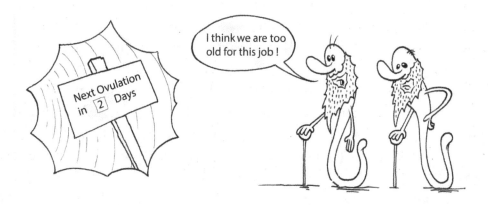

FATHER'S WEIGHT

Paternal weight is easily overlooked but it is equally as important as maternal weight. To underline this, research suggests a potential correlation of the worldwide obesity pandemic (40% of the world adult population have a body mass index (BMI) above normal) and the decline of sperm quality.

A meta-analysis from 21 studies (2012) concludes that men who are overweight or obese have a far higher risk of azoospermia (no sperm) or oligospermia (too little sperm).[50] Moreover, a newer study reports that obesity affects sperm morphology, vitality, motility and sperm DNA integrity.[51]

To give you some striking numbers: a study from 2006 indicates that male fertility decreases by 10% for every 10% of overweight. With every increase of 3 kg/m² of male BMI, the reduction in achieving a successful pregnancy diminishes by 12%.[52] This is due to many factors: lower sperm quality as seen in semen analysis but also impaired sperm functioning in terms of oocyte binding capacity and sperm mitochondrial functions, detrimental DNA integrity due to elevated ROS, epigenetic changes but also impaired sex hormones and elevated erectile dysfunction rates.[53] Fat tissue is a source of warmth, so obesity also leads to an increase in scrotal temperature.

Paternal weight and ART: Research shows a negative impact of male obesity on the outcome of IVF especially at the later stages of embryo development after activation of the embryonic genome. Then data showed a significant decrease in the proportion of expanded blastocysts as paternal BMI increased. This study demonstrated that paternal obesity at the time of conception is associated with reduced pregnancy rates and live-birth rates after ART treatment, IVF and ICSI respectively.[54] Although there is some debate about whether the negative impact can be seen in ICSI outcomes as well, research does agree on male obesity affecting IVF outcomes negatively.[55]

Paternal overweight causes a higher rate of miscarriage: There is a clear consensus in the current literature that male obesity is associated with higher levels of sperm DNA damage, which, as we know, is responsible for miscarriage.[56]

WANT TO KNOW MORE?

Obesity is part of the metabolic syndrome together with hypertension, high serum triglycerides, low HDL levels and high fasting levels of blood glucose. Metabolic syndrome has a correlation with male reproductive dysfunctions such as hypogonadism and erectile dysfunction. The negative impact on male fertility is due to the interference of metabolic hormones with the HPG axis. In fat tissue, androgens are transformed into oestrogens, which leads to low testosterone levels in obese men. Moreover, elevated oestrogen levels inhibit pulsatile GnRH and subsequent LH and FSH release from the hypothalamus and pituitary gland via a negative feedback mechanism. Obesity also leads to alterations in adipose tissue hormonal levels in serum such as leptin (which balances food intake and energy utilization) and ghrelin (the hunger hormone). Adipose tissue also works as a site of toxin deposit and exudes various hormones and inflammation markers such as adipokines.

Being underweight (BMI <20) is just as bad: Sperm concentration decreases (36% lower) according to a study done in more than 1500 Danish men.[57] Another research study concluded that men with a BMI at or below 18.5 kg/m² were found to have sperm counts which were 7% lower than men with normal BMIs. Men who were overweight had sperm counts that were 4% lower than men with normal BMIs.[58]

GENITAL TRACT INFECTIONS

Genital tract infections contribute considerably to the causes of male infertility. Globally, the presence of genital tract infection-related infertility varies between 10% and 20% in non-selected cases and up to 35% in a large study compromising more than 4000 patients consulting for infertility.[59]

Among the microorganisms causing an infection are bacteria such as *Chlamydia trachomatis*, *Neisseria gonorrhoeae*, *Mycoplasma hominis* and *M. genitalium* and *Escherichia coli*. The first two cause most of the sexually transmitted genital bacterial infections; the latter is the cause of 65–85% of non-sexually transmitted infections, particularly epididymo-orchitis and prostatitis. Genital infections not only increase scrotal temperature due to inflammation, but also lead to an attraction of leucocytes which are a common source of ROS and thus oxidative stress, generally affecting spermatogenesis and sperm functions negatively.

Chlamydia infections account for an estimated 92 million new urogenital infections per year. Due to its high asymptomatic nature, approximately 50% of men do not have symptoms. The bacteria cause prostatitis, epididymitis and urethritis.[60] Infections with chlamydia and mycoplasma lead to a notable increase of DNA fragmentation (as well as 80% more sperm anomalies and 10% lower motility). Several months of taking antibiotics (depending on the evolution of the symptoms) improved the DNA fragmentation rate and led to an increased pregnancy rate.[61]

Neisseria gonorrhoeae is the cause of one of the most common infectious diseases in men, leading to urethritis, prostatitis and epididymitis. Although its incidence is generally declining in the Western world, 78 million new infections worldwide have been recorded by the World Health Organization. In the USA and Europe, the numbers are trending up rather than down.[62]

Among viral infections causing orchitis, epididymitis and prostatitis, the mumps virus, coxsackie virus, cytomegalovirus (CMV), as well as herpes simplex (HPS), human papilloma virus (HPV) and HIV are the most common.

Thirty per cent of all male mumps patients who suffer from the disease post-puberty develop orchitis. This can lead to testicular atrophy and spermatogenic arrest, causing fertility problems as sperm parameters such as sperm concentration are impaired as well as overall sperm quality. In addition, orchitis may cause intratesticular obstruction leading to azoospermia. In fact, 15% of obstructive azoospermia are thought to be due to orchitis.[63]

The association between HPV positivity and male infertility was evaluated by a meta-analysis of case-control studies, including 5194 male participants. The overall prevalence of HPV DNA in semen was 11.4% in the general population (*n*=2122) and 20.4% in fertility clinic attendees (*n*=3072). HPV16 was the most common type, with a prevalence of 4.8% (95% CI=1.7–7.8%) in the general population and 6.0% (95% CI=3.8–8.2%) in fertility clinic attendees. A significantly increased risk of infertility was found for males with HPV positivity in semen. Results show that HPV DNA can be identified in every fraction of semen: spermatozoa, somatic cells and seminal plasma. Different samples can contain the HPV DNA in different fractions and several HPV genotypes can be found in the same fraction, especially impaired motility.[64]

SARS-CoV2

There is a possibility of testicular damage and subsequent infertility following Covid-19 infection, which is important as men are more prone to be infected by the virus. The testicular damage is caused by either direct viral invasion through binding of the SARS-CoV2 virus to ACE2 receptors or secondarily by the immunological and inflammatory response. Not only do the lungs contain ACE2 receptors, but the testicles also contain many such receptors. The four main testicular cell types showing expression of ACE2 mRNA are the seminiferous duct cells, spermatogonia, Leydig cells and Sertoli cells. Binding of the SARS-CoV2 virus with the ACE2 receptors enables its cellular entry and replication. Consequently, it may be perceived that cells with higher ACE2 expression are more susceptible to SARS-CoV2 infection. It is a breakthrough revelation in male fertility research that the testes show almost the highest ACE2 mRNA and protein expressions among the various body tissues.[65]

A possible mechanism might be as follows: SARS-CoV2 gains access to the reproductive system through the ACE2 and TMPRSS2 receptors present on testicular tissues. The immune response triggered by viral entry produces various inflammatory substances, such as cytokines, which induce oxydative stress in testicular cells, which in turn damages the DNA of developing spermatozoa. Various psychological stresses due to SARS-CoV2 infection may also lead to the production of ROS. SARS-CoV2 also causes damage to Leydig cells, lowering the production of testosterone, which may ultimately hamper the proper functioning of Sertoli cells. Impaired functioning of Sertoli cells may further disrupt the process of spermatogenesis. Studies suggest that normal testosterone levels may help combat Covid-19 infection in men.[66]

Conclusions: The sperm quality of patients who'd recovered from Covid-19 improved after a recovery time of nearly half a year, while the total sperm number showed an improvement after a recovery time of around 150 days. Covid-19 patients should pay close attention to the quality of semen and might be considered for medical interventions if necessary within about two months following recovery, in order to improve the fertility of male patients as soon as possible.[67]

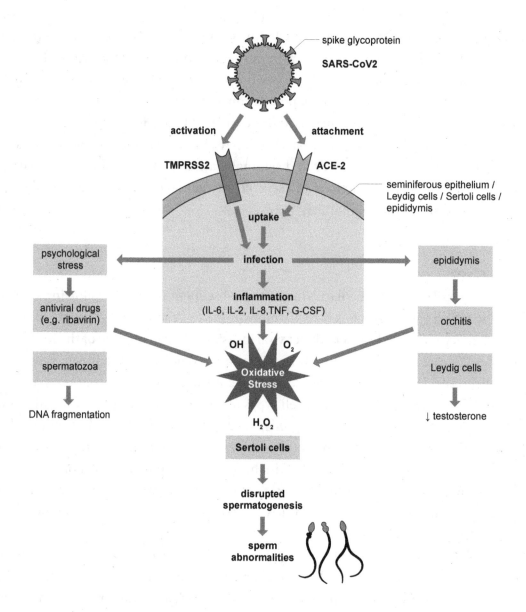

DIABETES

As diabetes mellitus (DM) is one of the most common medical conditions, with 8.5% of the world population suffering from it,[68] treatment of hyperglycaemia and uncontrolled diabetes should be considered for its impact on male fertility.

Diabetes decreases male fertility via different mechanisms, all resulting in changes in sperm parameters, decreased motility, density and abnormal morphology. Furthermore, it interferes with the vulnerable HPG axis, leading to lowered LH and FSH values, and thus decreased testosterone levels. Systemic illnesses such as DM lead to increased oxidative stress, which then causes DNA strand breaks with all the problems caused by fragmented sperm DNA. Crucially, the blood–testis barrier (BTB) also relies on glucose metabolism and hormonal control. Therefore, glucose dysregulation from DM negatively affects BTB function, which, as we already know, is essential to protect sperm from attack by the immune system, in addition to many other functions.

Research results indicated that diabetic plasma affect all sperm motility parameters with high HbA1c showing the most important deleterious effects. The direct impact of diabetic plasma on spermatozoa is revealed with overexpression of OS as the underlying mechanism.[69]

Both forms of DM harm male fertility for sure and it is assumed that type 1 and type 2 diabetes have slightly different underlying mechanisms contributing to the changes seen in sperm parameters. Sperm alterations in type 1 DM can be autoimmune-mediated whereas the changes in type 2 DM are likely to be multifactorial with metabolic syndrome and changes in testosterone.[70]

It should also be remembered that the number of diabetic male patients suffering from erectile dysfunction is three times as high as in the normal population, which has a secondary impact on fertility. Men with diabetes may have sexual disorders other than erectile dysfunction; examples include diminished sexual desire, lack of ejaculation with sexual climax (anejaculation or retrograde ejaculation) and premature ejaculation.[71]

SCROTAL TEMPERATURE

Spermatogenesis works best at 34°C and impairs with every degree of higher temperature.

We have already discussed conditions that cause the testes to overheat such as cryptorchism, infections, varicocele and obesity. In addition, the following should be avoided (beginning at least 2.5 months prior to desired conception date): saunas, hot baths, heat at work if possible.

Tight clothing should also be avoided. Given that the natural cooling methods for the scrotum rely on sweating and vasomotor changes, it is clear that clothing in combination with behaviour or posture can have significant effects. Normal scrotal temperature is approximately 34°C in a normally clothed man walking about or maintaining a loose stance, and it has been estimated that testicular temperature within the scrotum is 0.1–0.6°C higher than this. Clothing itself appears to contribute about 0.5–1.0°C, compared with being naked. Clothed and sitting down with thighs apart raises scrotal temperature to about 35°C, whereas sitting with thighs together quickly allows scrotal temperature to rise to above 36°C – that is, to abdominal temperature within the testis.[72] Knowing the impact of the correct clothing 'down below', research was conducted in Scotland which concluded that men should wear kilts to stay fertile![73] Another situation where scrotal temperatures become elevated is during sleep, when bedclothes and lack of movement prevent ventilation. Men with oligospermia or oligoasthenospermia who slept with a small apparatus that permitted nocturnal scrotal cooling showed significant improvements in semen quality over a period of 12 weeks.[74]

One lifestyle factor that may affect human fertility is driving a vehicle for a prolonged period, assuming that the driving position may increase the scrotal temperature. In a research study, the scrotal temperature in the driving position increased significantly after two hours of driving, reaching a value 1.7–2.2°C higher than that recorded while walking.[75] Temperature rises even more with the seat heating on! Placing a laptop on the lap increases temperature by 2.8°C and keeping a mobile phone in a trouser pocket also increases scrotal temperature. Wi-Fi also damages sperm, as shown in an experiment conducted by Japanese researchers. The study looked at the effect of electromagnetic (EM) waves from Wi-Fi devices on human sperm. It found that longer periods of direct exposure to a portable Wi-Fi router decreased the motility rate and increased the death rate of sperm from human samples. According to the researchers, Wi-Fi shields that intercept electromagnetic waves lowered the detrimental effects on sperm.[76]

Wearing plastic-lined nappies raised the scrotal temperature of babies by 1°C! So the future fertility of that baby can already be influenced negatively at that age. The cause of the temperature rise is the short distance of the gonads to the body as well as the fact that plastic allows no circulation of air.[77]

Certain occupations may also contribute to an increase in scrotal temperature – for example, welders, bakers, radiographers, train drivers, digger drivers, mineworkers (vibrations), farmers (chemicals), chemists, painters, lab workers (solvents).

SMOKING

Smoking reduces the fertile phase of life by 1–4 years. Research results indicate that cigarette smoking has detrimental effects on semen parameters. It negatively affected all conventional semen parameters in addition to sperm chromatin condensation and sperm viability. These abnormalities were also proportional to the number of cigarettes smoked per day and to the duration of smoking.[78]

If the male partner smokes during an ART phase, the success rate is impaired: intracytoplasmic sperm injection success (i.e. clinical pregnancy) in women with smoking male partners was 22% and was 38% with non-smoking partners. Similar results were seen for IVF, with 18% and 32% respectively. Multinominal logistic regression analysis revealed smoking in men to be a significant predictor of ICSI outcome.[79]

The male offspring of mothers who smoked during pregnancy have a higher risk for cryptorchism and hypospadias, their testes are smaller and they have a higher proportion of damaged spermatozoa.[80]

Within the first 15 weeks of embryo development, smoking seriously damages the gametes (stem cells, spermatogonia).[81]

ALCOHOL

Ethanol is a toxin for the testicles and as such influences sperm quality – from motility issues to azoospermia. But as Paracelsus said long ago, the dose makes the poison. To quantify the amount of alcohol intake, one should know that usually 1 unit = 125 ml wine or 330 ml beer or 30 ml spirits, all containing approximately 12.5 g of ethanol.

Dose-dependency is proven by an interesting study by Italian researchers: in a multivariate analysis, they found a relation between alcohol intake and semen volume, concentration and total count. Back-transforming semen volume and using men with < 1–3 units per week of alcohol intake as the reference group, they observed that men drinking 4–7 units per week had a significantly higher median semen volume, that men in both the 4–7 and ≥ 8 units per week groups had significantly higher sperm concentration, and that abstainers had higher median concentration as well. Total count was also associated with alcohol intake: men drinking 4–7 and ≥ 8 units per week had a higher total count than men drinking < 1–3 units per week) but without dose-dependent relation. No association emerged with sperm motility. That study did not investigate sperm quality of heavy or daily drinkers and the discussion behind the favourable effects of moderate alcohol consumption might be as concluded by the study's authors:

> A relation between alcohol drinking and semen parameter is biologically plausible. It is known that beer and wine contain polyphenols such as resveratrol or xanthohuminol, which were demonstrated to have a strong therapeutic and cell protective potential. Accordingly, it can be suggested that these compounds might stand behind the observed beneficial effects found in this study.[82]

To get a clue about a cut-off dosage, a large Danish study found that a habitual alcohol intake was associated with a reduction in semen quality from more than 5 units per week in a typical week, although the decreasing trend was most apparent for men with a typical weekly intake above 25 units. In addition, recent alcohol intake (for the week preceding the visit) was associated with an increase in serum testosterone and reduction in sex hormone binding globulin (SHBG).[83] Although sperm damage is dose-dependent, it is wise to recommend restricting alcohol consumption.[84] Sperm damage is more likely in regular drinkers than in occasional drinkers, which certainly has to do with the duration of sperm development over a period of approximately 72 days.[85] Interestingly, moderate alcohol intake appears to be positively associated with semen quality in male partners of infertile couples undergoing ART equal to the results for natural conception.[86]

CAFFEINE

Caffeine's effect on spermatogenesis is controversial. Ricci and colleagues attempted to perform a systematic review to assess the impact of caffeine intake on male fertility.[87] Although some evidence suggested a link between caffeine intake and decreased semen volume, sperm count and concentration, and increased DNA abnormalities, definitive conclusions could not be drawn. The only meta-analysis in the literature reviews two articles regarding coffee consumption, which concluded that the effects of coffee on semen parameters were statistically insignificant.[88] However, a recent study associated a paternal daily intake of 272 mg caffeine with reduced live-birth rates in ICSI cycles.[89]

As we know that caffeine forces hyperactivation of sperm, researchers looked at the usability of caffeine add-ons to sperm samples for ART. A recent paper concluded that as cryopreservation of sperm samples has negative effects on overall sperm quality and increases ROS production, a combination of caffeine and melatonin in pre-freeze and post-thaw sperm samples has proven to be a very effective and simple way to improve semen quality. This is particularly useful for initial low-quality semen samples, those which suffer the most from the freezing/thawing process.[90]

CANNABIS

Scientists at Duke University compared the sperm of 24 human men who smoked marijuana weekly versus a control group who used marijuana no more than ten times in their life and not at all in the past half-year and concluded that marijuana induced epigenetic changes. They demonstrated that cannabis use is associated with widespread DNA methylation changes in human sperm. Discs-Large Associated Protein 2 (DLGAP2), involved in synapse organization, neuronal signalling and strongly implicated in autism, exhibited significant hypomethylation at 17 CpG sites in human sperm, respectively.[91] Various research underscores the huge impact of marijuana use on the male epigenome, concluding that it causes significant changes to the sperm DNA methylome.[92]

Research by a fertility clinic in Boston – contrary to their hypothesis – observed that men who had never smoked cannabis had higher sperm concentrations (62.7 million sperm per ml of ejaculate), whereas their peers who had smoked cannabis at some point in their life had 45.4 million sperm per millilitre of ejaculate and total sperm count and generally lower prevalence of sperm parameters below the WHO reference value than men who had never smoked cannabis. In addition to that change in sperm parameters, FSH concentrations were lower in smokers, but significantly higher concentrations of testosterone, SHBG and inhibin B were found. The researchers sought to explain the unexpected result of their study findings with the critical role of the endocannabinoid system on spermatogenesis.[93] In contrast, a recent systematic review concluded that the strongest evidence of cannabis-induced alterations in male fertility is in the category of semen parameters. Research supports a role for cannabis in reducing sperm count and concentration, inducing abnormalities in sperm morphology, reducing sperm motility and viability, and inhibiting capacitation and fertilizing capacity.[94]

MEDICATIONS

Generally speaking, exogenous pharmaceutical intake has an effect on spermatogenesis. In addition, the quality of erection and libido can be affected. This is an overview of some of the most commonly used medications and their impact on male fertility and genital action.[95]

Antibiotics: Almost all of the major classes of antibiotics have adverse effects on sperm production and function, although we do not fully understand the mechanism.[96] The weakest negative impact seems to be from penicillin and cephalosporins. General effects include impaired spermatogenesis and motility, count and concentration.

Anti-inflammatories and salicylates: Long-term treatment over more than six months with acetylsalicylic acid and other nonsteroidal anti-inflammatory drugs (NSAIs) can cause a reversible, dose-dependent reduction in sperm motility, count and normal morphology.

Sulphasalazine use in therapeutic dosage over a period of more than two months leads to a decreased sperm count, motility and morphology, as well as a reduction in serum testosterone concentration. Alarmingly, ibuprofen disturbs testosterone production as seen in a recent research study with 31 men between the ages of 18 and 35 who took 600 mg a day of the drug for six weeks. Other volunteers were given a placebo. The net result was that overall testosterone levels remained constant, but the body was overstressing to compensate for the detrimental impact of the ibuprofen – a state called compensated hypogonadism – by increasing LH production.[97]

Corticosteroids: No known effect on spermatogenesis. In theory, indirect action on spermatogenesis is possible by inhibiting the HPG axis, but there is too little research to make specific recommendations; for now, it is not necessary to discontinue.

Immunomodulators: For monoclonal antibodies such as trastuzumab, alemtuzumab, rituximab, cetuximab, bevacizumab and omalizumab there is limited data in humans; on animals they didn't have a negative impact on the male reproductive organs.

Immunosuppressive drugs: Sirolimus can cause reversible alteration of sperm parameters such as decreased count, motility and morphology of spermatozoa as well as decreased testosterone levels; for ciclosporine and tacrolismus, there is too little data in humans, but in rats these drugs cause a decreased count and motility of spermatozoa; for azathioprine and mycophenolate, there is no known alteration of sperm parameters but they may have a mutagenic effect.

Diuretics such as spironolactone may cause impairment of sperm motility.

Testosterone and GnRH analogue: Testosterone causes azoospermia appearing on average four months after treatment initiation with recovery of initial sperm parameters in 3–7 months after discontinuation of treatment.

Anabolic steroids cause oligospermia up to cryptospermia (= cryptozoospermia) or azoospermia with testicular atrophy due to inhibition of spermatogenesis; effects are generally reversible in 4–12 months after discontinuation of treatment.

Antiepileptics: Decreased count, motility and morphology of spermatozoa are reported to be caused by treatment with valproate, phenytoin and carbamazepine.

Antidepressant therapy: Tricyclic antidepressants, selective serotonin reuptake inhibitors (SSRI) and monoamine oxidase inhibitors all potentially have an indirect effect on spermatogenesis by causing hyperprolactinemia. Some research shows that SSRIs cause decreased count, motility and morphology of spermatozoa but that is controversial, just like paroxetine causing increased sperm DNA fragmentation. Discontinuation or change of class is preferred for patients who want to conceive according to official recommendations.

Antihypertensive drugs: Here, the class of drugs makes a difference. Decreased sperm motility has been reported with beta blockers. In vitro experiments with calcium channel blockers show a decreased viability and motility of sperm as well as a reduced fertilizing ability of spermatozoa that could not be verified in vivo. ACE blockers may be potentially harmful for capacitation or acrosome reaction of spermatozoa, but findings remain controversial.

H2 blockers, especially cimetidine, cause a decreased sperm count. However, no negative impact is seen in humans with proton pump inhibitors, or H1 blockers (which might even improve motility).

Opioids affect dopamine secretion and potentially cause a reduction in testosterone level. Morphine at chronic doses causes fertility decline in rats. In people with chronic use of opioids, cocaine causes changes in sperm parameters such as decreased count, motility and typical morphology of spermatozoa. Guidelines recommend treatment discontinuation before conception.

5-a-reductase inhibitors such as finasteride, dutasteride and **alpha-blockers** such as tamsulosin, used in treatment of benign prostatic hyperplasia, showed a slight decrease in ejaculate volume and decreased count of spermatozoa for finasteride and utasteride, while tamusolin caused a reversible alteration of sperm parameters such as decreased count, motility and typical morphology of spermatozoa.

Antiviral drugs such as ribavirin cause a decreased motility and morphology of spermatozoa but an increase in sperm DNA fragmentation index up to eight months after drug discontinuation.

Cytostatics: Treatment of cancer with chemotherapy results in a decrease in sperm count, often to azoospermic levels, which may persist for several years or be permanent. The course of decline in sperm count can be predicted by the sensitivity of germ cells, with differentiating spermatogonia being most sensitive, and the known kinetics of recovery. Recovery from oligo- or azoospermia is more variable and depends on whether stem cells are killed and changes in the somatic environment that normally supports differentiation of stem cells. Of the cytotoxic therapeutic agents, radiation and most alkylating drugs are most effective in producing long-term azoospermia. Most of the newer biologic targeted therapies, except those used to target radioisotopes or toxins to cells, seem to have only modest effects, mostly on the endocrine aspects of the male reproductive system.[98]

SPORTS

Studies suggest that men who exercise are generally higher in sperm concentration – for example, physically active subjects from Spain have been reported to have higher numbers of motile spermatozoa and spermatozoa with normal morphology than sedentary controls.[99] Moreover, a higher level of physical effort has been associated with an increased sperm count and concentration among American students.[100] In addition, sperm concentration was reported to be 43% higher in men who engaged in moderate/vigorous exercise among a population of 231 men seeking infertility treatment. Exercising regularly – but not excessively – is clearly better than never or hardly ever exercising.

It is necessary to bear in mind that sports generally can cause an increase of scrotal temperature with some sports causing a greater increase in temperature than others (e.g. horseback riding, motor sports).

Furthermore, intense training (as with elite sportsmen) is correlated with decreases in the volume and number of spermatozoa, sperm concentration and the percentages of motile and morphologically normal spermatozoa. Moreover, very intense training (two hours a day, five days a week) leads to a decrease in testosterone levels by 40% and a reduction of total sperm count by 50%. Cycling (e.g. more than five hours a week) decreases sperm concentration and motility.[101] Cycling is one of the most detrimental activities for fertility due to the mechanical impact sustained from sitting on the saddle, gonadal overheating, wearing tight clothes and hormonal dysfunction (hypogonadism). In a number of studies (usually focused on road-bikers),[102] cycling has been associated with abnormal spermatozoa morphology and reduced motility. Running training also affects semen. It may be the result of disturbances in the hormonal milieu (e.g. gonadotropins and testosterone), the stress response (e.g. corticotropin-releasing hormone, adrenocorticotropin, cortisol and beta-endorphins), oxidative stress and scrotal heating.[103]

One study concluded that high-intensity exercise (running at either a moderate or high intensity for 120 minutes, five times a week, for 60 weeks) was correlated with decreases in sperm density, motility and morphology after 24 weeks of exercise, with a recovery period of 36 weeks for recovery to pre-exercise levels.[104]

SLEEP

Sleep problems have been associated with lower fertility for a long time. Studies have shown that men who sleep for less than six hours a night are 31% less likely to father a child than those who get between seven and eight hours of sleep. Men produce testosterone while they sleep, so sleeping too little reduces the release of testosterone. Compared to men with night sleep duration of 7.5–8.0 hours, men who slept less than six hours had lower total and progressive sperm motility of 4.4% and 5.0%, respectively.[105] Also, if you are exposed to light at night, a change of reproductive hormones will be the result alongside impaired sleep quality and prolonged time to fall asleep. It is recommended to avoid green or blue light from electronic devices as they disturb melatonin synthesis.[106]

STRESS

There are many studies on the connection between stress and reduced fertility. Stress has a huge impact on the HPG axis as it decreases the release of GnRH and furthermore the release of LH due to the increased secretion of the stress hormone cortisol, leading to decreased rates of testosterone excretion from Leydig cells, responsible for spermato-genesis. Glucocorticoids may also induce apoptosis of Leydig cells, thus reducing the total number of cells. A recent study found that stressful life situations can influence motility, shape and concentration of sperm. Interestingly, stress at work did not have an impact on sperm parameters; the study only found an association between high job strain and decreased levels of total testosterone, whereas private stress affects sperm parameters. The researchers propose that the cause of the sperm damage could be oxidative stress which has been shown to influence semen quality and fertility.[107]

SEX

Chances of conceiving are possible from six days prior to the egg release and end at the day after egg release. The 'hot spot' days are the four days prior to the egg release. The recommended frequency of intercourse within this time frame is daily – contrary to the opinion of lay people, daily sex does not harm the sperm! There is no study that would recommend a special sex position as being the best to conceive, but the degree of arousal (men are best aroused visually) makes a difference concerning sperm quality and even female arousal has an impact on the cervical mucus and lubricants that help sperm fertilize an egg. The context in which an ejaculate is produced is also important. For example, ejaculates produced during intercourse are generally superior to those produced during masturbation. They generally have higher ejaculate volume, total sperm number and grade of sperm motility than those obtained via masturbation. They also exhibit a greater percentage of motile and morphologically normal spermatozoa, and consequently perform better on various sperm function tests. The superior quality of ejaculates produced during intercourse may be attributable, in part, to the greater intensity and duration of sexual arousal that typically precedes copulatory ejaculation.[108]

Another research study concluded home-collected samples had statistically significantly higher values for sperm concentration, total sperm count, rapid progressive motility and total count of progressive motility than samples obtained in the clinic. There was no signficant difference with regard to semen volume, sperm morphology or markers of epididymal and accessory sex gland function.[109] Another research study tested whether ejaculate parameters change in response to the familiarity or novelty of the female stimulus used to induce sexual arousal. They showed men explicit films of the same woman six times with no significant changes in semen parameter and then changed to pictures of another woman that the men had not previously seen. The study concluded that ejaculate volume and total motile sperm count significantly increased when males were exposed to a novel female and time to ejaculate decreased.[110]

A study looking at the duration of sexual arousal and its impact on sperm parameters interestingly concluded that there was a significant positive relationship between the time taken to produce a specimen and sperm concentration. The duration of pre-ejaculatory sexual arousal is an important predictor of ejaculate quality for specimens produced by masturbation and the variation in the duration of pre-ejaculatory arousal may contribute to fluctuations in semen parameters over time.[111] A content analysis found support for the hypothesis that a man who spends more time performing cunnilingus produces an ejaculate with greater estimated volume.[112]

DENTAL HEALTH

You may wish to encourage your male clients to see their dentist. A research study with 85 men looked at the health of their teeth on the one hand and at their semen parameter on the other. Periodontitis was found in 75.3% of the examined patients, gingivitis in 24.7%. Out of the 85 patients, normospermia (= normozoospermia) was diagnosed in 20, oligospermia in 37 patients, and sperm submotility 65.[113]

DIET

An unhealthy diet has a negative impact on male fertility. But what kind of diet has the most positive impact on sperm? In 2017, a meta-analysis concluded as follows:

- **Positive:** A diet rich in omega-fatty acids, antioxidants (vitamins E and C, beta-carotene, selenium, zinc, cryptoxanthin and lycopene) and other vitamins such as vitamin D and folate has a positive effect on sperm parameter. (Nuts are perfect sources for all of the above.) Fish, shellfish and seafood, poultry, grains, vegetables, fruits and low-fat milk also have a positive impact on sperm.

- **Negative:** Foods to avoid include processed meat (ham, salami, bacon, sausages and canned luncheon meat), soya products, potatoes, full-fat dairy, cheese, coffee, alcohol, sweet drinks, sugar and saturated fat and trans-fatty acids.

In a nutshell, men are recommended to stick to the so-called Mediterranean diet (MedDiet).[114]

— CHAPTER 7 —

Diagnosis of Male Infertility: The Basics

Please note that any kind of medical examination mentioned in this chapter needs to be performed by a medical doctor; however, it is important to know about these tests and how and why they are done.

According to the 2021 guidelines published by the American Urological Association (AUA) and the American Society for Reproductive Medicine (ASRM) concerning diagnosis and treatment of infertility in men, the specific goals of the evaluation of the infertile male are to identify:

- potentially correctable conditions

- irreversible conditions that are amenable to assisted reproductive technologies (ART) using the sperm of the male partner

- irreversible conditions that are not amenable to the above, and for which donor insemination is a possible option

- life- or health-threatening conditions that may underlie the infertility or associated medical comorbidities that require medical attention

- genetic abnormalities or lifestyle and age factors that may affect the health of the male patient or of the offspring particularly if ART are to be employed.[1]

IS MALE FERTILITY A WINDOW TO A MAN'S HEALTH?

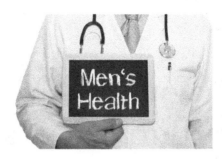

In addition to infertility treatment benefits, 1–6% of men evaluated for infertility have significant undiagnosed medical pathology, including malignancies, even when they have a so-called normal semen analysis.[2]

There is more and more evidence that male reproductive health and overall health are related. Additional concerns are being raised by emerging reports showing that infertile men carry a higher disease burden, with an increased risk of incident disease (including heart disease and cancer) and die younger compared with fertile men.[3] Male infertility has therefore been termed a 'harbinger of future morbidity and mortality'[4] and is a health problem of growing global importance.[5]

Moreover, male infertility has been suggested as a marker of future health, given that poor semen parameters and a diagnosis of male infertility are associated with an increased risk of hypogonadism, cardiometabolic disease, cancer and even mortality. Therefore, male fertility requires multidisciplinary expertise for evaluation, treatment and counselling. A large portion of the genome is involved with fertility, so the genes involved in reproduction may also be expressed in other cell types. In addition, epigenetic alterations may lead to global changes in expression, thus affecting spermatogenesis as well as other body functions.

WANT TO KNOW MORE?

Cancer risk

Several studies have suggested that male infertility is associated with an increased risk of cancer, thus acting as a potential biomarker. The cardinal example of this is the 20-fold increased risk of developing testicular cancer among infertile men with respect to a same-age and race-matched group of fertile men from the general population. In addition, other oncological malignancies have been found to be intertwined with male infertility, such as colorectal cancer, melanoma and prostate cancer.[6] There are several representative studies, including a Danish cohort study looking at more than 32,000 men over a 30-year period, which noted that low sperm concentration, decreased sperm motility and poorer sperm morphology were each independently associated with an increased incidence of testicular cancer.[7] Furthermore, a large American multi-centre cohort study of more than 51,000 infertile couples found that known male-factor infertility increases the risk of developing testicular cancer by nearly threefold.[8] In particular, those with lower semen quality had a higher risk of testis cancer.

The association between male infertility and prostate cancer has also been examined. Walsh *et al.* found that men with male-factor infertility were at higher risk of developing high-grade prostate cancer.[9] A Swedish study also demonstrated that infertile men conceiving with IVF or IVF with ICSI had high levels of prostate cancer incidence compared with men who conceived without assistance.[10]

A recent Italian study concluded that infertile men have higher PSA values than fertile individuals of comparable age. They found that serum PSA was higher while serum testosterone was lower in infertile than in fertile men. In participants younger than 40 years, 176 (27%) men had PSA greater than 1 ng/ml; of them, a greater proportion were infertile (28% infertile vs 17% fertile).[11]

Other malignancies

Male-factor infertility has also been associated with non-urological malignancies. In a cohort study including infertile and fertile patients and those who had undergone vasectomy, Eisenberg and colleagues showed that patients with male infertility had a 49% higher risk of being subsequently diagnosed with any cancer compared with fertile men, thus considering melanoma, bladder and thyroid cancer, as well as hematological malignancies.[12] Finally, in a study of 2238 infertile men linked to the Texas Cancer Registry, the authors assessed the association between azoospermia and the risk of cancer (any type) and found that men with azoospermia had a 2.2-fold higher risk of cancer compared with nonazoospermic men.[13]

Metabolic problems

Specific conditions included in the definition of metabolic syndrome have been found to be intertwined with male infertility. In this context, data from three large-scale epidemiological studies suggested that overweight and/or obese men have altered semen parameters and difficulties in fathering a child.[14] Additionally, other studies have confirmed the inverse correlation between BMI and total sperm count. The pathophysiological mechanism behind these alterations relies on the fact that obesity, insulin resistance and diabetes mellitus negatively influence androgen levels via the downregulation of serum levels of sex hormone binging globulin (SHBG). In this context, the European Male Ageing Study (EMAS) found that 73% of men with reduced testosterone (T) were overweight or obese.[15] Strengthening this, another study of the EMAS and a meta-analysis demonstrated that weight gain suppresses, and weight loss increases, serum T levels.[16] Likewise, a very recent study from Ferlin *et al.* found that men with low sperm count had higher BMI, waist circumference, systolic pressure, low-density lipoprotein cholesterol, triglycerides, insulin resistance and lower HDL cholesterol than men with a normal sperm count.[17]

Cardiovascular disease, hypertension and diabetes

Several cohort studies found that an infertility diagnosis was associated with an increased risk of comorbidity including hypertension. Eisenberg *et al.* found that men diagnosed with male-factor infertility had an increased risk of incident cardiovascular disease.[18] Additionally, Latif *et al.* found that men with a sperm concentration of less than 15 million/ml had a higher risk of cardiovascular disease.[19]

Male fertility may additionally be a marker for future diabetes risk. A US study demonstrated that infertile men are at a higher risk of incidence of diabetes in the years after an infertility diagnosis.[20] Two other large studies with more than 39,000 men within infertile couples and 744 infertile men showed a similar risk of developing diabetes.[21] Interestingly, Boeri *et al.* noted that up to 15% of infertile men may have undiagnosed diabetes or prediabetes.[22]

Mortality

Male infertility has also been associated with premature mortality. Certain habits and comorbidities – such as smoking, obesity and alcohol consumption – are not only associated with male infertility but are also risk factors for early mortality. Thus, they might act as potential confounders in studies, but there may be an independent association. While adjusting for current health status attenuating the association between semen parameters and mortality, men with two or more abnormal semen parameters still had a 2.3-fold higher risk of death compared with men with normal semen.[23]

Hypogonadism

Testosterone is important for male reproductive health, so alterations in its levels may lead to impairment of spermatogenesis. Additionally, testosterone deficiency can impair health in several ways such as elevated BMI, hypertension, dyslipidemia, elevated HbA1c and decreased bone mineral density. As such, detection of hypogonadism is important, and identification of male infertility could trigger testosterone testing and follow-up endocrine evaluation.[24]

Autoimmune conditions

Investigators have sought to find other associations of medical conditions with male fertility status as a potential biomarker. In a cohort of over 24,000 Danish men, Glazer *et al.* found that men with male-factor infertility had higher odds of having multiple sclerosis.[25] Using a US cohort, Brubaker *et al.* found that infertile men had a higher risk of autoimmune disease (e.g. rheumatoid arthritis, systemic lupus erythematosus, psoriasis, Grave's disease, multiple sclerosis).[26] Although the mechanism of the proposed association between infertility and autoimmunity remains unclear, there is some suspicion that androgens may play a protective role against autoimmunity, which may be compromised in the setting of hypogonadism.[27]

TO BEGIN

Initial evaluation of the male for fertility should include a reproductive history. This is to obtain insight into functional sexual, lifestyle and medical history including medications that can contribute to reduced fertility or sterility.[28]

Information about the following should be sought:

- former fertility and duration of current infertility period
- relevant childhood diseases
- systemic diseases and former surgery performed
- sexual anamnesis including sexually transmitted diseases
- exposure to gonadal toxins including heat
- family history
- medication.

Initial evaluation of the male should also include one or more semen analysis (SA).[29]

Men with one or more abnormal semen parameters or presumed male infertility should be evaluated by a male reproductive expert for complete history and physical examination as well as other directed tests when indicated.[30]

Physical examination should include:

- body habitus
- examination of the penis including urethra ostium
- measurement and palpation of the testes
- palpation of the epididymis (exclusion of a varicocele)
- inspection of the secondary sexual characteristics including body hair distribution and development of breasts
- digital rectal examination.

WANT TO KNOW MORE?

Body habitus

Body examination is essential to exclude the possibility of an endocrine abnormality causing delayed maturation seen by inadequate virilization. Look at the amount of body hair, breast enlargement (gynaecomastia) and general bodily appearance (tall/thin). Inspect the curvature of the penis and the angle and take a look at the opening of the urethra (meatus).

Examination of the penis including urethra ostium

Penile curvature or angulation should be assessed, as should the location of the urethral meatus (opening). Hypospadia is a common variation in foetal development of the penis in which the urethra does not open from its usual location in the head of the penis. It is the second-most common birth abnormality of the male reproductive system, affecting about one of every 200–250 males at birth.[31]

Unfortunately, the etiology of hypospadias in the majority of patients has remained unknown. Genetic and environmental factors are the main susceptibilities. Although androgen is known to be essential for sexual differentiation and penile development, only a small percentage of severe hypospadias can be explained by the genetic syndromes or defects involving the androgen receptor (AR) gene.[32]

If hypospadia comes along with cryptorchism, gonadal palpability is an important predictor of an intersex state. Likewise, the severity of hypospadia also has a strong positive correlation with an intersex state.

Measurement and palpation of the testes

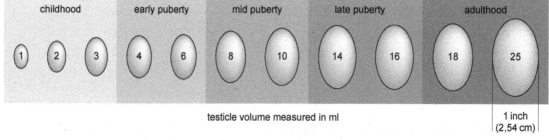

Orchidometer used to measure testicle size and track sexual development in boys

childhood | early puberty | mid puberty | late puberty | adulthood

1 2 3 | 4 6 | 8 10 | 14 16 | 18 25

testicle volume measured in ml

1 inch
(2,54 cm)

Testicular volume (TV) is considered a good clinical marker of hormonal and spermatogenic function. Boeri *et al.* concluded in their study that the median testicular volume was smaller in infertile than fertile men (15 ml vs 22.5 ml; $P < 0.001$). Testicular volume is positively correlated with total testosterone, sperm concentration and progressive sperm in infertile men. In conclusion, infertile men have smaller testicular volume than fertile controls.

Testicular volume thresholds of 15 ml and 12 ml had a good predictive ability for detecting OAT and non-obstructive azoospermia (NOA) status, respectively.[33] The measurement of testicular size using a Prader orchidometer is actually a simple but meaningful tool to explore fertility potential.

Varicocele

Up to 43% of the general adult male population, 7% of prepubertal males and 10–25% of postpubertal males have a varicocele.[34] Interestingly, 35% of men with primary and up to 80% with secondary infertility have varicose veins.[35] In healthy veins inside the scrotum, one-way valves move the blood from the testicles to the scrotum, and then they send it back to the heart. Sometimes the blood does not move through the veins as it should and begins to pool in the veinous plexus called plexus pampiniformis, causing it to enlarge. A varicocele develops slowly, and therefore the prevalence of varicoceles increases over time – it is estimated that a 10% rise in incidence occurs for each decade of life.[36] There are no established risk factors for developing a varicocele, and the exact cause is unclear, with varicocele formation likely to be multifactorial. An inverse relationship between the occurrence of varicoceles and body mass index seems likely, as well as intense physical activity over several years.[37] Varicoceles generally form during puberty and are more commonly found on the left side of the scrotum. The anatomy of the right and left side of the scrotum is not the same, resulting in a higher incidence of left-side varicoceles.

Digital rectal examination

A digital rectal examination is sometimes necessary to assess prostatic size as well as to rule out prostatic and/or seminal vesicular firmness, masses or cysts.[38] Clinicians should obtain hormonal evaluation including FSH and testosterone for infertile men with impaired libido, erectile dysfunction oligo- or azoospermia, atrophic testes or evidence of hormonal abnormality on physical examination.[39]

HORMONES

Sex hormones

The compendious name of the male sex hormones is androgens. They are mainly produced in the male gonads, although a small amount is produced in the adrenal cortex (such as androstenedione and dehydroepiandrosterone). These androgens are responsible for the development of reproductive organs and tissues as well as their maintenance. Among androgens, testosterone stands out as the most important one. It is produced by so-called Leydig cells, special interstitial cells of the testicles. In many androgen target tissues, testosterone needs to be converted in to its more active form which is calles dihydrotestosterone.

The enzyme that is responsible for that convertion is called 5-α-reductase. What are androgens for? In puberty they initiate the development of the male secondary sex characteristics such as the typical male body hair distribution, lengthening of the vocal cords to achieve a deep voice and of course they regulate any gonadal function.

WANT TO KNOW MORE?

Classification of androgens
Natural androgens

- From testes:

    - testosterone (5–12 mg daily)

    - dihydrotestosterone (more active) by 5 α-reductase.

- From adrenal cortex (weak androgens):

    - dehydroepiandrosterone

    - androstenedione (females testosterone: 0.25 – 0.5 mg/day (ovary + adrenals))

    - androsterone – metabolite of testosterone.

how hormones are made

Cholesterol

Pregnenolone ⟶ 17. OH Pregnenolone ⟶ DHEA

Progesterone ⟶ 17. OH Progesterone → Androstenedione

11 DOC (Deoxy-corticosterone)   11 Desoxycortisol   Testosterone

Corticosterone   Cortisol (Glucocorticold)   Estradiol (E2)

18 Hydroxy-corticosterone   Estrone (E1)

Aldosterone (Mineralocorticold)   Estriol (E3)

Testosterone is produced from cholesterol, primarily by Leydig cells in testes. Testosterone needs to be converted by 5 α-reductase to the more potent form called 5α-dihydrotestosterone (DHT), which is in charge of many of the responses to testosterone in the urogenital tract. It binds to and activates a single androgen receptor; these are present in many tissues including reproductive tissue, skeletal muscle, brain and kidneys.

It is secreted at adult levels at three stages of a male's life: in utero during the first trimester, during neonatal life and continually after puberty.

During foetal life, the testes are stimulated by chorionic gonadotropin from the placenta to produce moderate quantities of testosterone throughout the entire period of foetal development and for ten or more weeks after birth; thereafter, essentially no testosterone is produced during childhood until about the ages of 10–13 years. Then testosterone production increases rapidly under the stimulus of anterior pituitary gonadotropic hormones at the onset of puberty and lasts throughout most of the remainder of life, dwindling rapidly beyond age 50 to become 20–50% of the peak value by age 80.

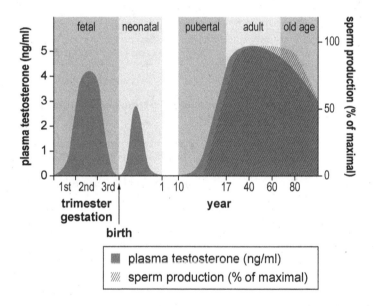

Testosterone androgenic effects

In the foetus, testosterone promotes the development of the male reproductive tract such as the internal genitalia, vas deferens, epididymis and external genitalia – generally speaking, it induces sex differentiation.

During puberty, testosterone promotes the development of:

- primary sexual characteristics (e.g. enlargement of penis, scrotum and testes)

- secondary sexual characteristics (e.g. male body shape, axillary/pubic hair, deeper pitch of voice, thickening of skin and loss of subcutaneous fat).

In adulthood, testosterone is in charge of baldness, development of benign prostate hypertrophy and in the worst case drives the development of prostate cancer.

In the testes, testosterone promotes spermatogenesis and maturation of sperm.

As the release of GnRH via the hypothalamus is a cyclic one, with peaks at night and in the morning, the production of testosterone also conforms to that rhythm. The highest testosterone levels in the daily profile are in the morning hours. Therefore, blood tests should be done in the morning.

Testosterone circulates in the blood 98% bound to protein. Approximately 40% is bound with high affinity to SHBG and approximately 60% is bound weakly to albumin. The testosterone fraction that is bound to albumin dissociates freely in the capillary bed, becoming available for tissue uptake. Only 2–3% of testosterone exists in the free state. All non-SHBG bound testosterone is considered to be bioavailable.

Reference range for total testosterone is 3–10 ng/ml in males.

Parameter	Normal range
Testosterone	3–10 ng/ml (10.4–34.6 mmol/L)
Dehydroepiandrosterone	2–5 µg/ml (5.4–13.4 µmol/L)
17-ß-Estradiol	10–50 pg/ml (36–180 pmol/L)
SHBG	13–55 nmol/L
DHT	16–108 ng/dl (55–370 nmol/L)
Free testosterone	9–47 pg/ml (31–163 pml/L)
Prolactin	3–14.5 ng/ml (40–290 mE/L)
Androstendione	0.57–2.65 ng/ml (1.99–9.25 nmol/L)

Pituitary hormones

An endocrine evaluation with serum FSH is indicated in oligospermia (< 10 million sperm/ml).

FSH is needed at the onset of puberty when spermatogenesis starts over, as it acts on the Sertoli cells promoting germ cell maturation. To maintain the whole spermatogenesis process, testosterone is necessary. Spermatozoa do not have a testosterone receptor but only androgen-binding protein (ABP) receptors. Therefore, to get them access to testosterone, they need the help of the Sertoli cells which do have a testosterone receptor and they can bind testosterone and produce the ABP for the spermatocytes. On top of that, FSH is also needed to convert testosterone into its more active form 5-α-dihydrotestosterone (5-α DHT).

Further evaluation of the male with LH is indicated for men with low serum testosterone

(< 300 ng/dl) as well as prolactin (PRL) evaluation for men with hypogonadotropic hypogonadism or decreased libido.

LH acts on the Leydig cells in the testes to stimulate testosterone production through the conversion of cholesterol. When testosterone levels accumulate, it sets a negative feedback effect at the pituitary to suppress the release of LH and at the hypothalamus to suppress GnRH production. Intratesticular testosterone levels are far higher than in the circulation.

Prolactin is a hormone secreted by the pituitary. A prolactin level of over 25 mcg/L is defined as hyperprolactinemia although at that mild elevated stage it seldom impairs fertility. A typical hormone profile for a man with clinical hyperprolactinemia is elevated prolactin levels with low LH levels and low testosterone. A pituitary MRI to check for a pituitary tumour should be considered when prolactin levels are 30 mcg/L or over; most experts order this test when prolactin levels are 50 mcg/L.

A prolactin level of between 25 and 100 mcg/L may be drug-related, caused by a microadenoma, or the result of pituitary stalk compression by a non-prolactin secreting tumour. A prolactin level over 250 mcg/L is usually consistent with prolactinoma, though some medications (such as reserpine or metoclopramide) can increase prolactin levels to over 200 mcg/L. A prolactin level above 500 mcg/L is diagnostic for macroadenoma.

WANT TO KNOW MORE?

When elevations of prolactin are found, check for reversible causes such as:

- hypothyroidism

- strenuous exercise

- high-protein meals

- nipple stimulation

- medications such as phenothiazines, tricyclic antidepressants, CNS-active drugs (antipsychotics, opiates, cocaine, sedative hypnotics, antidepressants), antihypertensives (alpha-methyldopa, reserpine, verapamil, labetalol) or other medications (cimetidine, ranitidine, anaesthetics, anticonvulsants, antihistamines, oestrogens, opiate antagonists).[40]

Thyroid hormones

Thyroid hormones act on the testes in multiple ways and exert their effect on different cell types, including Leydig and Sertoli cells and germ cells. An excess or deficit of thyroid hormones results in alterations of testis function, including semen abnormalities. More frequently, hyperthyroidism has been associated with reduced semen volume and reduced sperm density, motility and morphology, whereas hypothyroidism is associated with reduced sperm morphology. Therefore, thyroid function tests should be part of the diagnostic workup of the infertile man.[41]

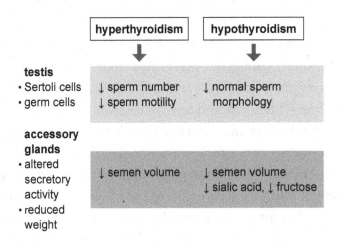

SEMEN ANALYSIS

It is important to bear in mind that:

> Semen is the most heterogeneous of biological fluids wherein parameters concerning the motility, concentration and morphology varies between regions, countries, individuals and between two samples in the same individual.[42]

Although a semen analysis is an important cornerstone to get an insight into the male reproductive function, it is just a snapshot taken at a certain moment and can never reflect the fertility potential of an individual on its own. Therefore, since we are going to dig further into the parameters that are examined in a semen analysis, it is always good to double-check the meaning of their outcome with caution and criticism.

WANT TO KNOW MORE?

As a warm-up, let's have a little bit of a history lesson. It was in the mid-17th century that Antony van Leeuwenhoek was able to improve on the rudimentary microscopes so that he could finally build a really 'potent' microscope that was able to magnify up to 300 times. That impressive magnification enabled him to assess a wide range of biological structures. A new microscopic world opened up for him, one that was previously unapproachable to the human eye. Leeuwenhoek later credited the discovery of spermatozoa to Johan Ham, a student from the Medical School of Leyden. Ham was the one to note male gametes in the semen of a man who was suffering from gonorrhoea. He called them animalcules spermatiques, as he assumed they were seminal parasites.

Since ancient times it was known that a pregnancy takes place by coupling between man and woman and that the man plays an important role within it. According to the Aristotelian theory, it was thought that the formation of the embryo relied on the combination of menstrual blood and semen. On the contrary, the Galenic theory assumed that it developed from the combination of both female and male semen.[43]

After the discovery of the sperm – historically credited to Leeuwenhoek – there began a debate lasting almost 100 years between the so-called spermists and the so-called ovists. Both sides believed that there was a preformed embryo in the gamete which would grow during pregnancy. The spermists believed that the sperm head could contain a miniature of a preformed embryo, whereas the ovists claimed the preformed embryo was contained inside the ovum.

In 1759, it was Caspar Friedrich Wolff who published a study that overthrew the Preformation theory. His famous explanation – known as epigenesis – stated that in the very beginning of its development, the germ is nothing but an unorganized material formed from each parent's sexual organ. After fertilization that material becomes organized. It took decades until Jean-Louis Prévost and Jean-Baptiste-André Dumas actually proved that spermatozoa were essentially necessary for the fertilization when it comes to reproduction.[44]

This was about 200 years after the discovery of spermatozoa, so it took a while to clarify its use.

Still, the basic mechanisms of human fertilization have been only fully understood since 1827, when the ovum was discovered. As a result, the interest in developing technologies for semen analysis arose from the early 1900s. Indeed, standard methodologies for semen analysis were designed mostly during the first half of the 20th century.

To highlight a few pioneers in the field:

William H. Cary was the first one to report a standardization for semen analysis in 1916, which became a historic milestone. Another researcher, Walter W. Williams, was a pioneer in reporting sperm morphology analysis in semen smears. By analyzing the semen of bulls, he described normal spermatozoon as having four basic structures: head, neck, body and tail – just as we do nowadays. He also reported the characteristics of the nucleus: acrosome (which he called cytoplasm), midpiece and tail. In conclusion, the sperm morphological characteristics and the association between abnormal sperm morphology and sterility as reported by these two men were essential for assessing sperm morphology in semen analysis after 1930.

Generally, as soon as the importance of the basic parameters of semen analysis (concentration, motility and morphology) was established, a more detailed analysis of seminal samples to evaluate a man's reproductive capacity became part of the routine investigation of sterility, chiefly in the early 1930s.[45]

Since then, although semen analysis has become the gold standard for evaluating sperm quality and production, there has been much criticism of its predictive value concerning a man's fertility. This has not been overcome during more than 90 years of laboratory practice.

WHAT IS SEMEN ANALYSIS AND WHAT IS IT FOR?

To give you a valid and evidence-based overview of the test, I would like to stick to the recently updated 6th Edition of the *WHO Laboratory Manual for the Examination and Processing of Human Semen* from 2021, which defines standard values of sperm parameters and guides examiners how exactly to do a high-quality semen analysis as well as further tests.

The introduction states:

Semen examination is important for different reasons:

- assessment of male reproductive function and genital tract patency to enable causal treatment for male subfertility and to monitor treatment response

- appraisal of fertility potential and choice of suitable treatment modality for an infertile couple

- measure efficacy of male contraception (e.g. vas occlusion and interventions including hormonal male contraception and other potential methods).

The clinical assessment of the male together with the semen analyses can guide the clinician to determine how to proceed with further investigation and management of the subfertile couple.[46]

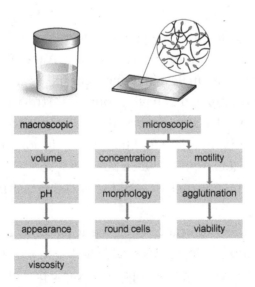

Semen analysis, falling into the category basic examinations, starts with retrieving ejaculate. For that purpose, there are certain recommendations given in the manual:

Sample collection:

- Before ejaculate collection, the specimen container should be kept at ambient temperature, between 20°C and 37°C, to avoid large changes in temperature that may affect the spermatozoa.

- The specimen container should be a clean, wide-mouthed container made of plastic, from a batch that has been confirmed to be non-toxic for spermatozoa.

- Ejaculate collection by masturbation is the primary recommendation.

- Coitus interruptus should only be recommended in exceptional cases due to the risk of incomplete collection and contamination with vaginal fluid and cells.

- Special condoms for fertility investigations may be an alternative under exceptional circumstances, but the entire ejaculate will not be available for examination and the specimen is likely to be contaminated by contact with the skin of the penis and to some extent also vaginal fluid and cells on the outside of the condom. Contraceptive condoms cannot be used due to the presence of spermicidal agents. Ordinary latex condoms must not be used for semen collection because they contain agents that interfere with the motility of spermatozoa.[47]

What really matters is that the ejaculate needs to be completely collected and the man should report any loss of any fraction of the sample.

To avoid the exposure of the semen to fluctuations in temperature and to control the time between collection and analysis it is recommended that the sample should be collected in a private room close to the laboratory. Ideally, investigations should commence within 30 minutes of collection, but at least within 60 minutes. In practice, it is often the case that ejaculate is brought from home, which, from a quality point view, might be better as sperm quality depends on arousal and time to produce ejaculate; on the other hand, this can present difficulties because the sample needs to be in the lab within a maximum of 60 minutes.[48]

On transport there are a few things to consider. As stated in the WHO manual:

- If not collected in the proximity of the laboratory, transport must not allow the sample temperature to go below 20°C, and not above 37°C.

- If the patient for any reason must collect the ejaculate at another place, the specimen container should be kept close to the body under the clothes – for instance, in the arm pit – during transport and should be delivered to the lab preferably within 30 minutes from collection and at least no longer than 50 minutes from the collection.[49]

Men need to be told that time and temperature are of the greatest importance – the initial reflex might be to put a sample in the fridge to keep it as fresh as possible, but that would certainly kill all spermatozoa.

So what can we examine in the test?

As discussed in Chapter 2, ejaculate is composed of spermatozoa (sperm cells) and a fluid named seminal plasma, which includes the secretions of the accessory glands (Cowper's glands, seminal vesicles and prostate). It is important to keep in mind that gametes (sperm cells) only account for 5% of the semen, whereas the vast majority is made up of secretions of the accessory glands.

The ejaculate is mainly examined for:

- volume (of ejaculate)

- sperm concentration (amount of spermatozoa per ml)

- sperm count (total amount of spermatozoa in the ejaculate)

- sperm motility (how many are fast, how many move at all)

- sperm morphology (percentage of normal-shaped spermatozoa)

- pH

- vitality of the sperm cells (how many viable spermatozoa are in the ejaculate).

SPERM PH

The pH of normal semen is slightly alkaline. Normal is 7.2 or greater. The pH at ejaculation depends on the relative contribution of acidic prostatic secretion and alkaline seminal vesicular secretion. A pH value under 7.2 may be indicative of a lack of alkaline seminal vesicular fluid.

LIQUEFACTION

Semen is a thick gel at the time of ejaculation and normally becomes liquid (i.e. thinner) within a few minutes at room temperature, at which time a heterogeneous mixture of semi-solid lumps will be seen in the fluid. As liquefaction continues, the ejaculate becomes more homogeneous and watery. Liquefaction time is a measure of the time it takes for the semen to liquefy. Complete ejaculate liquefaction is normally achieved within 15–30 minutes at room temperature but is considered to be normal up to 60 minutes.

VISCOSITY

Viscosity is measured after complete liquefaction has occurred. Viscosity is considered 'normal' if the liquefied specimen can be poured from a graduated beaker drop by drop with no attaching agglutinin between drops. If viscosity is abnormal, the drop will form a thread more than 2 cm long. The prevalence of semen hyperviscosity (SHV) is estimated to be between 12–29% and can lead to male-factor infertility both in vivo and in vitro.

WANT TO KNOW MORE?

Semen is composed of fluids secreted by the male accessory glands, which contain proteins essential to the coagulation and liquefaction of semen. More precisely, the prostate secretes the tumour marker known as prostate-specific antigen (PSA), the original purpose of which is the liquefication of the coagulated ejaculate. Hypofunction of the prostate but also of the seminal vesicles causes abnormal viscosity of seminal fluid. Infection and high levels of seminal leukocytes may also result in the development of SHV. Oxidative stress and biochemical and genetic factors can furthermore contribute to this condition. Hyperviscosity can impair normal sperm movement in the female reproductive tract and can lead to decreased sperm count.[50]

VOLUME

Normal volume is 1.5 ml or greater (2–6 ml). Precise measurement of volume is essential in any evaluation of ejaculates because it gives information on the secretory functions of the auxiliary sex glands. Precisely, the fluid volume is contributed by the various accessory glands. This reflects the secretory activity of the glands and the smooth muscle contractions that empty each gland. These activities are responses to autonomous nerve stimulation elicited by sexual arousal and as preparation for ejaculation.[51]

WANT TO KNOW MORE?

Hypospermia is a semen volume lower than 2 ml on at least two semen analyses. The etiologies of hypospermia are many and may be divided into two pathophysiologic subgroups: disturbances of ejaculation reflex leading to partial retrograde ejaculation (some of the semen is ejected through the urethra and some is directed towards the bladder) and anatomic and functional anomalies of the seminal glands and ducts.

The volume may also be low if a man is anxious when producing a specimen, if all of the specimen is not caught in the collection container, or if there are hormonal abnormalities (e.g. testosterone) or a very short abstinence time. Furthermore, volume decreases with age. Interestingly, the level and duration of sexual arousal have an impact, since the time spent producing a sample by masturbation also influences the ejaculate volume.

- **Total number of sperm (total sperm count):** 'The number of spermatozoa in the ejaculate is calculated from the concentration of spermatozoa and the ejaculate volume. For normal ejaculates, when the male tract is unobstructed and the abstinence time short, the number of spermatozoa is correlated with testicular volume [the size of the testicles, which influences the total number of spermatozoa produced per day and thereby indirectly output per ejaculate] and thus is a measure of the capacity of the testes to produce spermatozoa, the patency of the male tract and, potentially, the number of spermatozoa transferred to the female during coitus.'[52]

- **Concentration:** 'Sperm concentration is not a direct measure of testicular sperm output, as it is influenced by the secretion functioning of other organs… For example, sperm concentrations in ejaculates from young and old men may be the same, but total sperm numbers may differ, as both the volume of seminal fluid and total sperm output decrease with age, at least in some populations… The concentration of spermatozoa in the ejaculate, while related to fertilization and pregnancy rates, is influenced by the volume of the secretions from the seminal vesicles and prostate and is not a good measure of testicular function.'[53]

- **Motility:** 'The extent of progressive sperm motility is related to pregnancy rates. The total number of progressively motile spermatozoa in the ejaculate is of biological significance…' The velocity of motile spermatozoa is temperature-dependent, and therefore in the lab, a temperature of 37°C is recommended.[54]

In the new version of the WHO guideline, motility is divided into four categories, including the velocity of spermatozoa (in contradiction to the prior version).

Clinical data both from manual assessment of sperm motility as well as computer-aided sperm analysis demonstrate that the identification of rapidly progressive spermatozoa is important (Aitken *et al.*, 1985, Barratt *et al.*, 2011, Barratt *et al.*, 1992, Björndahl, 2010, Bollendorf *et al.*, 1996, Comhaire *et al.*, 1988, Eliasson, 2010, Irvine and Aitken, 1986, Mortimer *et al.*, 1986, Sifer *et al.*, 2005, Van den Bergh *et al.*, 1998). Therefore, the recommended categories are (with approximate velocity limits):

- **Rapidly progressive** (≥25 μm/s) – spermatozoa are moving actively, either linearly or in a large circle, covering a distance, from the starting point to the end point, of at least 25 μm (or ½ tail length) in one second.

- **Slowly progressive** (5 to <25 μm/s) – spermatozoa moving actively, either linearly or in a large circle, covering a distance, from the starting point to the end point, of 5 to <25 μm (or at least one head length to less than ½ tail length) in one second.

- **Non-progressive** (<5 μm/s) – all other patterns of active tail movements with an absence of progression, i.e. swimming in small circles, the flagellar force displacing the head less than 5 μm (one head length), from the starting point to the end point.

- **Immotile** – no active tail movements.

The extent of progressive sperm motility is related to pregnancy rates...[55]

WANT TO KNOW MORE?

A parameter that is of biological significance is the total number of progressively motile spermatozoa in the ejaculate.

The total number of progressively motile spermatozoa is obtained by multiplying the total number of spermatozoa in the ejaculate by the percentage of progressively motile cells. Methods of motility assessment involve computer-aided sperm analysis (CASA).[56]

More commonly used is the total motile sperm count (TMSC). This is the number of moving sperm in the entire ejaculate. It is calculated by multiplying the volume (cc) by the concentration (million sperm/cc) by the motility (per cent moving). This parameter is more predictive of infertility compared to concentration, volume and motility alone. There should be more than 40 million motile sperm in the ejaculate. It helps specialists to make clinical decisions. If the TMSC is over 10 million, there is a reasonable chance that taking the processed sperm and placing them directly into the uterus (IUI or intrauterine insemination) will be successful. If the TMSC, after maximizing the man's sperm production, is less than 10 million, most specialists feel that IVF is indicated. TMSC was recently proved to be a better predictor than total sperm count for ICSI outcomes compared to the classical WHO standard values.

How is sperm motility quantified?

There are two possibilities:

- **Manually** by using positive phase microscopy at x200 or x400 magnification. This version is very subjective, prone to errors and the test quality is much related to the training of the operator. Moreover, it takes several minutes.

- **CASA (computer-assisted sperm analysis):** CASA is a computer system which requires a high-resolution camera connected to a phase-contrast microscope. The analysis of a single view-field takes one second, so a complete analysis of sperm motility takes about a minute. CASA systems are best used for the kinematic analysis of spermatozoa, as they can detect and analyze motile cells. So, although CASA systems can perform varied functions including calculating concentration, assessing morphology and even fluorescent assays, a precise, repeatable motility analysis has become the primary feature relied on by many researchers. CASA can identify 50 motility characteristics including 8 kinematic parameters, and it is said to be objective and quantitative. According to a research study by Dearing *et al.* in 2019, computer-assisted sperm analysis (CASA) can reduce measurement uncertainty compared with manual SA.[57]

Simple overall motility gives no indication of the relative energy/ability/fertility potential of the sperm,[58] which is why the recent 6th edition of the WHO manual went back to taking into account the velocity of motile sperm.

WANT TO KNOW MORE?

If spermatozoa have a grade A motility (fast progressive), that says a lot about sperm quality and might be the number-one parameter for sperm quality according to some experts (e.g. Gerhard van der Horst of the University of the Western Cape, and David J. Smith of the University of Birmingham):

- If sperm are motile, they are alive.

- If they swim rapidly in a progressive way for a long time, most cell components such as the plasma membrane, mitochondria and the axoneme are obviously functioning properly. Also, the metabolite stores and metabolic processes required to produce ATP are functional.

- If they can penetrate cervical mucus and become capacitated and develop hyperactive swimming, a certain relationship with fertility is shown.

Often sperm with larger morphological abnormalities also have abnormal swimming patterns, such as the Dag defect. Dag defect sperm have an abnormal coiled tail morphology, are totally or almost totally immotile, and have severe abnormalities on the fibres in the axial filament.

Remember that in addition to motility, aspects such as hyperactivation relate strongly to fertilization rates and clinical pregnancy rates.

In humans, if a percentage of 20% of motile sperm is hyperactivated, that is a good prognostic factor in terms of fertilization potential.[59]

Generally, two basic types of 'good' motility have been characterized by observing spermatozoa motility in vitro:

- **Activated motility** (in vitro), to be found in:

  - freshly ejaculated semen

  - cervical mucus (up to utero-tubal junction).

  Typically the flagellum generates a symmetrical low-amplitude waveform and drives sperm in a relatively straight line. The head movement is low amplitude, linear and rapid.

- **Hyperactivated motility** (in vitro), to be found in:

  - sperm recovered from fallopian tubes or the site of fertilization

  - sperm incubated in media or artificially 'capacitated'.

  Typically, the flagellar beat is asymmetrical and of a higher amplitude. Characterized by 'starspin' or 'figure of 8' patterns.

  The head movement is high amplitude, circular, star spin, transition phase, linear phase.[60]

But how well do these observations in vitro relate to what sperm must do in real female physiology? The answer is: not very well.

There are certain physiological conditions that have a huge impact on sperm and its motility:

- Viscosity influences sperm selection.

- Observed in vitro 'marker' behaviour needs further thought.

- Sperm head morphology will affect their navigation/migration by directly affecting the flagellum.

- Female tract architecture will affect sperm navigation.

We are only just starting to know more about the journey through the female tract...

The average speed of a spermatozoa is 3 mm per minute. On average, it takes a sperm cell 15–40 minutes to reach the fallopian tube. Collectively, there are 50–500 million sperm cells, which delays movement – just like in a mass start of a cycling race where so many starters hinder themselves. That is why in reality it takes sperm about 1–1.5 hours to reach the ovum.

Morphology

Spermatozoa consist of a head and tail. The part of the tail that is connected to the head and the thicker part that contains mitochondria is called the midpiece. The rest of the tail consists of the principal piece (an axoneme or ciliary structure surrounded by outer dense fibres and a fibrous sheath with longitudinal columns) and endpiece. As the endpiece is difficult to see with a light microscope, the cell can be considered to comprise a head (and neck) and tail (midpiece and principal piece). For a spermatozoon to be considered without abnormalities, the head, midpiece, tail and cytoplasmic residue must be considered normal.[61]

The description for a good morphology of a spermatozoon has recently changed from 'normal' to 'ideal' as opposed to 'abnormal' if there is a visible defect. Defective spermatogenesis and some epididymal pathologies are commonly associated with an increased percentage of spermatozoa with abnormal shapes.[62]

The variable morphology of human spermatozoa makes assessment difficult, but observations on spermatozoa recovered from the female reproductive tract, especially in postcoital endocervical mucus […] and also from the surface of the zona […] have helped to define the appearance of potentially fertilizing (morphologically normal or, better, 'ideal' or 'typical') spermatozoa. By the strict application of certain criteria of sperm morphology, relationships between the percentage of 'normal' forms and various fertility endpoints (time to pregnancy, pregnancy rates in vivo and in vitro) have been established (Coetzee *et al.*, 1998, Eggert-Kruse *et al.*, 1996, Garrett *et al.*, 2003, Jouannet *et al.*, 1988, Liu *et al.*, 2003, Menkveld *et al.*, 1991, Toner *et al.*, 1995, Van Waart *et al.*, 2001), which may be useful for the prognosis of fertility.[63]

WANT TO KNOW MORE?

In general, the shape of the head appears to be more important than the exact size […] Abnormal spermatozoa generally have a lower fertilizing potential, depending on the types of anomalies, and may also have abnormal DNA. Morphological defects have been associated with increased DNA fragmentation (Gandini *et al.*, 2000), an increased incidence of structural chromosomal aberrations (Lee *et al.*, 1996), immature chromatin (Dadoune *et al.*, 1988) and aneuploidy (Devillard *et al.*, 2002, Martin *et al.*, 2003).[64]

Emphasis is therefore given to the form of the head, although the sperm tail (midpiece and principal piece) is also important to consider for understanding the male reproductive tract.

WANT TO KNOW MORE?

Head: The head should be smooth, regularly contoured and generally oval in shape. There should be a well-defined acrosomal region comprising 40–70% of the head area (Menkveld *et al.*, 1991). The acrosomal region should contain no large vacuoles, and not more than two small vacuoles, which should not occupy more than one fifth of the sperm head. The post-acrosomal region should not contain any vacuoles.

Midpiece: The midpiece should be slender, regular and about the same length as the sperm head. The major axis of the midpiece should be aligned with the major axis of the sperm head.

Tail: The principal piece should have a uniform calibre along its length, be thinner than the midpiece and be approximately 45 μm long (about 10 times the head length). It may be looped back on itself, provided there is no sharp angulation indicative of a broken flagellum.[65]

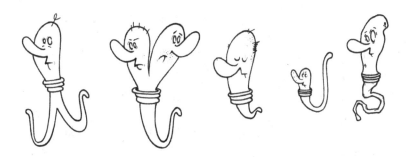

The percentage of normally shaped spermatozoa needed to fulfil the criteria of normal morphology within a sperm test has dropped dramatically. One reason is that the criteria were changed to using the so-called Kruger strict criteria for morphology. Those cut-off percentages for morphology were defined according to a research study performed by Kruger[66] on IVF results according to sperm morphology with the following results:

> For the stricter criteria, fertile men have > 14% normal forms in their semen and men with < 4% of normal forms are subfertile.

According to Kruger's criteria, IVF outcome was suboptimal when normal sperm morphology was less than 14% and worst if it was under 4%.

The sperm deformity index is a more reliable predictor of the outcome of fertilization in vitro than the proportion of normal sperm morphology.

The improved assessment of sperm morphology based on 'strict morphological criteria'[67] can be used to discriminate three categories in relation to the predicted outcome of standard IVF treatment:

- excellent prognosis (>14% morphologically normal spermatozoa)

- good prognosis (4–14%)

- and poor prognosis (<4%).[68]

(Grow *et al.*, 1994; Sukcharoen *et al.*, 1995)[69]

WANT TO KNOW MORE?

But why is it enough to have a small percentage of morphological normal spermatozoa for fertilization? What are all the malformed spermatozoa for?

In 1988, Robin Baker and Mark Bellis proposed their 'kamikaze sperm hypothesis', suggesting that different kinds of sperm might be adapted for different functions. They proposed that most are adapted for a 'kamikaze' role, to block the sperm of other males while only a few sperm in an ejaculate are 'egg-getters'.[70]

Abstinence

The ejaculate should be collected after a minimum of two days and a maximum of seven days of sexual abstinence.

This is what the WHO manual has to say about it:

> The time between the examined ejaculate and the most recent ejaculation before, 'abstinence time' (or period of sexual abstinence). As the epididymides are never completely emptied by one ejaculation (Cooper *et al.*, 1993), some spermatozoa remain from the time of the previous ejaculation. This influences the range of age and quality of spermatozoa in the ejaculate (Tyler *et al.*, 1982). Furthermore, extensive studies to determine the daily production of spermatozoa have indicated that 2–3 days of daily ejaculations is necessary to deplete the epididymal storage of spermatozoa (Amann, 2009, Amann and Howards, 1980). Thus, the recommendation, based on clinical experience, to ask men to collect the ejaculate to be examined, after a period of 2–7 abstinence days can contribute to variability and an indistinct limit between normal and subfertile results. The extent of this influence is difficult to ascertain, and it is rarely considered.[71]

So, even the authors of the manual point out that this wide range of recommended abstinence time might lead to some bias, but still it is in the updated guidelines.

What is important to know is that, first and foremost, whenever comparing two semen analyses, one needs to ensure that the ejaculates are both produced after the same abstinence time.

WANT TO KNOW MORE?

But how does abstinence time affect sperm quality?

Sobeiro *et al*. did a survey on this in 2005, examining the sperm of 500 men who were just about to undergo a vasectomy and concluded that the semen volume and sperm concentration increased according to how many days of sexual abstinence there were ($p < 0.05$). However, in patients with five or more days of sexual abstinence, a reduction in progressive motility ($p < 0.05$) was found. The sperm morphology did not vary with length of sexual abstinence.

Days of abstinence	Semen volume (%)	Sperm concentration (10 x 6/ml)	Sperm progressive motility (%)	Normal sperm morphology (%)
2	2.3 ± 1.1	105.1 ± 87.7	55.2 ± 16.5	16.4 ± 12.2
3	2.5 ± 1.3	104.8 ± 85.6	61.4 ± 15.3	17.1 ± 9.3
4	2.7 ± 1.3	105.4 ± 61.3	61.6 ± 13.5	18.4 ± 9.2
5	3.0 ± 1.6	127.1 ± 84.7	58.7 ± 15.6	18.0 ± 8.8
>5	3.3 ± 1.7	136.1 ± 82.1	56.3 ± 16.0	17.0 ± 9.1

Source: Based on Sobreiro et al. (2005)[72]

Levitas *et al*. did a research study in 2005 on over 9400 men, dividing them into four groups (three with oligospermia of different severity and one group with a normal amount of sperm) and investigated the changes within the groups according to abstinence time.[73] Their results could give us a practical guide to what abstinence time could be an advantage.

Among oligospermatic ejaculate they observed a consistent reduction of normal morphology as well as the percentage of motile sperm which were both inversely related to the duration of abstinence. These samples also showed an increase in total sperm count and total motile sperm count for up to four days of abstinence.

Moreover, abstinence of only one day or even skipping (the usually recommended) abstinence resulted in the best sperm quality among all probes.

Interestingly a different outcome was observed when looking at sperm probes from normospermic men. Within this group the morphology stayed constantly steady up to 10 days of abstinence, whereas the percentage of motility increased from day 0 to day 7. No real change was observed when looking at the total motile sperm count and the total sperm count in these men.[74]

Similar results come from a survey investigating two semen samples taken on consecutive days in order to perform a double intrauterine insemination. Semen volume, sperm concentration and total motile spermatozoa were significantly reduced in day 2 raw and prepared samples, whereas normal morphology, motility characteristics and percentage of acrosome-reacted spermatozoa increased significantly in day 2 inseminated samples as compared with day 1. Oligospermic, asthenospermic and teratospermic samples showed a significant improvement in concentration, various motility characteristics and normal morphology of spermatozoa in day 2 samples as compared to day 1.[75]

Interestingly, even the so-called acrosome index benefits from a short abstinence time according to a research study from 2006.

An improved fertilization rate in conventional IVF correlated with a so-called high acrosome index (percentage of sperm with normal acrosome morphology – cutoff value > or =10%). Again, comparing semen of oligospermatic and normospermatic men showed that the peak of the acrosome index was different in these two groups. Oligospermatic men achieved the best results at only one day of abstinence whereas normospermatic men had their peak value on day 2 and day 5 of abstinence. In a nutshell: for men with oligospermia, a short or even very short abstinence duration is recommended.[76]

So, in summary: oligospermic men should be advised to stick to abstinence times from 1–4 days, not longer, especially when the ejaculate is further used for insemination or IVF.

Round cells

The ejaculate invariably contains cells other than spermatozoa, called round cells, without further differentiating them into leucocytes or immature germ cells. This could be because of the difficulty in identifying and differentiating those cells under the microscope (in an unstained wet preparation). They could be either inflammatory cells, most commonly leucocytes, or cells of immature spermatogenic series.

WANT TO KNOW MORE?

The WHO manual advises that if the round cells are more than 1×10^6/ml, they should be differentiated to examine for leucocytes. To know whether these round cells are of spermatogenic or non-spermatogenic origin is important for a more accurate semen report. There have been several research studies investigating the average distribution among those round cells being either leucocytes or immature germ cells and whether that correlated with fertility issues. On average, the proportion was as follows: 80–90% were immature germ cells and 10–20% were leucocytes. The prevalence of leucocytospermia more than 10^6/ml was seen in approximately 10–20% of patients of male infertility and the presence of white blood cells can affect sperm function. Those having leucocytospermia can be subjected to further investigations such as reactive oxygen species or immunofluorescence microscopy.

Some patients are subfertile even when the sperm counts are normal and may have high immature germ cell counts. The counting of these cells could be a good indicator of a dysfunction at the testicular level. It may give us information about germ cell maturation arrest which is associated with increased shedding of germ cells from spermatogonia to spermatocytes and spermatids in semen. These patients can be segregated and further analyzed for cytogenetic studies for sperm DNA damage or DNA fragmentation index which may be the cause of subfertility.[77]

Sperm vitality

Sperm vitality, estimated by assessing the membrane integrity of the cells, can be determined routinely on all ejaculates, but is not necessary when at least 20–40% of spermatozoa are motile. In samples with poor motility, the vitality test is important to discriminate between immotile dead sperm and immotile live sperm.

WANT TO KNOW MORE?

The percentage of live spermatozoa is assessed by identifying those with an intact cell membrane, by dye exclusion (dead cells have damaged plasma membranes that allow entry of membrane-impermeant stains) or by hypotonic swelling.[78]

Sperm agglutination

This means that sperm adhere to one another in various kind of ways. Typically, they have a frantic shaking motion, as they want to move but cannot. Hence, being agglutinated means that their motility is hindered. The presence of agglutination is not sufficient evidence to deduce an immunological cause of infertility but is suggestive of the presence of anti-sperm antibodies; further testing may be required.

Anti-sperm antibody testing

If the blood–testis barrier is violated (e.g. by testicular surgery, torsion or varicocele), an immune response to sperm in the form of anti-sperm antibodies (AsAb) might be the result. Those autoimmune antibodies stick on to the spermatozoa causing an agglutination, thus hindering its motility in general and its ability to penetrate the cervical mucus as well as sperm and egg-fusion in particular. AsAb are deemed to be an important factor for impaired fertility and are seen in approximately 10% of infertile men versus 2% of fertile men.[79]

WANT TO KNOW MORE?

Anti-sperm antibodies (AsAb) in semen belong almost exclusively to two immunoglobulin classes: IgA and IgG. IgM antibodies, because of their larger size and main function in the acute phase of infection, are rarely found in semen. IgA antibodies may have greater clinical importance than IgG antibodies but more than 95% of cases with IgA sperm antibodies are also positive for IgG. Both classes can be detected on sperm cells or in biological fluids in related screening tests.[80]

There are two commonly used tests to detect antibodies on spermatozoa ('direct tests'):

- Sperm mixed antiglobulin reaction test (MAR): detects IgG and IgA antibodies against sperm surface in the semen sample.

- Immunobeat (IB) tests: detects IgG, IgA and IgM antibodies; also demonstrates the specific area of the sperm that is affected by the antibodies.

The MAR test is performed on a fresh semen sample while the IB test uses washed spermatozoa.

The 6th Edition of the WHO manual on semen analysis has changed sperm parameter standard values into ranges:[81]

Characteristic	Units	Normal	Borderline	Pathological
Volume	ml	2.0–6.0	1.5–1.9	< 1.5
Sperm concentration	10^6/ml	20–250	10–20	< 10
Total sperm count	10^6/ejaculate	≥ 80	20–79	< 20
Motility	% motile	≥ 60	40–59	< 40
	% progressive	≥ 50	35–49	< 35
	% rapid	≥ 25		
	progession grade	3 or 4	2	1 or 0
Morphology	% typical forms	≥ 14	4–13	< 4
Vitality	% vital (alive)	≥ 60	40–59	< 40
Leucocytes	10^6/ml			> 1.0
Anti-sperm antibodies	% binding	< 50	50–79	≥ 80

Based on WHO Laboratory Manual for the Examination and Processing of Human Semen, 6th Edition. Geneva: World Health Organization; 2021. Licence: CC BY-NC-SA 3.0 IGO.

Note: As the interpretation and validation of something as important as new standard values in semen analysis should be performed by absolute experts, the following paragraphs cite an article on the 6th Edition written by several leading andrologists. It gives an overview of news and changes of the 6th Edition compared to the 5th Edition that was used from 2010 to July 2021.

Comment on the new 6th edition and its changes quoted in extracts[82]

I. USE OF DECISION LIMITS TO IDENTIFY ABNORMAL EJACULATES

The most important change proposed in the 6th edition is the adoption of decision limits to differentiate normal from abnormal ejaculates. The editors of the 6th edition acknowledge that the reference ranges described in the 5th edition should be abandoned as they are of limited value in differentiating fertile from infertile men. The 5th edition WHO manual utilized a population of 1,800 fertile men to obtain the reference distributions for semen parameters. The lower 5th percentile was used to define the reference values for normal semen parameters. While the 5th percentile is commonly utilized as a statistical approach to determine cut-off norms in medical tests, this resulted in much controversy when applied to male fertility. It has been argued that the 5th percentile is not applicable to assign normality in this case and proves unable to discriminate between fertile and infertile patients. Several studies reported a shift of fertility status from abnormal to normal in 15% to 44% of patients by just using the 5th edition norms instead of the 4th edition.

The editors of the 6th edition have acknowledged these limitations (Appendix 8.1 of the manual) and stipulated that semen examination cannot strictly differentiate between pathological and normal samples. Moreover, they recognize that using the lower 5th percentile is not the correct approach to identify normal or abnormal semen samples, and that semen analysis alone cannot predict fertility as this depends on multiple variables, particularly, female factors. Hence, the 'normal' reference values of the 5th edition have been replaced by 'decision limits' in the 6th edition. These are classified 'normal', 'borderline', and 'pathological'. A 'normal' concentration is $\geq 20 \times 10^6$/ml, 'borderline' lies between 10 to 20×10^6/ml, and 'pathological' is the various groups will help refine these limits. The creation of a 'borderline' group will have significant clinical implications as many men whose sample would previously have been labelled as normal using the 5th edition criteria, will now be classified as 'borderline' and be eligible for therapeutic interventions. Clinicians can still offer hope for natural pregnancy in these cases before opting to pursue ART. The impact of this classification shift will likely be significant in clinical practice. If we now apply the new criteria and deem men with parameters below the new 'normal' threshold ('borderline'+'pathological') as infertile, we will suddenly increase the number of infertile men in our practices.

2. CHANGE IN MOTILITY GRADING SYSTEM

A criticism of the 5th edition was the decision to eliminate the reporting of rapidly progressive motility, and the editors of the 6th edition have now reverted back to a four-category classification as follows:

- Rapidly progressive: ≥ 25 μm/s, or at least half tail length per second.

- Slow progressive: 5 to < 25 μm/s, or at least one head length to less than half tail length/sec.

- Non-progressive: < 5 μm/s, or less than one head length.

- Immotile: no tail movement.

A return to the earlier classification of the 4th edition of WHO manual for sperm motility is a welcome improvement as it allows a better characterization of motility and may provide additional prognostic information.

3. SPERM DNA FRAGMENTATION TESTING

The editors of the 6th edition should be commended for introducing tests of sperm DNA fragmentation (SDF) in the manual...

4. REACTIVE OXYGEN SPECIES (ROS) TESTING

The 6th edition recognizes the increasing clinical relevance of seminal oxidative stress by dedicating a section to the methods assigned for ROS testing. Possibly due to the limited availability of such testing, this assessment has been incorporated under 'Advanced Examination' section, suggesting that this should still be considered a research tool...

— CHAPTER 8 —

A Deeper Look Inside: An Overview of Add-on Examination Opportunities

Often a normal semen analysis is not enough to judge the quality of the sperm as it doesn't tell us anything about the sperm's genetic material – the DNA.

Not only does DNA damage influence male fertility negatively and decrease the chance of a pregnancy, but recent research shows that there is a connection between DNA fragmentation and the rate of recurrent early miscarriage.[1] That has led to a new awareness of sperm integrity, casting doubt on the idea that ICSI is the solution for any male-factor problem, as believed by many reproductive endocrinologists for a long time.

Sperm DNA abnormalities have an impact on every single fertility checkpoint:

- poor embryo development

- failure of fertilization in IVF

- failure to implant in ICSI

- post-implantation loss and malformations

- increased miscarriage rate

- poorer childhood health.[2]

WANT TO KNOW MORE?

To underline the clinical relevance of sperm DNA damage, here are some more facts, perfectly summarized by Esteves at the ESHRE Congress 2019:

- Sperm DNA damage is common in infertile men and male partners in couples attending ART programmes.

- It leads to reduced fecundability (longer time-to-pregnancy) and recurrent pregnancy loss.

- Unfortunately it also impairs the reproductive outcomes of IUI and ART.

- Transferring sperm genetic defects via ART might potentially affect the health of the resulting offspring.[3]

The problem with sperm DNA damage is that neither the sperm cell itself nor the secretions and contents in the semen can repair it. Only the oocyte has the potential to do so. This ability requires a healthy and preferably young oocyte, which leads us to the problem of 'elder' women whose oocytes are no longer capable of repairing sperm DNA damage.

In a nutshell, sperm DNA is all that matters post-fertilization.

The condition of the DNA cannot be examined with a simple sperm analysis but must be done with special tests that are rarely done in the routine treatment of an infertile couple.

Generally speaking, those tests make the broken DNA visible by different methods and then calculate a so-called DNA fragmentation index (DFI).

DNA FRAGMENTATION – WHAT HARMS THE SPERM?

There are physical (heat, trauma), chemical (smoking, medication), anatomic (varicocele) and infectious causes that lead to string breaks in the DNA of sperm. Sperm with damaged genetic material are rarely able to fertilize an egg. If they manage to do so, those pregnancies are more likely to end in an early miscarriage. In men with unfulfilled fatherhood, approximately 25% with a pathologic semen analysis and even 10% with a normal sperm test have a raised amount of DNA fragmentation.

The most common external factors leading to elevated DNA fragmentation are:

- environmental factors such as phalate exposure, radiation, temperature, drugs

- diseases such as varicocele, genital tract infections, especially accessory gland infections, systemic inflammation and fever

- lifestyle causes such as obesity, diabetes and smoking

- age

- prolonged stasis of the spermatozoa in the epididymitis or in transit

- immature/abnormal spermatozoa.

All of the above lead to elevated oxidative stress which harms the sperm cell and thus leads to DNA damage.[4]

Oxidative stress is one of the main causes of sperm DNA damage; others are apoptosis during sperm maturation in the testis and epididymitis, as well as protamination failure (deficient replacement of histones to protamines during spermatogenesis).[5]

WHAT DNA INTEGRITY TESTS ARE AVAILABLE AND WHAT DO THEY INVESTIGATE?

	Test	Principle	Advantage	Disadvantage
[1]	AO test	Metachromatic shift in fluorescence of AO when bound to single strand (ss)DNA. Uses fluorescent microscopy	Rapid, simple and inexpensive	Inter-laboratory variations and lack of reproducibility
[2]	AB staining	Increased affinity of AB dye to loose chromatin of sperm nucleus. Uses optical microscopy	Rapid, simple and inexpensive	Inter-laboratory variations and lack of reproducibility
[3]	CMA3 staining	CMA3 competitively binds to DNA indirectly visualizing protamine deficient DNA. Uses fluorescent microscopy	Yields reliable results as it is strongly correlated with other assays	Inter-observer variability
[4]	TB staining	Increased affinity of TB to sperm DNA phosphate residues. Uses optical microscopy	Rapid, simple and inexpensive	Inter-observer variability
[5]	TUNEL	Quantifies the enzymatic incorporation of dUTP into DNA breaks. Can be done using both optical microscopy and fluorescent microscopy. Uses optical microscopy, fluorescent microscopy and flow cytometry	Sensitive, reliable with minimal inter-observer variability. Can be performed on few sperm	Requires standardization between laboratories
[0]	SCSA	Measures the susceptibility of sperm DNA to denaturation. The cytometric version of AO test. Uses flow cytometry	Reliable estimate of the percentage of DNA-damaged sperm	Requires the presence of expensive instrumentation (flow cytometer) and highly skilled technicians
[7]	SCD or Halo test	Assess dispersion of DNA fragments after denaturation. Uses optical or fluorescent microscopy	Simple test	Inter-observer variability
[8]	SCGE or comet assay	Electrophoretic assessment of DNA fragments of lysed DNA. Uses fluorescent microscopy	Can be done in very low sperm count. It is sensitive and reproducible	Requires an experienced observer. Inter-observer variability

[1] Acridine orange (AO) stains normal DNA fluoresces green; whereas denatured DNA fluoresces orange-red. [2] Aniline blue (AB) staining showing sperm with fragmented DNA and normal sperm. [3] Chromomycin A3 (CMA3) staining: protamine deficient spermatozoa appear bright yellow; spermatozoa with normal protamine appear yellowish green. [4] Toulidine blue (TB) staining: normal sperm appear light blue and sperm with DNA fragmentation appear violet. [5] Terminal deoxynucleotidyl transferase dUTP nick end labeling (TUNEL) assay fluorescent activated cell sorting histogram showing percentage of SDF. [6] Sperm chromatin structure assay (SCSA): flow cytometric version of AO staining. [7] Sperm chromatin dispersion (SCD) test: spermatozoa with different patterns of DNA dispersion; large-sized halo; medium-sized halo [2]; very small-sized halo. [8] Comet images showing various levels of DNA damage.

WANT TO KNOW MORE?

Let's go through them one by one to understand how they work and which one might be preferable to the others.

1. Sperm Chromatin Structure Analysis (SCSA) testing

The test uses fresh ejaculate (2–7 days of abstinence). Sperm is stained with a special technique, so sperm with intact double-strand DNA is visible as green and those with broken (fragmented, single-strand) DNA appear as red. Then the relation between green and red spermatozoa is calculated (about 5000 spermatozoa are examined) and a so-called fragmentation index is worked out.

Classification of DFI (DNA fragmentation index):

a) Excellent to good (less than or equal to 15% DFI)

b) Good to fair (greater than 15% to less than 25% DFI)

c) Fair to poor (greater than or equal to 25% to less than 50% DFI)

d) Very poor (greater than or equal to 50% DFI)

Interestingly there is some research concluding that this kind of DNA fragmentation test can be used as a predictor for IUI outcomes.

2. TUNEL assay (terminal deoxynucleotidyl transferase dUTP nick end labelling)

At the free ends of broken DNA, fragments of certain hydroxygroups (3'-OH-groups) can be attached with the enzyme TdT which is marked with nucleotides that can be made visible via fluorescence in the microscope.

3. SCD (sperm chromatin dispersion test) or 'halo' test

Sperm with intact DNA have 'halos'. These halos represent dispersed chromatin without strand breaks. Sperm with fragmented DNA do not have halos, so haloless sperm cells represent those with DNA damage. A normal result would show less than 20% of cells with fragmented DNA.

4. COMET test

This is the only test to measure double-strand breaks separately.[6] It is based on the capacity of negatively charged loops/fragments of DNA to be pulled through an agarose gel in response to an electric field, appearing like a 'comet'. In the comet structure, the undamaged DNA nucleoid part is referred to as the 'head' and the trailing damaged DNA streak is referred to as the 'tail'. The percentage of DNA in the tail is directly proportional to the percentage of DNA damage that has occurred in a particular cell. There are two types of COMET test: the alkaline COMET test and the neutral COMET test.

Are the results of the tests comparable with each other?

There is a huge debate about which DNA fragmentation test is the one, but also about the standard values of the results of the tests; some still have no definition of a 'normal' result. It is also difficult to compare the tests. DNA fragmentation tests differ in their fertility predictive value and that is the most important reason to undertake the tests. There are some studies on that topic, such as that by Javed *et al.* in 2019, with the aim to compare the ability of the five most widely utilized methods of measuring DNA fragmentation to predict male infertility and reactive oxygen species by Oxisperm kit assay. They concluded that the alkaline comet test showed the best ability to predict male infertility, followed by the TUNEL assay, the SCD test and the SCSA, while the neutral comet test had no predictive power.[7]

According to Jackson Kirkman-Brown, one of the leading researchers in andrology, the TUNEL and the COMET tests have the most evidence for proper test results after recurrent miscarriage.[8] In any case, he strongly recommends thinking the test results over and always naming the type of test with which the DNA fragmentation was measured.

Why is it important to also be able to measure not only single-strand breaks (SSB) but also double-strand breaks (DSB) of the DNA?

single-strand break (SSB) and double-strand break (DSB) have different mechanisms of damage

SSB: Oxidative Stress attack from outside

high impact during epididymal transit

DSB: dysfunction inside sperm

Topoisomerase or endonuclease dysfunction mechanical stress on chromosomes

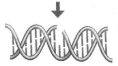

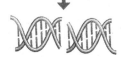

more toxic; irreparable by oocyte post fertilization

can't be protected by antioxidant supplementation

Sperm with DNA fragmentation still have fertilization ability and developmental potential. Depending on the level of sperm DNA fragmentation, three situations can be expected.

In some cases, the oocyte repair machinery is not sufficient to repair DNA damage, and the embryo may fail to develop or implant in the uterus or may be aborted naturally at a later stage (uncompensable damage).

In other cases, the oocyte repairs the DNA strand breaks before the initiation of the first cleavage division, and this sperm is then able to generate normal offspring (compensable damage).

In the worst and last scenario, deletions or sequence errors may be introduced because of partial oocyte repair, and abnormal offspring may then result (partial compensable damage). It has been reported that 80% of de novo structural chromosome aberrations in humans are of paternal origin.[9]

Therefore, it is up to the capacity of the oocyte to fix the sperm DNA problem: it is believed that DNA repair in the newly fertilized embryo relies entirely on the maternal mRNAs and proteins which are deposited and stored in the oocyte before ovulation.

Of course, the extent to which the sperm DNA is damaged will be important: Ahmadi *et al.* suggest that the oocyte has the capacity to repair DNA damage of sperm when it is damaged by less than 8%.[10] The ability of the oocyte to repair DNA damage in the fertilizing spermatozoon will also depend on the type of sperm DNA damage. As indicated previously, sperm DNA fragmentation can be classified as single-stranded and double-stranded. In general, single-stranded DNA damage is easier to repair than double-stranded DNA damage, although there is evidence that polymerases can also repair double-stranded DNA damage.[11]

Who should be tested for sperm DNA fragmentation? Why don't we include DNA tests in the standard lab work?

New in the 6th Edition of the WHO manual is the recommendation that DNA fragmentation testing is used as an add-on test in certain situations.

Due to cost issues, it is not advised to test every man for his DNA integrity. Currently, the official recommendation is to test the following:

- men with clinical varicocele

- men with unexplained infertility

- men with repeated IUI failures

- male partner of women with recurrent pregnancy loss

- men with IVF and/or ICSI failures

- borderline abnormal or normal semen parameters with risk factors.[12]

What to do with a high DFI?

- **Antibiotics** in the co-existence of an infection.

WANT TO KNOW MORE?

Studies have shown that the use of oral antibiotic and anti-inflammatory agents over a given period of time, depending on the infection's cause, significantly reduces sperm DNA fragmentation, and their administration to patients prior to IVF may be beneficial, especially in men with a high percentage of sperm with DNA damage.[13]

- **Lifestyle changes:** drugs, smoking, environment and obesity.

WANT TO KNOW MORE?

Exposure to environmental and lifestyle factors has far-reaching implications on male fertility. Current data has consistently associated smoking with higher SDF values when compared to non-smokers. There are also numerous environmental factors such as air-borne pollutants, ionizing radiation and pesticides that have been linked to increased SDF values. Several studies have demonstrated higher SDF in obese men, yet a recent meta-analysis found no robust association between BMI and SDF.[14]

- **Diet and supplements:** fresh foods, particularly those containing antioxidants or vitamin C and E, are preferable when it comes to helping the body repair DNA damage naturally.

WANT TO KNOW MORE?

A recent study found out that the combination of healthy eating and the intake of micro-nutrients leads to a twofold higher pregnancy rate in men with an initially high DFI (> 15%) than diet changes alone.[15]

- **Varicocoele repair.**

WANT TO KNOW MORE?

A review from 2018 including 21 studies and a total of 1270 participants confirmed the effectiveness of varicocelectomy as a means of both reducing oxidatively induced sperm DNA damage and potentially improving fertility. Varicocele repair should be offered as part of treatment options for male partners of infertile couples presenting with palpable varicoceles.[16]

- **Short abstinence time:** The negative impact of prolonged ejaculatory abstinence on DNA fragmentation has been reported without significant detrimental effect on conventional semen parameters.

WANT TO KNOW MORE?

Short-term recurrent ejaculation may be a simple non-invasive manoeuvre to improve SDF. Although the beneficial effect of short abstinence time on natural conception is unclear, application of the technique to assisted reproduction may have value. In addition to higher pregnancy rates in ICSI, recurrent ejaculation has been associated with a significantly lower DNA fragmentation rate.[17]

What is meant by short abstinence time? Three hours abstinence had a lower level of sperm DNA damage than 24 hours.[18] One day was better than 5–7 days of abstinence[19] and men with high DNA damage decreased to normal in 1–3 subsequent samples after one day of abstinence.[20]

- **Testicular aspiration of sperm:** DNA damage occurs at the post-testicular level; therefore, testicular sperm may have a better DNA integrity than ejaculated sperm.

WANT TO KNOW MORE?

Testicular sperm has been explored as a treatment option for high SDF based on the finding of lower SDF in testicular sperm than ejaculated sperm and better ICSI outcome. Hence, studies suggest that TESTI-ICSI is an effective option to overcome infertility when applied to selected men with oligospermia and high ejaculated SDF levels.[21]

- **ICSI** rather than IVF.

WANT TO KNOW MORE?

A meta-analysis showed a significant increase in miscarriage after ART in patients with high DNA damage compared with those with low DNA damage risk ratio (RR) = 2.16.[22] Therefore, any type of additional sperm selection is advisable. In men with a DFI > 30%, ICSI should be performed rather than IVF, as shown in a study from 2007 showing that ICSI leads to a 42% pregnancy rate compared with 26% in IVF in men with a high DFI.[23] The reason might be the prolonged culture in IVF compared with ICSI. It is known that sperm DNA fragmentation increases with longer cultivation time as well as with temperature (incubation). Additionally, the oocyte cytoplasm with its DNA repair tools favours ICSI.[24]

- **Testicular retrieval of sperm.**

If there is either azoospermia in the ejaculate or a high percentage of DNA fragmentation, there are some options how to retrieve sperm cells from the testis or epididymitis directly.

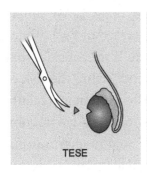 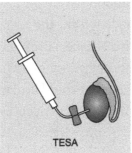 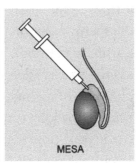 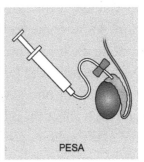

- **TESA (testicular sperm aspiration):** Using local anaesthesia, a needle is inserted in the testicle to aspirate tissue/sperm. TESA is most commonly used in men who have an adequate amount of sperm throughout the testicles.

- **TESE (testicular sperm extraction):** This procedure means a surgical biopsy under local anaesthesia or sedation. The goal is to retrieve tissue from the testicle that contains sperm. In the best case, this tissue to be extracted has already been identified through mapping techniques prior to the biopsy. The tissue is extracted through a small incision. It can either be done with sedation or local anaesthesia.

- **MESA (microepididymal sperm aspiration):** This procedure is used in men who suffer from vasal or epididymal obstruction. Using an operating microscope, MESA is performed under general anaesthesia. Aim is an extensive collection of mature sperm.

- **PESA (percutaneous epididymal sperm aspiration):** PESA is used in men who suffer from obstructive azoospermia either from a prior vasectomy or an infection. It is performed under local anaesthesia, inserting a needle into the epididymis.

- **microTESE (microdissection TESE):** Performed under general anaesthesia, a transverse cut is made through the skin in the centre of the testicle, followed by 'pulling out' the inside of the testicle. Using the help of a surgical microscope, the seminiferous tubules can now be examined for sperm to be retrieved.[25]

Sperm selection methods

After intercourse, from the millions of spermatozoa ejaculated, only a small number – a few hundred – make it to the region of the oviduct, where they encounter the egg and fertilization takes place. It is likely that this subpopulation has been selected through the oviduct so that only those with the highest fertilization capability and the best features for supporting embryo development get the opportunity to fertilize the egg. The relatively low efficiency of ARTs might be explained by the fact that we currently lack an effective methodology to separate this specific sperm subpopulation for its use in ARTs. We simply don't know enough of the sperm selection mode within the female tract and we cannot imitate it with scientific artificial methods. This is especially relevant if we consider that both IVF and ICSI bypass the sperm selection operating in vivo, increasing the risk of fertilizing the oocyte with defective spermatozoa that could lead to developmental failure and even affect the offspring in the long run. In natural conception, only a small fraction out of the millions of sperm make it close to the ovum, whereas in IVF 50,000 sperm are put in the petri dish together with the egg cell. Moreover, in ICSI one single sperm is selected by the embryologist and injected into the oocyte.

WANT TO KNOW MORE?

That is why sperm-selecting methods gain more and more importance in ART. Both the very simple but commonly used ones and the modern and more sophisticated techniques are introduced here.

Swim-up is one of the most commonly used migration techniques for sperm preparation. The sperm are selected on their motility and capability to swim out of the seminal plasma. Therefore, 1 ml of semen is placed in a tube and covered with 1.3 ml of cultural media. The tubes are then put in an incubator, inclined at an angle of 45° and incubated at 37°C for 30–60 minutes. The tube is then returned to the vertical position and 1 ml removed from the tube, aspirating the selected sperm from the upper meniscus with a sterile pipette.[26]

Density grade centrifugation (DGC): This is the most popular procedure to select spermatozoa in ART. Gametes are forced to cross a gradient made of colloidal silicon and are separated based on their density. 'DGC yields sperm populations with higher motility, better morphology and maturity with respect to whole semen. However, recent evidence indicates that DGC may increase sperm DNA fragmentation (SDF) levels, a parameter that negatively impacts reproductive outcomes after ARTs. In particular, one group of researchers reported that DGC increases SDF in about 50% of infertile couples treated by IVF/ICSI. More importantly, these subjects experienced a 50% lower pregnancy rate with respect to those showing a decrease of DNA damage during selection.'[27]

These two standard methods for sperm selection face several problems. First, the optimal time for sperm selection is about 10 minutes for 1 ml of sample containing 100 million/ml sperm. The density gradient technique separates about 36% of sperm from 0.5 ml raw semen in about 30 minutes, whereas swim-up selects about 12% of the sperm population from 1 ml in about one hour.[28] Thus, the process takes too long to avoid harming the sperm in terms of DNA fragmentations. Several studies conclude that both swim-up and DGC enhance SDF. One recent study, for example, concluded that DGC and swim-up increase SDF in viable spermatozoa in, respectively, about 60% and 40% of the subjects.[29]

That is why new methods with lower artificial DNA damage have been introduced, such as:

IMSI (intracytoplasmic morphologically selected sperm injection): This is an add-on technique to the common ICSI procedure. The main difference is the microscope used. During IMSI, a magnification of 6000–8000x is used (400x in ICSI). This gives the embryologist the opportunity to examine the sperm cell and especially the head's morphology very carefully. This method is also called MSOME (motile sperm organelle morphological examination). As there is a significant correlation between DNA damage and sperm head morphology, as well as between morphological scoring and chromatin decondensation, intense examination of the head is a proper tool for sperm selection. A large study including over 9000 treatment cycles with either ICSI alone or IMSI concluded that the fertilization rate and blastulation rate were both significantly higher in the IMSI than the ICSI group. Moreover, in an adjusted model, the IMSI group obtains better pregnancy and live-birth rates, although only the pregnancy outcome reached statistical significance: an IMSI cycle was 1.17 times more likely to result in a clinical pregnancy than an ICSI attempt. The population most likely to benefit from IMSI was that with the poorest sperm. IMSI was twice as likely to result in a live birth for female partners of 30–40 years of age. The authors suggest that IMSI should be considered as a first-line procedure for severe male-factor infertility and as a second-line procedure in cases of ICSI failure or when a previous attempt has demonstrated a lack of blastulation.[30]

PICSI (physiologically selected intracytoplasmic sperm injection): This technique is based on the fact that the mature sperm head has a specific receptor that allows it to bind to hyaluronic acid (HA), the main component of the *cumulus oophorous*; this is in contrast to the immature spermatozoa, which do not have this ability to bind to HA. Thus, they have a whole DNA and low frequency of aneuploidies and miscarriages. In this way, the genomic contribution of the spermatozoa to the zygotes can be compared to that of the spermatozoa that are selected by the *cumulus oophorous* during natural fertilization.[31] The major difference between the ordinary ICSI procedure and the PICSI procedure is the actual dish with the hyaluronan. The sperm binding to the dish allows the lab to have criteria for selection more than just visualization. In the HAB-select study from 2019 including 2772 couples, the authors observed a significant reduction in miscarriage with PICSI compared with standard ICSI, but there was no effect on clinical pregnancy rate or preterm live-birth rate.[32] According to Jackson Kirkman-Brown, one of the authors, selecting sperm may alleviate oocyte ageing.[33]

MACS (magnetic-activated cell sorting): MACS can be used to separate apoptotic sperm with high proportions of fragmented DNA from the rest, thus improving the overall quality of the seminal sample. The MACS process involves the use of very small magnetic particles. These particles have an antibody known as protein annexin. The antibody fastens itself to sperm with high DNA fragmentation, which are more likely to undergo apoptosis or programmed cell death. The semen sample is then passed through a column with weak magnetic fields around it. The apoptotic sperm get drawn towards the walls while the healthy ones pass through the channel.[34]

Zeta sperm selection: The electrical potential between the sperm membrane that is negatively charged and its surrounding is called zeta potential. Sperm with high negative surface electrical charge – that is, high zeta potential – are mature and more likely to have intact chromatin. On the other hand, zeta potential is lower in sperm with DNA damage. This property can be used to select sperm with intact DNA.[35]

Microfluid separation of sperm: This is the latest technology to separate sperm. Micro-fluidics provides the opportunity to sort sperm cells in a faster, gentler way that more closely mimics the natural selection processes and avoids some of the most detrimental elements of current sperm-sorting techniques. Generally speaking, this technique consists of a radial network of channels which separates sperm into left, straight and right swimmers. Motile sperm move and flow through the microchannel in the medium that mimics the viscosity of the reproductive tract fluid. Dead or immotile sperm are retained in the inlet; motile sperm are collected from the microchannel outlet. The additional separation using sperm's swimming direction selects those with intact DNA swimming left or right whereas sperm with strand breaks tend to swim straight ahead. In this procedure, 1 ml of semen could be processed in less than 20 minutes, resulting in over 80% improvement in selected sperm integrity.[36] Sorting sperm cells based on their motility is beneficial for three main reasons: (1) it is a natural way to separate them from somatic cells and debris in semen; (2) dead and damaged sperm cells are also selected against; (3) high motility is required for successful fertilization in IUI or IVF.[37]

When to use which method?

That is a difficult question causing a lot of debate in the research world.

One interesting prospective randomized trial from 2020 including 413 ICSI cases concluded that PICSI and MACS are efficient techniques for sperm selection in cases with abnormal sperm DNA fragmentation. However, MACS is preferred when the females are younger than 30 years, while PICSI is preferred in older females.[38]

PART II

Chinese Medicine

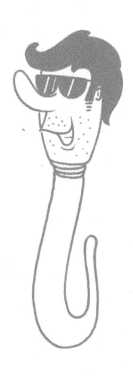

CHAPTER 9

Chinese Medicine Anatomy of the Male Genital Area

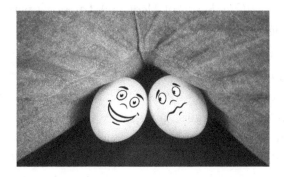

Books that deal exclusively with Chinese Medicine andrology ('Nan Ke') are rare. Those that do exist are relative recent, as Chinese andrology – as a specialist field within Chinese Medicine – doesn't have a long history; in fact, it has only been established over the past few decades.

Certainly, in the old books and in many of the famous Chinese Medicine Classics, diseases of the male and their cure with acumoxa and herbs had their relevance. In particular, the maintenance of erectile function was of great interest in the culture of ancient China and therefore in ancient Chinese Medicine. In almost every dynasty there were books on the preservation of erectile function.

What might be new to most readers is the fact that, according to Western biomedical medicine, in Chinese Medicine there are specific terms and names for the anatomic structures and organs of the male urogenital tract.

However, that has nothing to do with the supposedly precise knowledge of human anatomy by the ancient Chinese. In fact, they had a hard time figuring out the proper anatomy of a human body as Confucianism forbade dissections. Accordingly, dissections were forbidden from the Han dynasty (202 BC to 220 AD) onwards.[1] Of course, this couldn't completely stop the curiosity of the Chinese concerning the inner workings of the human body.

Historically, the first official dissection – of a convicted rebel – was ordered by emperor

Wang Mang 王莽 in the 16th century. His inner organs were measured and bamboo canes were put into his blood vessels to follow them and to achieve a better understanding of pathomechanism and the treatment of diseases. Similar dissections for anatomic reasons are described in the *Huangdi Nei Jing Ling Shu* 黃帝內經靈樞 (Ling Shu Jing 靈樞經), chapter 12 Jing-Shui 經水, which are astonishingly precise.[2]

Despite rare correct descriptions like the one mentioned above, the generally rather infantile anatomic knowledge within ancient Chinese Medicine hasn't really changed. Although during the Qing dynasty attempts were made to update anatomic knowledge through dissections on people sentenced to death or by investigating dead bodies in epidemic areas.

Wang Qingren (1768–1831) was a Chinese physician who lived in the Qing dynasty and wrote a book trying to correct the anatomy described in the *Nei Jing*. Entitled *Yi Lin Gai Cuo* (*Correcting the Errors in the Forest of Medicine*), the book was published in 1831 and included a lot of knowledge from autopsies.[3]

To be fair, the anatomic inaccuracy within Chinese Medicine is only to be seen for inner organs and structures. For organs and tissue on the surface there are often many names as the Chinese were good observers – for example, there are various names for the penis.

It is an achievement of the so-called integrative Chinese–Western Medicine that the anatomic structures known from our biomedical anatomy books actually do have Chinese names. Integrative Medicine is based on the fact that diseases that are not described as such in the Chinese Medicine classics, such as prostatitis, have been categorized nowadays by doctors for Chinese Medicine and classified according to pattern discrimination. This is possible because even in China, doctors of Chinese Medicine receive a dual education – that is, they are trained in both Western and Eastern Medicine.

This method of re-classifying Western diagnosis into Chinese Medicine patterns is called reframing. It enables us to put Western diseases into Chinese Medical drawers, although they never occur in any classical book of Chinese Medicine. Reframing modern diagnosis into Chinese Medicine terminology is the foundation of modern 'Nan Ke' and gives us the opportunity and understanding to treat them according to the Traditional Chinese Medicine way with acupuncture and herbs.

Having a brief knowledge of the Chinese terminology and an understanding of the male urogenital anatomy helps a lot in understanding male infertility problems. So let's take a look.

In Suwen, the first book of the Yellow emperor (*Huangdi Nei Jing*), genitals were generally called 'Yin'. The translation for this kind of Yin is 'hidden' or 'in the dark', but scholars, students, doctors and knowing readers knew it was the codename for something sexual. 'Yin' also means the hidden and forbidden body structures such as the scrotum, penis, anus and certain parts of the urogenital system.

Do not mistake this sexual Yin (淫) with the Yin (陰) that we know from Yin-Yang theory. In pictograms they are totally different and so is their meaning!

First of all, the whole genital region is divided into two parts:

- the front Yin region, consisting of lower abdomen, scrotum, testes and the penis

- the back (dorsal) Yin region, including anus and the dorsal part of the perineum.

The whole genital region (front and back) is directed by the Kidney – this dominance is reflected by the fact that many names for structures include the word Kidney. The following explanations have their source in Bob Damone's fabulous book on TCM andrology.[4]

TESTIS AND EPIDYMIDIS

Western Medicine: Responsible for production of testosterone and spermatogenesis respectively the storage of the maturing sperm cells.

Chinese Medicine: The testis and epidymidis are taken together and called:

- Kidney's child (Shen Zi)

- egg semen (Luan Zi)

- external Kidney (Wai Shen).

A specific name for either the testis or the epidymidis doesn't exist; they coexist together as one structure in the Chinese Medicine perspective.

Channels: The testes and epidymidis have a close relationship to the:

- Liver channel (runs around the genital region)

  - main channel

  - luo-connecting channel

  - divergent channel

  - tendino-muscular channel.

  They all have a relationship to the male genitals, respectively.

- Kidney channel (also passes genital region):

  - main channel

  - luo-connecting channel

  - tendino-muscular channel.

SCROTUM

Western Medicine: Covers and protects testes and epidymidis and helps in regulation of the temperature.

Chinese Medicine: It is called:

- Yin sac (Yin Nang)
- Kidney sac (Shen Nang)
- sac (Nang).

Channels: According to their courses, the same meridians as above are on duty:

- Liver
- Kidney.

DUCTUS DEFERENS AND SEMINAL VESICLES

Western Medicine: The main function of the ductus deferens is the transport of the mature sperm cells with the ejaculate. The seminal vesicle also produces an alkaline secretion that helps the sperm cells to survive in the acid climate of the vagina. It also nourishes the spermatozoa on their way.

Chinese Medicine: The ductus deferens and seminal vesicle together are called:

- Path of semen (Jing Dao).

SPERMATIC CORD

Western Medicine: This cord consists of the ductus deferens, veins, arteries, nerves and muscles.

Chinese Medicine: It is called:

- seminal tie (Jing Zi Xi).

Channel:

- Liver.

PENIS

Western Medicine: Consists of three spongy bodies with a tunica albuginea (connective tissue) wrapped around them and holding them together. The filling of those spongy bodies is the main mechanism of an erection.

Chinese Medicine: There are many different names for the penis:

- jade stem (Yu Jing)

- stem (Jing)

- ancestral sinew (Zong Jin).

According to Chinese Medicine anatomy, the penis can be divided into three parts: (from distal to proximal):

- head of turtle

- body

- root/foot of the penis.

Channels: Almost all the channels have a relevance for the penis:

- Liver and Kidney channel, due to their course

- Spleen and Stomach channel, due to course and function of producing Blood and energy

- Small Intestine channel, in its function of controlling the urination process

- Ren Mai, Du Mai and Chong Mai, all of them run somewhere near the penile region or have branches running along.

Importantly, from a Chinese Medicine point of view, the tunica albuginea (made of connective tissue) is part of the so-called 'Huang membranes' from which all are influenced by the Chong Mai. So, in a nutshell, the Chong Mai is *the* spongy body meridian!

PROSTATE

Western Medicine: As the biggest gland, its main function is to absorb secretion. This special prostate secretion is the main part of semen and improves the sperm's chance of surviving and ameliorates motility.

Chinese Medicine: The prostate is the most important organ in andrology. Therefore, it is named:

- Essence chamber (Jing Shi)

- in Nan Jing the prostate is part of the Gate of Life (Ming Men)

- room/chamber of semen/sperm according to the uterus being the room/chamber of Blood.

For those readers who ever asked themselves what the man's equivalent to a woman's uterus is, the answer is most likely the prostate. This is due to the fact that the Chinese word 'Bao' – as we know it, from the uterus – consists of a character that shows a container and a radical that means organ. So the correct translation of Bao would be a hollow organ filled with liquid: in men filled with semen/sperm, in women filled with blood.[5] According to the Daoists, Bao is located in the lower Dan Tian (lower abdomen). Interestingly, Dan Tian means cinnabar field located 3 cun below the umbilicus, which refers to the Alchemists who thought that cinnabar would allow alchemical transformation to achieve immortality.[6] Actually, calling the lower Dan Tian a transformation centre nails it because, similar to menstrual blood, sperm is a kind of Tian Gui – heavenly water. This Gui is so special because it is built directly from Essence (Jing) – that's what makes it heavenly (Tian). In short, Bao has a connection to the Ming Men as well as with blood. Su Wen I, chapter 33 points out the communication between the Heart and the uterus via a vessel called Bao Mai.[7]

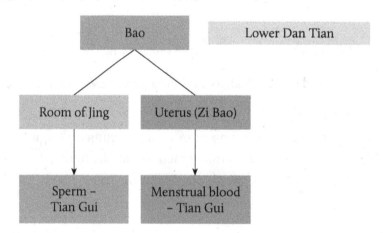

Channels: Du Mai, Ren Mai, Chong Mai – they all originate from the prostate in men and therefore have an obvious connection to it.

Some structures that are described in Chinese Medicine do not refer to a Western anatomic structure – for example, the Essence Gate (Jing Guan). This is defined as the barrier that regulates the discharge of the semen. It is described as 'a gate that is felt to open in ejaculation' by Zhang Jie-Bin. Signs such as seminal efflux (loss occurring day and night) and seminal emission (loss at night) and premature ejaculation are attributed to 'insecurity of the Essence Gate' due to Kidney diseases.[8]

The same applies to the term 'Zong Jin', which causes some debate concerning its exact meaning. As Franconi summarizes in her book, there are several possible interpretations.

In Chapter 13, the Ling Shu states that the locomotor apparatus consists of 12 Jing Jin (sinew channels) and one Zong Jin. Although the role of the Zong Jin remains unclear in the Ling Shu, the Jing Jin represent a set of muscles with their pathway corresponding to the 12 channels.

Looking at the pictogram of the word, we have the term 'Zong' meaning 'ancestors, clan' with the best explanation being the great connector between an individual and its environment.

'Jin' roughly means 'sinew, tendon'. It has the radical for bamboo in the upper part and the radical for flesh as well as the radical for power and strength in the lower part.

Zong Jin, with the two terms put together, is widely translated as ancestral sinew.

In the Huangdi Nei Jing the Zong Jin is kind of a strategic intersection of the Chong Mai, Du Mai and the Dai Mai with the Stomach/Yang brilliance conduit.

Giovanni Maciocia, on the other hand, refers to the penis and the rectus abdominis muscle, whereas Jeffrey Yuan states that Zong Jin can either refer to the genitals, the diaphragm or the abdominal rectus muscle.[9]

Part and names	Pinyin name
Scrotum (sac) Kidney sac Yin sac	Nang Shen Nang Yin Nang
Testes (often grouped with epididymis and called Kidney seed)	Shen Zi
Vas deferens and seminal vesicles (seminal pathway)	Jing Dao
Prostate (Essence chamber or life gate)	Jing Shi or Ming Men
Spermatic cord (seminal tie)	Jing Zi Xi

CHAPTER 10

Causes of Disease and Pathomechanism

Unlike in Western Medicine, where after one year of unprotected intercourse with no pregnancy, infertility or at least subfertility is suspected, in Chinese Medicine male infertility is likely to be seen as an issue after two years of not conceiving when female causes can be ruled out.

As always with Chinese Medicine, there is not only one term for male infertility but several, such as:

- Bu yu – male infertility

- Wu zi – childlessness

- Nan zi nan ci – male difficulty in (producing) an heir.[1]

Under the influence of Western Medicine, the most commonly used term nowadays in andrology books is nan xing bu yu zheng – male infertility.

In Chinese Medicine, there are several prerequisites for a man to be fertile:

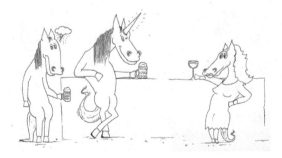

- There must be enough Kidney Jing. Semen is called Sheng Zhi Zhi Jing (reproductive Essence) and is stored in the Kidneys which are a kind of master of reproduction. Therefore, in Chinese Medicine everything concerning fertility or infertility goes back to the Kidneys.

- His Ming Men fire must be warm enough to trigger the transformation of Kidney essence into semen and sperm. Semen is made of Tian Gui (heavenly water – an equivalent of menstrual blood in women) that is derived from the original Qi of the father and the mother. 'At two times eight, fertility arrives', the Suwen states. This means that Tian Gui arrives. It enables the Ren Mai to flow to the testis, the Chong Mai fills and circulates, and spermatogenesis is possible.

- His Liver Qi must move freely to enable the Kidney Qi's transformation and ensure a proper ejaculation: a smooth flowing Liver Qi affects all kind of sexual secretions as well as the ejaculation of sperm. Moreover, every transforming process needs Qi to promote it. This makes Qi and its free flow extremely worthy.

- He must be free of substantial obstructions such as stasis or phlegm to guarantee that the spermatic duct permits a normal ejaculation: Phlegm blocks the passage of Essence as well as of Qi and therefore has a huge negative impact on male fertility, as does Blood stasis. In the worst scenario, those two unite to form something called phlegm stasis which is the foundation of everything you don't want to suffer from (e.g. cancer).

- He must be free of damp-heat or heat-toxins in the Essence chamber: however damp-heat developed, it always pours downwards, affecting the Lower Burner and thus the Essence chamber. Any type of heat damages sperm, just as we know from the Western Medicine perspective. It dries fluids and semen is a Yin substance that is easily harmed by drying heat.

- There must be enough Qi and Blood, (post-heaven Jing) to be added to the pre-heaven Jing in the Kidneys: if one manufactures more Qi and Blood than one consumes in a day, at night, during sleep, this excess Qi and Blood is transformed into acquired Jing which is also stored in the Kidneys. Therefore, Qi and Blood vacuity can also lead to infertility due to a lack of acquired Jing nourishing and supporting the congenital Jing.[2]

Most textbooks say that if two or more of these prerequisites fail, a man becomes infertile.

HOW SPERM IS MADE

All four of the Chinese Medicine organs described in Chapter 9 are needed to form sperm.

- The Kidneys produce the Tian Gui which is the direct origin of sperm.

- The Postnatal Qi and Blood of the Spleen and Stomach indirectly supplement the Tian Gui (by being postnatal Jing as possible add-on to the prenatal Jing producing Tian Gui).

- The Liver stores the Blood contributing to the production of Tian Gui.

- Heart Yang descends to meet Kidney Yin to produce Tian Gui, also the physiological Fire of the Heart warms the sperm.[3]

In particular, Kidney and Heart need to communicate with each other. The Water of the Kidneys and the Fire of the Heart need to nourish each other. While the Kidney Essence is the origin of sperm in men, the Heart plays an important role in erection, orgasm and ejaculation. They both depend on the descending of Heart Qi. To perform these functions, Heart Qi descends to communicate with Kidney Qi. Kidney Water needs to ascend towards the Heart and Heart Fire (the physiological Emperor Fire) needs to descend towards the Kidneys to assure a normal sexual function in men.[4]

From a TCM perspective, healthy sex – as an essential tool for fertility – depends on three basic things:

- **The connection of the Heart-Bao-Kidney axis via the Bao Mai and Bao Luo:** Proper communication between the Heart and Kidneys is needed to get aroused (upwards movement) and to have an ejaculation (downwards movement). Note that the 'Bao' (uterus in women) is known as the 'room of sperm' in men.

- **The ascending of Kidney water and the downbearing of Heart Fire:** Emotions cause arousal which stirs the Minister Fire, which flares up to the Heart and Pericardium, which in turn discharges it downwards to enable orgasm.

- **A connection between the Ren Mai (Conception vessel) and Du Mai (Governing vessel):** This connection is at the mouth and genitals of both partners, which enables a free circling flow of Qi through these two extraordinary vessels.

As practitioners, our job is to ensure proper function and nourishment (Jing, Qi, Blood) of these vessels and that they are connected to each other (i.e. no obstructions in the genital/mouth areas).

Aetiology and pathogenesis of male infertility can be summarized in six main points.

1. Inherited weakness or acquired constitutional weakness of Kidney Essence

As we know, the Kidneys store the Essence (both-pre- and post-heaven Essence) and govern growth and reproduction.

Essence is the most important raw material as it can be transformed into many other substances (Qi, Blood, body fluids, semen and sperm).

The quality and quantity of sperm are directly linked to quality and quantity of Jing. Hence, if a man is born with a lack of Kidney Essence or he wastes it due to his lifestyle, diminished fertility or infertility may result. As Jing is the essential raw material for sperm creation, all sperm parameters are negatively affected when being diminished: volume and concentration, morphology, viscosity and liquefication time.

Note that in Chinese Medicine conceiving while drunk is a main reason for low inherited prenatal Essence – maybe we in the West should think about that. Other reasons for a lack of prenatal Jing according to old textbooks are the parents marrying too early or giving birth to too many children, as well as being relatives. Sun Simiao recommends staying away from medicines and tonics that promote fertility if less than 40 years old. Furthermore, the Classics rule that it is better to abstain from sexual activity at a full or new moon, during a storm, before having digested a heavy meal, after great efforts, with wet hair or after a tiring journey as well as before the healing of a drained wound.[5]

2. Life gate fire debility (Ming Men fire debility) with vacuous and cold essential Qi

Normal life gate fire provides the warmth and activation for the entire body and especially for all the reproductive and sexual functions of the Kidney. If the life gate fire is sufficient, it catalyzes the transformation of Kidney Essence into Kidney Qi and helps with the transformation that is needed to create sperm and semen.[6]

If one is sexually overactive (e.g. by masturbating heavily during adolescence), over time this consumes Kidney Yang and impairs Kidney Qi and the Essence chamber (room of sperm), resulting in 'vacuous and cold essential Qi'. This, of course, affects the reproductive capacity as well as the sexual capacity of a man negatively.

In a nutshell, a proper life gate fire is responsible for a normal sperm morphology (spermatogenesis) and motility and ensures that the seminal fluids are not too cold (i.e. too watery and dilute). Some authors say that the Kidney Yang is responsible for the liquefication; for others the life gate fire mentioned above is crucial.

3. Phlegm and Blood stasis obstruct the Essence pathway

Constitutional Spleen Qi vacuity as well as excessive consumption of sweet, greasy food can disturb the Spleen's ability to transform and move. Hence, fluids and dampness accumulate, resulting in food stagnation, and if that congeals, it becomes phlegm. With its typical tendency of pouring downwards, phlegm blocks the Essence pathway (vas deferens), leading to fertility problems due to obstruction. Phlegm, as a Yin evil, over time leads to Blood stasis, and if Blood stasis and phlegm stick together, phlegm-stasis results as the worst thing that could happen (causing e.g. cancer). Whatever the origin of static blood is, either due to trauma, long-lasting Qi stagnation or enduring illness into the Luo vessels, it blocks the Essence chamber and the Essence pathway just as phlegm does. Both static evils – either alone or in concert – lead to diminished volume, low density, increased liquefication time, abnormal morphology as well as anti-sperm antibodies (AsAb)

4. Liver Qi stagnation

As the Liver channel runs around the genitals, a free flow within that channel is highly important for the reproductive organs to function properly. In particular, the seven emotions (joy, anger, melancholy, worry, grief, fear and fright) can easily cause Liver Qi stagnation. Of these seven emotions, massive grief has the hugest impact on sexuality in general.[7] A lack of free flow can result in a decrease of sperm production or hinder its further transport. In particular, when stagnation leads to heat that may enter the Essence chamber, fertility issues that have to do with decocting fluids result – for example, low volume, increased viscosity, prolonged liquefication time, low density and abnormal morphology.

5. Damp-heat pouring downward

Bad eating habits (alcohol, greasy fried food and sugar) weaken the Spleen. In particular, the Spleen's function as a detoxifying organ that can get rid of dampness may be disturbed by those dietary failures. If that dampness gets stuck, it provokes food stagnation. An easy rule in Chinese Medicine is that every stagnation or stasis (no matter of which substance) leads to heat over time. This damp-heat resulting from the weakness of the Spleen pours downward to the Lower Burner (often with the Liver channel) and is a cause of obstruction and blockage. When entering the Essence chamber, this damp-heat scorches the Essence and blocks the Essence pathway just as phlegm and/or Blood stasis do. The results can be seen in the semen analysis as diminished volume, increased viscosity, prolonged liquefication, abnormal morphology or low density.

6. Vacuity of both Qi and Blood

A lack of Qi and Blood (vacuity) always has some impairing effect on Jing. According to Chinese Medicine Classics, 'liver and kidney share the same source'. In other words, later heaven Essence and early heaven Essence mutually transform into one another. If surplus Liver Blood can be transformed into Essence and stored in the Kidneys, it can supplement early heaven Essence and make it abundant.[8] Remember that Essence is the raw material from which semen and sperm are made. The goal of a healthy lifestyle should always be to achieve such a surplus as to be able to fill up the Essence reserve. Vacuity of Qi and Blood can result from a weak Spleen not being able to produce enough of these two treasured substances, or from constitutional weakness or long-term illness. In terms of sperm, vacuity of both leads to the same changes in sperm tests as Jing deficiency does, namely affecting volume and concentration, morphology, viscosity and liquefication time.

CHAPTER 11

The Most Important Organs in Chinese Medicine Andrology

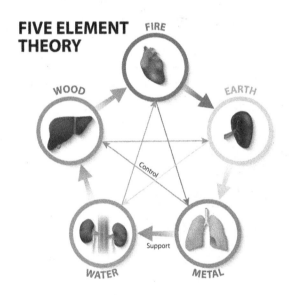

THE LIVER IN ANDROLOGY

According to *Ling Shu* chapter 10: 'The liver is the uniting place of the sinews. Its sinews gather at the Yin organs (i.e. the penis and scrotum) and its vessel nets at the root of the tongue.'[1]

And according to *Zhen Jiu Jia Yi Jing*: 'During sleep, blood returns to the liver. When the liver receives blood, one can see. When the feet receive blood, one can walk. When the hands receive blood, one can grasp.'[2] (We all know what happens if the penis receives blood...)

The Liver is therefore responsible for the 'sinews'. The penis is the meeting point of the hundred tendons/sinews, also called the 'sinew of the ancestors'. The name underlines the importance of the Liver as an organ in andrology. In addition, the Liver channel leads directly around the genital area in its outer course and thus supplies it with Qi and Blood.

In order to fully understand the enormous importance of the Liver for a functioning sex life, we need to take a closer look at some of the basic functions of the Liver from the point of view of potency.

We know how the Liver works to hoard and store Blood. If the Blood reservoir is empty, not enough Blood will reach the 'tendons' of the penis as a result. For a proper erection, the penis must be sufficiently filled with Blood. For this, on the one hand, there must be enough Blood in the Liver as the storeroom; on the other hand, the Blood must be able to flow freely into the penis.

The Liver Blood is also used for the production of Tian Gui – the ejaculate. The Liver is also responsible for an undisturbed flow of Qi and Blood. Constricted Liver Qi can obstruct the free flow of blood and Qi and can thus impair erectile function. The intact Yang component of the Liver is responsible for erectile function.

We often forget that the Liver Yang not only causes pathology, but is also physiological and performs important functions.

The Kidneys, but also – and this is less well known – the Liver, are in charge of the ministerial fire. This is especially important for the Liver in the form of Liver Yang to ensure three functions that are important for erectile function:

- to keep Blood from getting too cold – even the Liver can get too cold. There is not only fire in the Liver!

- to let the Liver Qi flow in the right direction

- to ensure the highest possible degree of free Qi flow.

Chinese herbs that warm the Liver Yang are mostly herbs to warm the Kidney Yang.

At first glance this is confusing, but it becomes understandable when you consider the interaction between the ministerial fire and the Liver Yang. The ministerial fire has to warm the Liver; otherwise, Liver Yang cannot develop and all of the above-mentioned functions that are dependent on Liver Yang fail.

I like to compare the Liver with a central railway station. All trains – loaded with blood and Qi – depart from there. As the station master, the Liver is in charge of coordinating the trains so that they all reach even the remotest regions of our 'rail network' – our body. The only problem is when the station master gets stressed. The Liver is not capable of multitasking. As soon as it has to cope with stress, it forgets about its original function – the distribution of Qi and Blood.

This explains why stress can lead to the stagnation of Liver Qi, contrary to the stereotype, in both men and women. One should never underestimate the emotions of the Liver which can block the free flow of Qi and which are often the cause of lack of libido and erectile dysfunction.

Suppressed anger or troubles – and, most importantly, unfulfilled desires and longings – are emotions that most of us are only too familiar with.

THE SPLEEN IN ANDROLOGY

According to Suwen chapter 21: 'The spleen governs the movement and transformation of water and grain essence.'[3] And: 'The spleen moves and transforms water-damp.'[4]

We know that the Stomach–Spleen axis is the postnatal source of Qi and Blood which is obtained from food. I always see it as a factory in which Qi and Blood are built from food. The better our diet, the better our 'factory' can work and the higher quality it can produce.

In any case, insufficiency of the Spleen and our factory can be a cause of erectile dysfunction. If there is not enough Qi and Blood, the penis will not erect because it is not supplied. In contrast to Liver problems, this is a case of an under-supply due to deficiency, not due to distribution disorders.

The Spleen is also the source of pathological moisture such as dampness and phlegm. Usually, its job is to separate what is clear and what is murky, and to send what is clear up to the Lungs and to dispose of what is murky via the intestines or the bladder.

The Spleen should therefore actually work according to the 'Cinderella principle' (the good ones go into the pot, the bad ones go into your crop). If it does not, murky elements accumulate, forming moisture and dampness which sinks and can reach the genital region via the Liver channel. As a sluggish, adynamic substance, dampness is predestined to generate heat. And heat in the Liver channel is one of the main causes of many itchy or inflammatory diseases of the genital region.

As already mentioned, the Spleen and Stomach are the source of the postnatal Essence. The prenatal Essence, as we know, is stored in the Kidneys. In the Western world, we often teach that there is no way to increase the prenatal Jing – that is, the prenatal Essence. The following fact is often forgotten. When so much postnatal Essence is produced that a surplus remains at the end of the day, this surplus is stored in the Kidneys in the form of Liver Blood, merges with the prenatal Essence and stocks it up (according to Jing Yue Quan Shu).

This also explains the often incomprehensible use of herbal formulas that tonify the Spleen and Stomach to treat Kidney deficiency. The simple strategy here is to produce so much postnatal Essence that there is still some left at the end of the day which then can be used to stock up the prenatal Kidney Essence.

Emotions such as worries and brooding, learning and mental overload in the form of overstimulation weaken our Spleen and they therefore reduce the productivity of our factory. All are feelings that are constantly present in our life and thus have a massive influence on our potency and libido.

THE HEART IN ANDROLOGY

According to *Su Wen* chapter 44: 'The heart governs the body's blood vessels.'[5] And in chapter 10 it says: 'All blood belongs to the heart.'[6] *Ling Shu Xie Ke* chapter 71 states: 'The heart is the great monarch of the five viscera and the six bowels, it is the residence of the essence-spirit.'[7]

These three quotations give us a rough overview of the important functions of the Heart in relation to everything concerning blood. Since adequate Blood flow in the penis is naturally important for achieving and maintaining an erection, this explains the importance of the Heart in Chinese andrology.

In Chinese Medicine, the Heart is not only the governor of the Blood and the blood vessels, but it also plays an important role in the production of Blood. According to the five-phase theory, it is responsible for the red colour of the Blood (Hua chi). The independent Heart Fire turns the Gu-Qi and the clear Qi into red, life-enabling Blood. That Blood is able to nourish, moisturize and enrich the body.

Blood supplies all organs and enables them to function. When there is enough Blood, all the Zang-fu organs can work well; when there is a lack of Blood, the organs and the mind cannot work properly. This also applies to the anterior Yin region.

In addition, the Heart also has a physiological Heart Fire.

This is sent down to the Kidneys in order to produce Tian Gui together with the Kidney Yin/Kidney water. As we know, Tian Gui – the heavenly water – denotes the ejaculate in men and it is 'brewed' from both Heart Fire and Kidney Yin.

Consequently, all the male fertility disorders are caused by the Heart and the Kidneys, among other things. The Heart also houses and rules the Shen spirit.

The correct translation of Shen has been the subject of many discourses. Most plausible to me is the idea that Shen is what we commonly refer to as our 'soul'. It is Shen that allows us to communicate with others; it makes our eyes shine and sparkle and can be read from the shine of the tongue. If you want to know what Shen is, just watch people of all ages who are newly in love.

The Heart needs a tight leash to keep this bustling Shen spirit under control – the leash in this picture would be vessels totally filled with blood. The more the vessels are filled with blood, the stronger is the leash to control Shen. In the Classics, you can read that Blood anchors Shen.

In the case of too little Blood, the Shen becomes independent and does what it wants. Insomnia, mental disorders, and outbursts of emotion are examples of a Shen out of control. Accordingly, the emotions of the Heart, such as massive fear, are important pathogenic factors for the development of male pathologies.

When the Heart does not work properly, due to deficiency or stagnation, this can lead to various diseases of the male genital system.

A satisfactory erection requires enough Qi and Blood and that they reach the anterior

Yin region, remaining there for a sufficiently long time. Here the Heart plays an important role as it rules and forms the Blood and also transports it to the prostate (room of sperm) and the penis. In case of a Heart Qi weakness or a lack of Heart Blood, the anterior Yin region is not supplied with sufficient Blood and erectile dysfunction as well as infertility can result.

Both can also result from hyperactive Heart Fire. Too much Heart Fire consumes the Heart's Blood – as blazing fire boils away water – and thus a situation like this can also lead to a lack of Heart Blood. When such a hyperactive Heart Fire is directed down to the ministerial fire (the Kidneys) and stirs it up, then that fire disturbs the chamber of sperm (the prostate) and wet dreams or bloody ejaculate may occur.

THE KIDNEY IN CHINESE ANDROLOGY

According to *Su Wen* chapter 1: 'When a male is eight years old, his kidney qi is replete and his teeth are fully developed. At 16 years old, his kidney qi is exuberant, his heavenly tenth (tian gui) arrives, his essential qi flows, his yin and yang are harmonious, and he is able to produce a child.'[8] And in chapter 9: 'The kidney governs hibernation, is the root of sealing and storage, and is the dwelling place of essence. Its bloom is in the hair, and its fullness is in its bones. It is the yin within lesser yin and it flows to the qi of winter.'[9]

The great importance of the Kidney for andrology will surprise no one. We all know the important functions of the Kidney with regard to its Essence. The Kidney is the home of the prenatal Essence. This is the one that is created when the egg and sperm cells fuse. This corresponds to our backpack, so to speak, that we take with us for our journey through life.

Whenever our factory – the Spleen – cannot create enough postnatal Essence, our body uses its 'emergency power generator', the backpack in the form of prenatal Kidney Essence. Of course, this cannot happen all the time. According to the TCM philosophy, a person dies as soon as his Essence is used up. The prenatal Essence must therefore be used sparingly.

In addition, one should try, at least from time to time, to produce a surplus of postnatal Essence to fill up one's prenatal Essence, and thus one's backpack (see the Spleen section above).

However, it is important to know that the term Essence (Jing) has two meanings in relation to andrology.

On the one hand, it means the Essence from which all the important body substances are derived – the Qi, the Blood and the body fluids, so the Essence as raw material for everything that supplies the Zang-fu organs.

On the other hand, the term Essence also means reproductive Essence, something that corresponds to the Western term 'genetic' and means genetic material (DNA) that is necessary for conception. Bob Damone, author of the book *Principles of Chinese Medical Andrology*, even asks whether the Kidney Essence could in some way correspond to a stem cell.[10] An even more recent approach would be to compare Essence with the telomeres at the end of our chromosome arms. Both analogies underline once again the importance of the Kidney for all male reproductive and sexual functions.

As already described with the role of the Heart, Kidney Yin together with Heart Fire is needed to form Tian Gui – semen.

Kidney Qi deficiency and the inability of the Kidney to seal, preserve and store often lead to premature ejaculation, whereas a lack of Kidney Essence is either inherent or caused by reaching into the 'backpack' too often. A delayed onset of puberty, a reduced shaping of the sexual organs and, of course, infertility are typical symptoms.

A weak Kidney Yang always causes a lack of warmth and power and can manifest itself in a lack of libido, impotence, cold genitals, urinary retention or incontinence and, of course, infertility.

CHAPTER 12

Channels That Significantly Influence the Male Sexual Organs

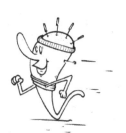

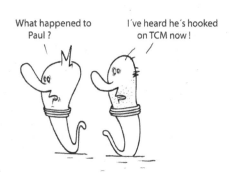

What happened to Paul?

I've heard he's hooked on TCM now!

A generally intact channel system is, of course, the optimal requirement for any good reproductive outcome. However, some channels have a special relationship with the male genital organs, and we should have a closer look at them.

To summarize before diving deeper: all Yin channels of the lower limb (Spleen, Liver and Kidney channels) have a relationship with the genital organs, including the divergent channels. Also the three Yin sinew channels of the foot pass the genital system and are inserted in the region between CV 3 and CV 4.

Among the Yang channels, only those of the Stomach and Gallbladder are connected with the genitals. As we don't consider them further in later sections, we will consider them briefly now. On the Stomach channel, the point St 29 is traditionally considered to be a useful point for genital problems in general. The classic approach of using the point has recently been proved by research as stimulation with electroacupuncture (10 Hz) increases testicular blood flow.[1]

The second point often used on the Stomach channel is St 30, a point where the Chong Mai enters the surface and therefore a point on the very important extraordinary channel as discussed below. It is also called 'junction of Qi' to indicate the passage of Qi in the pelvic region. The Gallbladder channel houses the front-mu point of the Kidney – Gb 25 – which is often included in protocols for male infertility due to Kidney Yang vacuity, according to Jane Lyttleton.[2] Moreover, some Gallbladder points also lie on the Dai Mai (girdle) vessel, which is the only horizontal vessel and runs around our waist, hence covering the location of the reproductive tract.

To keep things easier, I love using 'best of' hitlists.

Concerning male fertility, my hitlist would be the following, including:

2 primary channels	3 extraordinary channels
Liver channel	Ren Mai
Kidney channel	Du Mai
	Chong Mai

Of the 12 primary channels, the Liver and Kidney channels are of particular importance for the genital system. It is essential to emphasize that it is not only the primary channels with their mostly known external courses and lesser-known internal courses that are responsible for the influence on the genitals. It is an often forgotten fact that each channel, in addition to its primary channel, also has a network channel (Luo vessel), a sinew channel (tendino-muscular channels) and a divergent channel. These channels are also responsible for supplying the genital organs.

This is crucial to understanding why certain channels are of particular importance in the treatment of male fertility problems.

In most cases, readers will be proud that they know the exact external course of all the primary channels. However, hardly any readers will have knowledge of the exact inner course of the primary channels, the Luo vessels, the sinew channels or the divergent channels. But you will see that it makes perfect sense and really helps to understand why certain spots on certain channels work so well for male infertility treatment.

Before we have a closer look at the channels, I would like to introduce some general information on special features and functions of these very special channels – repetition is always helpful.

SPECIAL CHANNEL CATEGORIES[3]

Luo-connecting vessels (Luo Mai) – network vessels

Each of the 12 primary channels has a Luo-connecting vessel that branches off at the so-called Luo point of the primary channel. The network vessels connect the Yin-Yang-paired channels with one another and strengthen their connection.

After they have connected to the paired pathway, they usually follow their own course.

FUNCTIONS OF THE LUO MAI

- Connection of the channels and organs within the same element.

- With their small connections, they ensure balance between the primary channels of the elements.

- Extension of the primary channels.

- Local distribution of Qi and Blood; there are many small ramifications (in the depths) and on the surface.

Divergent channels (Jing Bie)
(Note: Bie means 'branch off'.)

- They are branches of the 12 primary channels.

- They serve as the expansion of the primary channels.

- They run deeper in the body than the primary channels.

- They connect with the internal organ and thus strengthen the relationship between the channel and the internal organ.

- They connect the Yin-Yang-paired channels.

- They have no acupuncture points of their own.

- They have internal connections/courses that the primary channels do not have.

The sinew channels (Jing Jin), synonym: tendino-muscular channels (TMM)

- They are connected to the primary channels and take their name from them.

- They roughly follow the course of their assigned primary channel but are wider.

- They are shallow and follow the lines of the primary muscles, muscle chains, fascia, tendons and ligaments.

- They carry Qi and Blood and especially Wei Qi to the surface.

- It is in them that the first contact between Wei Qi and the invading pathogenic factor takes place.

- All originate at the ting points of the extremities.

- The ting points connect the primary channels with the associated sinew channels (tendino-muscular meridian (TMM)).

- They run upwards to the head (Yang TMM) and chest region (Yin TMM).

- They have no specific acupuncture points of their own.

- Treating Ashi-points, using techniques on the surface of the skin such as cupping, massage, Gua Sha or the plum blossom hammer, primarily influences these sinew channels.

- They are primarily used against pain, spasms, stiffness and restricted mobility, and for the rapid elimination of pathogenic factors that have just entered (e.g. flu-like infections).

- The ting points are also outlet valves for pathogenic factors, for which you can prick them with a lancet.

PRIMARY CHANNELS

The Liver channel

Both the Liver primary channel pathway and the Liver Luo-connecting vessel as well as the sinew channel of the Liver are related to the male genital region and thus exert an important influence on the reproductive tract. In the *Ling Shu*, chapter 10, it says: 'The Liver-channel joins the tendons and the tendons assemble at the genitals.'[4]

COURSE OF THE PRIMARY CHANNEL OF THE LIVER
It arises on the lateral side of the big toenail at the point Liv 1, runs over the foot to Liv 4 (1 cun in front of the medial malleolus), then runs upwards along the medial lower leg where the Liver channel crosses the Spleen pathway at point Sp 6.

The Liver channel runs in front of the Spleen channel up to an area 8 cun above the medial malleolus, then crosses it and runs behind the Spleen channel up to the knee and to the medial part of the thigh. There the primary Liver channel runs to the groin and flows around the genitals. The outer course finally passes the abdomen and ends in the 6th ICR on the nipple line with the acupuncture point Liv 14.

So far, all of this is well known. Let us continue with the inner courses of the Liver channel.

The inner part of the Liver primary channel runs via acupoints Sp 12 and Sp 13 to the pubic area where it circles the genitals. Then it rises to enter the lower abdomen. There it crosses the Conception vessel (Ren Mai) at Ren 2, Ren 3 and Ren 4 and goes around the Stomach before entering the Liver as an organ and connecting with the Gallbladder. It crosses the diaphragm and spreads out in the rib region and in the hypochondrium, runs along the neck to the nasopharynx to connect with the tissues that surround the eye. And finally, it runs to the vertex over the forehead and meets at Du 20 with the Governor vessel.

The Liver primary channel connects to the following Zang-fu organs: Liver, Gallbladder, Lungs, Stomach.

The Liver primary channel meets other primary channels:

- with the Spleen channel at points Sp 6, Sp 12 and Sp 13

- with the Conception vessel at points Ren 2, Ren 3 and Ren 4

- with the Pericardial channel at Pc 1

- with the Governor vessel at Du 20.

THE LUO-CONNECTING CHANNEL (LUO VESSEL) OF THE LIVER

The Liver Luo-connecting vessel separates from the primary channel at point Liver 5 on the medial lower leg and connects to the Gallbladder channel. Similar to the primary Liver channel, it also runs up to the genitals.

Location of the Luo point Le 5: 5 cun above the peak of the medial malleolus, on the dorsal edge of the tibia.

THE SINEW CHANNEL OF THE LIVER

Like the primary channel, it arises on the back of the big toe and runs upwards to connect to the anterior part of the medial malleolus. It eventually runs up the medial thigh to the genitals where it connects to the sinew channel of the Spleen.[5]

The Kidney channel

According to the *Systematic Classic of Acupuncture and Moxibustion* (Zhen Jiu Jia Yi Jing), the Kidney channel is connected with the Governor vessel, which in its course in men follows the penis to the perineum. In addition, the *Ling Shu*, chapter 38, describes the path of the lower branch of Chong Mai when it enters the 'great Luo' of the Kidney channel, presumably at the level of Kidney 4, providing a link between these channels. The Chong Mai joins the ancestral tendon (*Su Wen I*, chapter 44) and this is another reason that justifies the use of the points of the Kidney channel to treat andrological problems.[6]

THE KIDNEY PRIMARY CHANNEL

It starts beneath the little toe (on the ball of the foot) and crosses the sole of the foot to point Ki 1. The primary channel then comes to the front at Ki 2 and reaches the surface below the navicular tuberosity and runs behind the medial malleolus to acupoint Ki 3. From there the primary channel descends to the heel, then rises again to Ki 6 below the medial malleolus, runs up along the medial part of the leg, crosses the Spleen pathway at Sp 6,[7] runs along the medial side of the leg along the posterior edge of the tibia to the medial knee joint fold (between musculus semimembranosus and musculus semitendinosus) as far as acupuncture point Ki 10 and continues over the inside of the thigh to the middle of the coccyx and reaches the perineal region.

The outer course now continues between the ventral median line and the Stomach channel over the abdomen, in the section of the abdomen and thorax to Ki 21 each 0.5 cun lateral to the median and then ascending parasternal from Ki 22 upwards, to end with the point Ki 27 at the sternoclavicular joint.

INNER COURSE OF THE PRIMARY KIDNEY CHANNEL
(DIRECTION: FROM BOTTOM TO TOP)

From point Bl 67, an inner course runs over the sole of the foot to Ki 1. The loop that the outer course forms around the inner ankle is related to the heel and penetrates into it. From point Ki 11 this branch connects with the points Ren 3 and Ren 4.

An inner branch of the primary Kidney channel crosses the Du Mai in Du 1, then penetrates the spine and the Kidneys and connects internally with the bladder.

A deep, inner branch rises from the Kidney, penetrates the Liver and the diaphragm, enters the Lungs and runs up to the throat, where this inner branch ends at the root of the tongue.

Another internal branch detours in the Lungs, connects with the Heart, and spreads across the chest to join the pericardial pathway and Ren 17.[8]

The primary Kidney channel is connected to the following Zang-fu organs: Kidney, Bladder, Liver, Lungs, Heart.

The primary Kidney channel meets other channels at the following points:

- with the Spleen channel at the point Sp 6

- with the Conception vessel (Ren Mai) at points Ren 3, Ren 4, Ren 7 and Ren 17

- with the Governor vessel (Du Mai) at point Du 1.[9]

THE LUO-CONNECTING CHANNEL OF THE KIDNEY:

The starting point of the Luo-connecting Channel is Ki 4, from here it continues around the Achilles tendon to finally flow into the primary channel of the bladder. Another branch of this Luo-connecting Channel of the Kidneys runs further upwards and around the pericardial area and then traverses the lumbar region of the spine. According to Van Nghi, the longitudinal Luo vessel ends at the point Ming Men (Du 4).

Location of the Luo point Ki 4: medial to the insertion of the Achilles tendon on the calcaneus.

THE SINEW CHANNEL OF THE KIDNEY

It starts beneath the little toe and connects to the sinew channel of the Spleen at the lower part of the medial malleolus, narrows in the heel area, then runs up the leg together with the sinew channel of the bladder. It narrows at the medial condyle of the tibia, connects with the sinew channel of the Spleen on the medial surface of the thigh, joining the genitalia.

A branch of the sinew channel runs to the vertebral bones, climbs the inner part of the spine up to the neck, where it connects with the occipital bone and converges with the sinew channel of the Bladder.[10]

THREE EXTRAORDINARY CHANNELS

Ren Mai, Du Mai and Chong Mai

The three extraordinary channels are Ren Mai, Du Mai and Chong Mai.

The extraordinary channels linked to the pelvic region are the ones that according to classical texts originate from the Ming Men – namely, Ren Mai, Du Mai, Chong Mai and Dai Mai. The Ming Men is the site of the destiny of a person, and the so-called 'first generation' extraordinary meridians must protect and fulfil the mandate. Moreover, these meridians are connected to the seas, according to *Nan Jing* 28th difficulty: Sea of Yin and Sea of Qi with the Conception vessel (Ren Mai), Sea of Twelve Meridians and Sea of Blood with the Penetrating vessel (Chong Mai), Sea of Yang and Sea of Marrow with the Governor vessel (Du Mai) and Sea of the Ming Men with the Girdle vessel (Dai Mai).[11]

FEATURES AND FUNCTIONS OF THE EXTRAORDINARY CHANNELS

- They serve as a reservoir for Qi and Blood. They can remove excess Qi and Blood from the primary channels when there is a surplus, just like a reservoir absorbing water from the canals when it rains. When there is no Blood or Qi, the extraordinary vessels open and give off Qi to the primary channels.

- They connect the 12 primary channels. The Du Mai connects all Yang channels at Du 14 and is known as the 'Sea of Yang'. The Ren Mai connects all Yin channels and is known as the 'Sea of Yin'. The Chong Mai (Penetrating vessel) connects the Stomach and Kidney channels and also strengthens the connection between Ren Mai and Du Mai. The Penetrating vessel is called the 'Sea of Blood'.

- They protect the body. Ren Mai, Du Mai and Chong Mai circulate the Defence Qi (Wei Qi) through the thorax, abdomen and back, and thus help to protect the body from external pathogenic factors (e.g. wind, cold).

- They do not have an assigned Zang-fu organ. Moreover, only the Ren Mai and the Du Mai have their own acupuncture points; the other six extraordinary vessels borrow points from other primary channels.

- They connect the prenatal (pre-heavenly) hereditary Essence which is determined when the egg and sperm cells are united with the postnatal (post-heavenly) acquired Essence which we produce by food intake. Both together form the Kidney Essence (Jing) which is transported through the body via extraordinary channels.

- They have a close relationship with Kidneys, Yin, Yuan Qi, constitution (and thus with growth, reproduction and development).

- They control the seven-year cycle for women and eight-year cycle for men.

- They distribute Jing (essence), Ying Qi and Wei Qi to the body regions they supply.

- They supply the six extraordinary Fu organs with Jing and are closely related to them. The six extraordinary Fu include: brain, marrow, bones, vessels, uterus/room of sperm and Gallbladder.

- They have their own passage points: each extraordinary channel has an opening point and a coupled point.

APPLICATION OF THE EXTRAORDINARY CHANNELS

- In cases of weak/low Jing.

- In early childhood diseases, prenatal and early-rooted diseases including psychological trauma.

- In cases of chronic illnesses (chronic illnesses lead to the consumption of Yin and Qi).

- In persistent, long-lasting, complicated cases.[12]

SPECIAL FEATURES OF THE EXTRAORDINARY CHANNELS

There are eight extraordinary channels, two of which (Ren Mai and Du Mai) have their own internal and external course and have their own acupuncture points.

We know that Qi flows in the primary channels, more precisely the so-called Ying Qi. In the 24 hours of a day, this Ying Qi flows through each channel for exactly two hours, starting at the Lung channel and ending at the Liver channel.

After the Ying Qi has passed the Liver channel, it flows via an inner connection to the upper lip and from here it reaches the Du Mai, flows along the channel course of the Du Mai down the spine to the perineum, passes into the Ren Mai there and flows upwards along the Ren Mai back to the face. The Ying Qi now flows back to the Lungs via an inner branch, where the cycle begins again.

The other six extraordinary channels have no course of their own and no points of their own; they use points from other primary channels.

Extraordinary channels have no relation to the Zang-fu organs and cannot be attacked by external pathogenic factors. However, after a long time of existence, pathogenic factors can be transferred to the extraordinary vessels via the primary channels.

Unlike the primary channels, the eight extraordinary channels have a rather shallow/superficial course. However, one must not forget that the origin of the extraordinary channels lies in the depths of the Kidneys. Their special function is to transport Jing (Essence) through the body. They nourish the tissues of our body and control the cycles of our development (seven-year cycle for women, eight-year cycle for men).[13]

So let's have a closer look at those three extraordinary channels that have a special relevance to male fertility.

Ren Mai

OUTER COURSE OF THE PRIMARY CHANNEL

There is disagreement about where the origin of Ren Mai lies.

- According to *Suwen* chapter 60 and *Nan Ching*, the Ren Mai originates at Ren 3.

- If you consult *Ling Shu*, chapter 65, then the Ren Mai begins in the lower pelvis (Lower Dantian, literally Bao) or in the uterus (in men we now know that it begins accordingly in the room of sperm, the prostate).

- Nguyen Van Nghi (translator of many classical texts and an author himself), claims that the Ren Mai arises from the Kidneys and from there runs to the genital organs.

However, there is agreement that the Ren Mai comes to the surface at point Ren 1 and thus Ren 1 is in any case the beginning of the outer course of the Ren Mai.

From there it runs along the body's median front line over the pubic area (Ren 2) via Ren 4 (3 cun below the navel), which is a very special point as it is related to the ancestral energy, to the navel (Ren 8), continues along the abdomen and chest up to the throat (Ren 23), from there to the chin, ending its outer course at Ren 24.[14]

INNER COURSE OF THE PRIMARY CHANNEL

Starting from Ren 24, small vessels run around the lips and gums. At point Du 28, the Ren Mai connects with the Du Mai. Also starting from Ren 24, another branch of this branch runs over the corners of the mouth and cheeks to the point St 1. This branch links up with the Stomach channel at St 4 and St 1.

Another inner branch runs from the perineum to Du 1.

REN MAI LUO-CONNECTING VESSELS

From point Ren 15, a network of small lanes flows like a swallowtail into the upper abdomen. A deep branch of the Ren Mai goes from Ren 3, Ren 4 and Ren 5 directly to the uterus/room of sperm.

- Opening point: Lu 7

- Connecting point: Ki 6

SPECIAL POINTS ALONG THE PRIMARY CHANNEL

Six of the alarm points (front-mu points) are on the Ren Mai: Ren 3 as the alarm point of the Bladder, Ren 4 as the alarm point of the Small Intestine, Ren 5 as the alarm point of the Triple Burner (San Jiao), Ren 12 as the alarm point of the Stomach, Ren 14 as the alarm point of the Heart and Ren 17 as the alarm point of the Pericardium.[15]

WHY IS REN MAI SO IMPORTANT FOR THE MALE GENITAL SYSTEM?

Since, depending on the source, the Ren Mai arises in men either in the room of sperm or moves from the Kidneys up to the genital organs, this channel plays an important role simply because of its course in the lower abdomen. As is well known, the channel runs along the front of the body and thus also runs over the external genitalia.

Ren Mai as the 'Sea of Yin' not only controls Yin, but also transports Nutritional Qi, Defence Qi and Jing (Essence). A lack of Jing means that Ren Mai cannot supply the genital organs with sufficient Essence. As a result, the 'room of sperm' becomes or remains empty. This also affects sexual functions such as ejaculation and erection as well as all the reproductive functions. If Ren Mai is empty, there is naturally also a lack of Kidney Yin. This can make the Kidney Yang overpowering, which in men can lead to excessive sexual desire and premature ejaculation.

Du Mai

The Governor vessel is called the Sea of Yang as it connects with all six primary channels at the point Du 14 and is distributed mainly in the Yang region of the body. Its other name is Sea of Marrow, which needs some explanation. In the embryo, the Governor vessel is responsible for the formation of the nervous system and for cranial/caudal development. That explains the name Sea of Marrow as this extraordinary vessel regulates the brain and marrow and their relationship with the reproductive organs.[16]

OUTER COURSE OF THE PRIMARY CHANNEL

Again, we have disagreement among the various Classics regarding the exact origin of Du Mai.

- In *Suwen* chapter 60, it says that Du Mai arises in the lower part of the abdomen, more precisely in the centre of the pubic bone and runs to the vagina in women, via the Luo vessel around the vagina, flows on to Ren 1 and from there to Du 1. In men, Du Mai circulates around the penis trunk, from there to Ren 1 and on to Du 1. Further internal and external processes start from Du 1.[17]

- In the *Golden Mirror of Medicine* (*Yizong Jinjian*, 1742) it is said that the Governor vessel arises in the lower abdomen, externally in the abdomen and internally in the

'Bao' which is also called Dantian in men and women; for women it is the uterus, for men it is the room of sperm.[18]

- In *Nan Jing* (difficult question 28), on the other hand, it simply claims that Du Mai has its origin in point Du 1 and from there it runs to Du 16 along the spine, penetrates the brain there and continues to flow to the vertex and point Du 20. From there it continues to the philtrum, passing the forehead and the tip of the nose and in the frenulum of the upper lip its superficial course ends at Du 28.

SECONDARY VESSELS OF DU MAI

To understand the function and importance of Du Mai, its inner courses and secondary vessels are more important than the course of the primary channel.

Abdominal vessel: An inner branch of Du Mai branches off at the level of the genitals, which comes to the surface at Ren 2 where it divides into two further lanes:

An ascending branch follows the sinew channel of the Spleen, penetrates the navel, goes deeper there, climbs up the inner abdominal wall and enters the Heart together with the sinew channel of the Spleen.

It comes to the surface at St 12 and St 13, connects there with the sinew channel of the Bladder and runs up to neck and face where it enters the middle of the eye and ends at Bl 1.

The second branch runs down the body, via the genitals to the rectum, runs around the buttocks, joins the sinew channel of the Bladder and runs across the head and finally penetrates Bl 1 where it terminates.

Dorsal vessel: From Du 1 the dorsal vessel passes the buttocks and close to the sinew channel of the Bladder it runs up to the head, where it penetrates Bl 1. The Du Mai dorsal vessel then follows the primary channel of the Bladder as far as the neck, continues to Bl 23 along the back and finally enters the Kidneys.

THE LUO-CONNECTING VESSEL OF DU MAI

It starts at Du 1, climbs up to Du 16 next to the spine, spreads across the cranium, descends to the shoulders, connects with the Bladder channel, penetrates deep into the muscles, and runs into the genital area, where it unites with the Kidney channel.[19]

- Opening point: SI 3

- Connecting point: Bl 62

WHY IS DU MAI SO IMPORTANT FOR THE MALE GENITAL SYSTEM?

Du Mai is also known as the 'Sea of Yang' and therefore monitors the entire Yang and also all Yang channels in our body. It serves as the Yang reservoir and can therefore be used to strengthen the Yang of the body in general and the Kidney Yang in particular. As we know, Yang is a warming and energizing force. That is also important for sexual arousal and erection but also for the composition and creation of semen.

These functions are dependent on sufficient Yang Qi (which comes from the Ming Men fire) and particularly on its supply through the Du Mai. Insufficiency leads to a sub/infertility, a lack of libido and potency problems. Deficiency in Kidney Yang and Minister Fire is a common cause of male issues in men of all ages. Yang deficiency can result from either too much exercise or hard physical work. As a result, the Du Mai is also weakened and gets empty. The disorders in the course of Du Mai as described – with regard to the male sexual organs – express themselves in the form of impotence, premature ejaculation, infertility (especially due to a lack of sperm motility) and a lack of libido.[20]

Chong Mai (Penetrating vessel)

Here, too, there is different information in the various sources about where the Chong Mai comes from.

- In *Suwen* chapter 60 as well as in *Nan Jing*, St 30 is described as the starting point.

- In *Ling Shu* chapter 65, however, we can read that the Chong Mai has its origin in the uterus/room of sperm. In chapter 62 of the same work, on the other hand, it is claimed that the Chong Mai begins in the Kidneys. Nguyen Van Nghi, Giovanni Maciocia and Barbara Kirschbaum share this opinion.

- The Chong Mai flows from the Kidneys into the genital region. The vessels originating from the left and right Kidneys unite at point Ren 1 and then divide into primary and secondary courses (a total of five branches).[21]

Dorsal branch: A deep branch runs from Ren 1 along the abdomen to the spine and rises along it. Via the point Du 4, it is connected to Du Mai and to Dai Mai (Girdle vessel).[22]

Ventral branch: Another branch follows the course of Ren Mai from Ren 1 to Ren 4, enters the primary channel of the Kidney at Ki 11 and runs across the abdomen to Ki 21. From there it runs to Ki 27, passing the rib cage, and during its course gives off numerous small branches that flow into the intercostal spaces. From Ki 27, the Chong Mai continues to the throat, joins Ren 23, rises up to the face and circles the lips.

Downwards secondary vessels: At Ki 11 a secondary vessel branches off which runs along the inside of the thigh and lower leg, runs behind the inner ankle and spreads out in the sole of the foot.

Another secondary vessel runs from Ki 11 via St 30 on the inside of the thigh to the inside of the calf, flows further to the malleolus medialis and via the inner edge of the foot to the big toe, which it circles, before returning to malleolus medialis.[23]

- Opening point: Sp 4

- Connecting point: Pc 6

The Chong Mai meets other channels at the following points (connecting points):

- Ren Mai (Conception vessel) at points Ren 1 and Ren 7

- Stomach channel at Ma 30

- Kidney channel at Kidney points 11, 12, 13, 14, 15, 16, 27, 18, 19, 20, 21.[24]

WHY IS THE CHONG MAI SO IMPORTANT FOR THE MALE GENITAL SYSTEM?

There are seven good reasons, described mainly on the example of the penis:

1. Chong Mai is the 'Sea of Blood' and as such is also responsible for the Blood flow of the erectile tissue of the penis, especially the corpus cavernosum; if this erectile tissue is well supplied with Blood, an adequate erection takes place. So, quite simply, a normal erection depends on the healthy state of the Chong Mai. Apart from that, the proper production of spermatozoa in the tubuli of the testicles requires Blood.

2. The penis is often referred to as the 'ancestral muscle' in ancient literature, and it is this ancestral muscle that is influenced by the Chong Mai.

3. The Chong Mai controls all network pathways, and the penis as an external and therefore 'superficial' structure is very rich in Luo-connecting vessels. Those are, of course, also of great relevance when it comes to spermatogenesis, which, from a Chinese perspective, takes places in such a network vessel formation.

4. The Chong Mai also controls all membranes (Huang). The penis consists to a large extent of connective tissue – as do the testicles – which in Chinese Medicine is assigned to the membranes. Thus, Chong Mai also controls the connective tissue of the penis and the testes.

5. Chong Mai is connected to the postnatal Qi (which we obtain through food and is provided by the Spleen/Stomach) via St 30 which is located near the base of the penis. In addition to the Blood, it also provides the Qi necessary for an erection and for the production of sperm.

6. Chong Mai is also connected to the prenatal Qi (which is located in the Kidney) via the points Ren 1, Ren 4 and Ki 13, and can therefore also provide the Essence necessary for reproduction.

7. Chong Mai connects the Heart and Kidneys and thus contributes significantly to the communication between these two organs. For the erectile function but also the reproductive function, it is important that the Heart Blood and the Heart Qi can descend to the room of sperm and the penis and can connect to the Kidneys. If this communication is disturbed and the connection blocked, the Chong Mai must be treated for male-factor infertility and erectile dysfunction.[25]

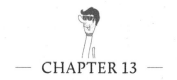

— CHAPTER 13 —

The Short Guide

KNOW YOUR PATIENTS, PATTERNS, POINTS AND PRESCRIPTIONS

This section presents the most common patterns involved in male subfertility and infertility, along with sketches of the typical patient, and the main points and herb prescriptions to use. Keep in mind that this chapter is for those in a hurry and only represents the most important facts in a nutshell. Readers who really want to study male fertility treatment with TCM are advised to jump forward to the subsequent chapters.

The medical history

It is important that the TCM practitioner does not skip uncomfortable questions about the couple's frequency and timing of intercourse, likes and dislikes, and whether libido is lacking in either partner. To get an honest answer, it is recommended to consult with both partners separately and assure them that it is only possible to help if you know the truth. During the man's consultation, as well as questions about libido, it is necessary to ask about the health of the genital region to identify the appropriate pattern and treat it accordingly (e.g. to check for eczema, itching, swelling, discharge, history of sexually transmitted diseases, pain on ejaculation or urination).

From a TCM perspective, healthy sex – from attraction to orgasm – depends on three things:

- **The connection of Heart-Bao-Kidney axis via the Bao Mai and Bao Luo:** Proper communication between the Heart and Kidneys is needed to get aroused (upwards movement) and to have an ejaculation (downwards movement). Note that the 'Bao' (uterus in women) is known as the 'room of sperm' in men.

- **The ascending of Kidney water and the downbearing of Heart Fire:** Emotions cause arousal which stirs the minister fire, which flares up to the Heart and Pericardium, which in turn discharges it downwards to enable orgasm.

- **A connection between the Ren Mai (Conception vessel) and Du Mai (Governing**

vessel): This connection is at the mouth and genitals of both partners, which enables a free circling flow of Qi through these two extraordinary vessels.

As practitioners, our job is to ensure proper function and nourishment (Jing, Qi, Blood) of these vessels, and that they are connected to each other (i.e. no obstructions in the genital/mouth areas).

KIDNEY YIN VACUITY

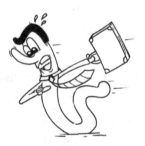

This is often the overworked, restless businessman who is always on the run and thus 'overheating his engine'. He may complain of back or knee pain, tinnitus, poor memory, poor sleep, feeling hot at night, and there is typically a red tongue (if there is vacuity heat) and a rapid pulse. Vacuity heat tends to lead to an increased libido but with an insufficient erection and/or premature ejaculation.

Main points

- To tonify Kidney Yin: *Taixi* Ki 3, *Zhaohai* Ki 6, *Guanyuan* Ren 4

- To tonify Kidney Qi: *Henggu* Ki 11, *Dahe* Ki 12, *Zhongji* Ren 3, *Qihai* Ren 6, *Shenshu* Bl 23, *Zhishi* Bl 52

- To clear empty-heat: *Rangu* Ki 2

- To support fluids: *Zusanli* St 36

- To increase Blood flow in the testicles: *Guilai* St 29, *Sanyinjiao* Sp 6 (with electrostimulation at 2 Hz joining same side points for 5–20 minutes)

- Local points to move Qi and Blood in the testes and improve sperm quality Bl 31, Bl 32.

Representative herbal formula: Zuo Gui Wan (Restore the Left (Kidney) Pill)

Shu Di Huang *Rx. Rehmanniae Preparata*
Shan Yao *Rx. Dioscoreae*
Gou Qi Zi *Fr. Lycii*
Shan Zhu Yu *Fr. Corni*
Chuan Niu Xi *Rx. Cyathulae*
Tu Si Zi *Sm. Cuscutae*
Lu Jiao Jiao *Colla Cervi Cornus*
Gui Ban Jiao *Colla Plastrum Testudinis*

This formula nourishes Yin, tonifies the Kidneys without overheating or overloading and supplements Jing.

KIDNEY YANG VACUITY

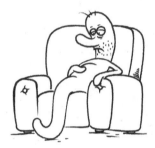

This is the tired, puffy-looking 'couch potato', who typically presents with fatigue, cold and/or painful back or knees, frequent urination at night, a pale, coated tongue, and a slow, soft pulse. Sexually, he tends to present with weak orgasm and ejaculation, low libido, erectile dysfunction, premature ejaculation and watery semen.

Main points

- To warm and tonify Kidney Yang: *Shenshu* Bl 23, *Zhishi* Bl 52, *Ming Men* Du 4 (use moxa)

- To warm the Lower Burner, promote Kidney Yang: *Guilai* St 29, *Shenque* Ren 8, *Ciliao* Bl 32, *Qichong* St 30, *Guanyuan* Ren 4 (use moxa)

- Raise Yang Qi: *Baihui* Du 20

- To increase Blood flow in the testicles: *Guilai* St 29, *Sanyinjiao* Sp 6 (with electrostimulation at 2 Hz joining same side points for 5–20 minutes).

Representative herbal formula: You Gui Wan (Restore the Right (Kidney) Pill

Shu Di Huang Rehmanniae Rx. Preparata
Shan Yao Dioscorea Rh
Shan Zhu Yu Corni Fr
Gou Qi Zi Lycii Fr
Du Zhong Eucommiae Cx
Tu Si Zi Cuscutae Sm
Fu Zi Aconiti Rx lat. prep
Rou Gui Connamomi Cx
Lu Jiao Jiao Cervi Cornu gelat.

This formula warms and tonifies Kidney Yang, replenishes Essence and Blood and Ming Men fire.

QI AND BLOOD STASIS

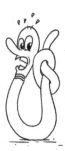

This patient may have a strong body, but presents with a dark complexion, purple lips, purple tongue, spider veins on the skin and may report sensations of distension, heaviness and pain in the scrotal/perineal area, burning inguinal pain during ejaculation, erectile dysfunction and pain in the testicles. They may have been diagnosed with varicocele (traditionally described as a scrotum that feels like a 'bag of worms').

Main points

- Move Qi and Blood in the genitals and Lower Burner: *Dadun* Liv 1, *Taichong* Liv 3, *Ligou* Liv 5, *Zhongdu* Liv 6, *Sanyinjiao* Sp 6, *Diji* Sp 8

- Local points to invigorate Qi and Blood in the genital region and ease pain: *Ciliao* Bl 32, *Guilai* St 29, *Qichong* St 30, *Zhongji* Ren 3, *Dazhu* Ki 11

- Invigorate Blood: *Geshu* Bl 17, *Xuehai* Sp 10

- To increase Blood flow in the testicles: *Guilai* St 29, *Sanyinjiao* Sp 6 (with electrostimulation at 2 Hz joining same side points for 5–20 minutes).

Representative herbal formula: Xue Fu Zhu Yu Tang (Decoction for Removing Blood Stasis in the Chest)

Dang Gui *Rx. Angelicae Sinensis*	12 g
Sheng Di Huang *Rx. Rehmanniae Glutinosae*	9 g
Chi Shao *Rx Paeoniae Rubrae*	6 g
Chuan Xiong *Rx. Ligustici Chuanxiong*	6 g
Tao Ren *Sm. Persicae*	12 g
Hong Hua *Fl. Carthami*	9 g
Chai Hu *Rx. Bupleuri*	3 g
Zhi Ke *Fr. Citri seu Ponciri*	6 g
Chuan Niu Xi *Rx. Cythulae*	9 g
Jie Geng *Rx Platycodi Grandiflori*	6 g
Gan Cao *Rx. Glycyrrhiazae*	3 g

This is another very well-known formula that invigorates Blood but also dispels Blood stasis, spreads Liver Qi and unblocks the channels. Most modern texts replace *Niu Xi* (*Rx. Achyranthis Bidentatae*) with *Chuan Niu Xi* (as in our formula above).

DAMP-HEAT IN THE LOWER BURNER

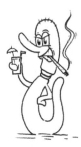

This is the heavy drinking, cigar-smoking, curry-loving 'gourmand'. He may complain of delayed ejaculation, priapism or an inability to ejaculate at all, distension and pain in the genital region after sexual activity, swollen genitals, genital itching, red, overly warm, moist and malodorous genitals, genital eczema, and may present with prostatitis or cystitis. The tongue is red with yellow slimy fur, and the pulse is slippery and stringlike.

Main points

- Eliminate damp-heat and Lower Burner: *Dadun* Liv 1, *Xingjian* Liv 2, *Taichong* Liv 3, *Ligou* Liv 5, *Ququan* Liv 8, *Rangu* Kid 2, *Jaoxin* Ki 8, *Yinggu* Ki 10, *Sanyinjiao* Sp 6, *Yinlingquang* Sp 9, *Quchi* Ll 11

- Local points to remove damp-heat from the genitals: St 28, St 30, Bl 28, Ren 3, Bl 35 and Ren 1, Bl 27, Bl 28.

Representative herbal formula: Bi Xie Fen Qing Yin (Dioscorea Separating the Clear Decoction)

Bi Xie Rhiz. *Dioscorea*	12 g
Yi Zhi Ren Fr. *Alipinae Oxyphyllae*	9 g
Wu Yao Rx. *Linderae Strychnifoliae*	9 g
Shi Chang Pu Rhiz. *Acori Graminei*	9 g

Bi Xie drains Damp from the urogenital system and *Shi Chang Pu* opens orifices to facilitate this draining. *Yi Zhi Ren* and *Wu Yao* warm the Bladder and Kidney to facilitate efficient excretion of fluids.[1]

WANT TO KNOW MORE?

Remember to include what I call 'GPS' points in your prescriptions to direct the effect to the required area: such as *Sanyinjiao* Sp 6 for the reproductive region. In herbal therapy, the guiding herbs to the testicles are *Wang Bu Liu Xing* (*Vaccariae Semen*) and *Lu Lu Tong* (*Liquidambaris Fructus*).

— CHAPTER 14 —

Pattern Differentiation

Successful treatment with Chinese Medicine is rooted in an appropriate and exact analysis of the presenting pattern. When the correct pattern is found, it is not that difficult to treat effectively. The much harder work is to solve the puzzle to get to that point. Unfortunately, our patients rarely have a well-behaved, single pattern, sticking to the textbook description, but far more often present with mixed patterns.

This chapter works as kind of a 'mastermind process guide' that will help you find your way through the maze to get the pattern diagnosis right.

As with the start of every journey, the most important decision you have to make is the very first one: is it a deficiency pattern or is it a repletion pattern? In our labyrinth analogy, that would mean choosing to start going right or left.

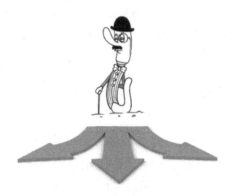

If you get your first direction decision correct, it would be perfect if you found out about the exact Chinese substance that is in deficiency (Blood, Yin, Yang...). But even if you get that 'second level' decision wrong at the first try, with a little detour, you'll get to the destination in the end.

But if you start treating your patient as having a deficiency pattern while the truth is that he suffers from a repletion pattern, you will make his symptoms (and root) worse and need to completely correct your path.

Let's start with an overview of possible patterns for male infertility:

Deficiency	Repletion	Mixed
Kidney Yin	Qi stagnation	Spleen deficiency with…
Kidney Yang	Cold stagnation	Damp-heat pouring downwards
Kidney Jing	Blood stasis	Damp-phlegm blocking
Spleen deficiency (Qi and Blood)		

Furthermore: male infertility patterns include syndromes of the following organs:

- Kidney

- Liver

- Spleen.

It is important for me to explain that none of these pattern discriminations is my own invention or genius idea – it is more like a gallery with me as the curator. My job is to collect all these commonly used patterns from various sources and put them together as an exhibition you can learn from.

In some pattern names, the literature is in agreement; in others, there are differing views. In the same way, some patterns are described in every textbook, whereas other patterns can only be found in one author's.

To keep it as simple as possible, but to still give you the full picture, the patterns that are rarely cited are marked with the Professor Sperm symbol.

DEFICIENCY PATTERNS

Kidney Yin deficiency

Generally speaking, Yin has an impact on fluids, so the dominant adjectives in this pattern are dry, stiff and an impaired cooling ability of the body, and thus the tendency to overheat.

- **Sex signs:** Often there is vacuity heat meaning a hyperactive ministerial fire not being controlled by Yin, which leads to increased libido but often with an insufficient erection and/or a premature ejaculation and seminal emission.

- **General signs:** Back pain or knee pain, tinnitus, poor memory, sleeplessness. If there is vacuity heat as well: feeling hot at night, dry stools, dry mouth and throat, pain in the heels (this reflects insufficient nourishment to the Kidney channel).[1]

- **Semen analysis:** Sticky and thickened seminal fluid, low volume, decreased sperm count, prolonged liquefication time and a high percentage of sperm with abnormal morphology.

- **Tongue:** Red tongue with scanty fur or lack of fur.

- **Pulse:** Fine, rapid pulse (if there is empty-heat).

Kidney Yang deficiency

The Kidney Yang has to warm the 'Bao' (room of sperm), which is the source of reproduction. If it fails, that sperm factory gets too cold and fertility is reduced. In traditional textbooks this is mainly caused by excessive sexual activity and/or frequent masturbation (even if only during adolescence). Nowadays, stress can practically be considered an 'equivalent' of sexual excess.[2] The main adjectives of that pattern are cold and slow.

- **Sex signs:** Weak orgasm and ejaculation, low libido, erectile dysfunction, premature ejaculation, cold and damp in the genital region.

- **General signs:** Cold and/or pain in back or knees, frequent urination at night, early morning diarrhoea, fatigue, aversion to cold that does improve with exposure to warmth.

- **Semen analysis:** Low motility, cold, thin and watery semen, prolonged liquefication time, abnormal morphology, azoospermia.

- **Tongue:** Pale, enlarged tongue with thin white, moist fur.

- **Pulse:** Sinking, fine, forceless pulse.

Kidney Essence vacuity

Essence is the most fundamental raw material which can be transformed into various other substances such as Qi, fluids, Blood and, of course, semen and sperm. The quality and quantity of semen and sperm depend massively on the quality and quantity of Jing. When reframing Kidney Essence into Western terminology, it is often compared with stem cells or, more recently, with telomeres.

- **Sex signs:** If there is a lack of prenatal Jing, the genitalia are underdeveloped, as well as the secondary sexual characteristics; low or no libido if only the post-heaven Jing is lacking, indicating an acquired essence deficiency; genitalia and secondary sexual characteristics are normal, but there are signs of premature ageing.

- **General signs:** Chronic back pain, weak knees, poor healing of the bones or bone pain, poor and bad teeth, vertigo, tinnitus, poor memory, loss of hair, fatigue.

- **Semen analysis:** Low volume, low total sperm count, abnormal morphology, prolonged liquefication time.

- **Tongue:** Small, thin, eventually pale reddish tongue without coating.

- **Pulse:** Sinking, fine, forceless pulse.

Spleen vacuity

As the Spleen is the Qi- and Blood-producing factory, as well as the root of the acquired Jing (postnatal), Spleen deficiency can lead to a lack of both of those very important substances.

- **Sex signs:** Weak ejaculation, poor libido, erectile dysfunction, premature ejaculation.

- **General signs:** Pale face, weakness, fatigue, poor sleep with heavy dreaming, poor appetite (as most of our patients suffer from the opposite, keep in mind that poor appetite can also be defined as desire to eat, but not knowing what to choose in front of the full refrigerator),[3] vertigo, blurry vision, lazy speakers (taciturn), pale tongue, pale fingernails, fragile hair, shortness of breath, abdominal distension, loose stools.

- **Semen analysis:** Low density, 'clear and cold semen', low motility, low count.

- **Tongue:** Pale tongue with scanty fur, sometimes swollen with tooth marks.

- **Pulse:** Deep, fine or soft pulse.

WANT TO KNOW MORE?

Vacuity of Liver Blood/Liver Yin

As described in some books, is the result of Spleen vacuity or Kidney Yin vacuity and is therefore not discussed separately.

Kidney and Spleen Qi vacuity

This is described as an extra pattern by some authors. It is a logical combination of the above vacuity patterns.

REPLETION PATTERNS

Liver Qi Stagnation

A proper and free flow of Qi and consequently Blood is essential for the organs to function properly. The Liver channel goes around the genitals and therefore a free flow within that channel is highly important for the work of the reproductive organs. A lack of free flow can result in a decrease of sperm production or hinder their further transport. In particular, emotions such as unfulfilled desires and repletion of emotions in general can easily cause Qi stagnation. So can a lack of exercise and stress as a common lifestyle pathogen. That lack of free flow certainly has an impact on ejaculation.

- **Sex signs:** Decreased force of ejaculation up to an inability to ejaculate, painful ejaculation, weak erection.

- **General signs:** Frequent sighing, moodiness, irritability, depression, supressed anger, intercostal and flank tension, chest oppression, plum pit feeling in the throat.

- **Semen analysis:** The greater the stagnation leading to heat that may enter the essence chamber, the bigger the impact on sperm quality. Low volume, increased viscosity, prolonged liquefication time, low density and abnormal morphology.

- **Tongue:** Normal in colour.

- **Pulse:** Tight or wiry.

Blood stasis

Growing older in combination with a lack of exercise (especially in the pelvic area) and a poor diet leads to a 'hard and stiff abdomen', which affects the Qi and consequently the Blood flow in that area negatively. Bear in mind that Qi needs to invigorate Blood, as Blood itself is a static substance that needs to be moved by Qi. Therefore, Blood stasis can either be the result of a long-term Qi stagnation or could also be due to the action of internal pathogenic factors or a result of a trauma.

- **Sex signs:** A scrotum that feels like a 'bag of worms' (varicocele), feeling of distension, heaviness and pain in the scrotal and perineal area, burning inguinal pain during ejaculation, erectile dysfunction, pain in the testicles, nodules in the testes.

- **General signs:** Fixed pain in the lower abdomen (especially at night), long medical history (often with periods of relapse and remission), purple lips, purple tongue, spider veins, varicose veins, ageing spots, haemorrhoids.

- **Semen analysis:** No spermatozoa or a low density, poor motility, high amount of abnormal morphology, high percentage of red blood cells in the semen, AsAb (anti-sperm antibodies).

- **Tongue:** Purple tongue with purple spots; thick, visible tongue veins.

- **Pulse:** Sinking rough pulse or fine rough pulse.

WANT TO KNOW MORE?

Cold stagnating in the Liver channel

In times of heated homes, climate change and a lifestyle that generally tends to cause overheating problems, this pattern can easily be overlooked. Nevertheless, it has relevance as cold finds its way into the body and especially the Liver channel through exposure to cold. Pastimes such as surfing, boating, swimming (water sports in general are prone to cause cold in the Liver channel as they often require the lower body being in the cold water for some time) open the door for this pathogen. Cold as a Yin evil always causes stagnation and congelation.

- **Sex signs:** Clear and cold semen, distension and/or pain in the testes, swelling, pain in the lower abdomen that worsens after sexual activity, coldness and dampness of the scrotum worsening after exposure to cold, often accompanied by retraction and pain of the scrotum, scrotal hydrocele and scrotal hernia.

- **General signs:** Occasionally feeling exhausted, limb soreness and pain, aversion to cold, cold feet and legs in particular, sombre white facial complexion.

- **Semen analysis:** Low motility, cold, thin and watery semen, prolonged liquefication time.

- **Tongue:** Pale or light red tongue with toothmarks and a thin white fur.

- **Pulse:** Stringlike tight or stringlike moderate.

MIXED PATTERNS

Repletion patterns of the Spleen also result from a weak Spleen, which is why we call it a mixed pattern. In short, if the drainage function of the Spleen breaks down, in modern terms 'no detox function' results and the evil factor dampness can therefore easily pour downwards in the Lower Burner following gravity and can there transform into damp-heat and/or phlegm.

Damp-heat in the Lower Burner

Often caused by excess consumption of greasy and spicy food, smoking and drinking, as well as unresolved infections (especially in the genital tract) or chronic inflammation.

- **Sex signs:** Delayed ejaculation, priapism or inability to ejaculate at all, distension and pain in the genital region after sexual activity, swollen genitals, genital itching, red, overly warm and moist genitals with possible malodour, genital eczema, tendency towards prostatitis or cystitis.

- **General signs**: Heaviness and soreness of the lumbus with heavy sensations in the legs, fatigue, heavy head, dry mouth with the desire for cold drinks, unsmooth bowel movements that are sticky and smelly, difficult, painful and turbid urination, dark urine, irritability, epigastric and chest fullness.

- **Semen analysis:** Thick yellowish and turbid semen, high percentage of white blood cells in the semen, pus, prolonged or missing liquefication, low volume, high percentage of dead spermatozoa (low viability), low motility, low density.

- **Tongue:** Red with yellow slimy fur, swollen lingual frenum.

- **Pulse:** Slippery, stringlike rapid pulse.

Damp-phlegm blocking

A high intake of sugary and fatty foods can overwhelm the Spleen's ability to transform and transport in any men, but particularly in those who are already overweight or even obese. As a consequence, dampness and food stagnation will result, both easily turning into phlegm. Phlegm is a Yin evil that blocks the passage of Essence, hence causing obstruction in the male genital region and hindering reproduction.

- **Sex signs:** Inability to ejaculate, nodules in the testicles, swollen testes.

- **General signs:** Obesity, vertigo, nausea, oppression in the chest, heaviness of the limbs, heart palpitations.

- **Semen analysis:** Low volume, low density and motility, low viability, azoospermia.

- **Tongue:** Enlarged tongue with white slimy fur.

- **Pulse:** Sinking slippery pulse.

CHAPTER 15

Treatment Options from the Chinese Medicine 'Bag of Tricks' – Acupuncture

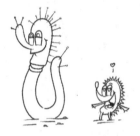

FREQUENCY OF ACUPUNCTURE

At a very minimum, once a week for at least ten weeks; if possible, twice a week. When treating twice a week, the patient lies on the back on the first treatment of the week and on the abdomen for the second treatment of the week. When treating once a week, I prefer to put the patient in the lateral position.

BASIC ACUPUNCTURE PROTOCOLS

These protocols can be used as the foundation of a point prescription, with individual points based on the patient's very individual needs, added as appropriate.

Several authors give us an overview of their ideal basic protocols, so I am presenting some of them here at the beginning of this chapter before delving into the pattern-based point selection later.

Main points according to Peter Deadman[1]

Bl 32, Bl 35, Ren 4, St 30, Sp 6

EXPLANATION OF THE POINTS USED

Bl 32: Bl 31–34 together are called the Baliao group (eight gaps). They have quite a similar effect that consists mainly of treating different diseases of the Lower Burner. Bl 32, as suggested, is used the most, as it has the biggest impact on the urogenital system. For treating male fertility issues, one needs to needle deep, approximately 1.5–2 cun through the second sacral foramen. When needled correctly, a strong De-Qi sensation should pour through the abdomen and should even be recognized in the genital area.

Bl 35: The main point for male sexual disorders, and therefore also used for infertility. Always a good choice in male indications but fits perfectly in cases of Yang vacuity or damp-heat patterns. It is recommended to insert the needle up to 1.5 cun to achieve a strong De-Qi sensation going downwards to the perineum and the genitals.

Ren 4: Meeting point of the Conception vessel (Ren Mai) and the three Yin channels of the lower extremities. All three of them (Spleen, Liver and Kidney) have a huge impact when it comes to the treatment of male genital problems in general. It has a close relationship to ancestral energy (pre-heaven). It can be used in any pattern but fits well especially when there are Kidney vacuity patterns. Needle deeply to achieve a strong sensation down to the penis. Tell the patient to empty their bladder before the acupuncture session to ensure the bladder will not be painful.

St 30: Meeting point of the Chong Mai (Penetrating vessel) and the Stomach channel. As we know, the Chong Mai is a very important vessel for the treatment of the genital region. Even due to its location, St 30 is perfect for the treatment of genital diseases. It is perfect to use as soon as there is any sign of pain or swelling in the genital region or in the lower abdomen, because pain always indicates stagnation or stasis. The point is closely related to the acquired energy (post-heaven). Acupuncture should be performed carefully and not with a very deep needle insertion, in order to keep away from the spermatic cord. Insertion direction should be downwards (caudal) and medial, to achieve a De-Qi sensation that pours downwards to the testicles.

Sp 6: Meeting point of the three Yin channels of the leg. A very important and useful point for any kind of sexual dysfunction including male infertility, since disharmonies in at least one of these three channels and organs are very likely to harm male fertility. Moreover, in acupuncture manuals it is ranked as one of the main points for treating sexual, urological and andrological diseases.

Main points according to Anna Lin[2]

Bl 23, Bl 32, Ren 4, St 30 (St 36, Liv 3, Du 4, Hua Tuo Jia Ji points)

EXPLANATION OF THE POINTS USED

Bl 23: Back-Shu point of the Kidneys and as such an important point for the treatment of Kidney weakness in general, be it Kidney Qi vacuity, Kidney Essence deficiency, Kidney Yin or Kidney Yang deficiency.

Bl 32: Bl 31–34 together are called the Baliao group (eight gaps). They have a quite similar effect that mainly consists of treating different diseases of the Lower Burner. Bl 32, as suggested, is used the most as it has the biggest impact on the urogenital system. For treating male fertility issues, one needs to needle deep, approximately 1.5–2 cun through the second foramen sacrale. Needled correctly, a strong De-Qi sensation should pour through the abdomen and should even be recognized in the genital area.

Ren 4: Its name 'Gate of the Original Qi' underlines the main function of this point: tonifying and strengthening. Ren 4 strengthens the original Qi and supports the Essence, tonifies and strengthens the Kidneys and regulates the Lower Burner. It is located in the so-called lower Dantian (lower cinnabar field), a special centre of the deepest energies of the body, which extends from Ren 7 to Ren 4. The feeling of De-Qi should be directed towards to the outer genitals. The point strengthens the Bao, hence the genital system in men in general. It has a close relationship to the ancestral energy (pre-heaven).

St 30: Meeting point of the Chong Mai (Penetrating vessel) and the Stomach channel. As we know, the Chong Mai is a very important vessel for the treatment of the genital region. Due to its location, St 30 is perfect for the treatment of genital diseases. It is perfect to use as soon as there is any sign of pain or swelling in the genital region or in the lower abdomen as pain always indicates stagnation or stasis. Acupuncture should be performed carefully and not with a very deep needle insertion in order to keep away from the spermatic cord. Insertion direction should be downwards (caudal) and medial to achieve a De-Qi sensation that pours downwards to the testicles.

For malformation of the sperm (Teratospermia) add:

St 36: This point tonifies Qi, nourishes Blood and Yin, strengthens the Stomach and Spleen and can clear dampness. As it stimulates Spleen and Stomach, it enhances the production of postnatal Qi which can be stored with prenatal Essence in the Kidneys. All these functions are essential for fertility.

Liv 3: Important in its function as a Qi distributing point, it also suppresses Liver Yang rising and nourishes Liver Blood and Yin and regulates the Lower Burner. It can be used with the same effectiveness for both full and empty patterns.

Du 4: This point is called Ming Men (gate of vitality), with its location being exactly where the ministerial fire is commonly assumed to be (although that understanding has changed in different eras). It is precisely that ministerial fire that it can stir up, if necessary. Conversely, Du 4 also has the ability to discharge heat in the body that 'feels like fire'. The Classics of Difficulties quote that Ming Men is the residence of the Essence and stores semen in men. Du 4 further strengthens the Kidneys, but also influences Du Mai as the most important Yang meridian, which also runs around the genitals with its anterior course.

Hua Tuo Jia Ji points along the spine: These classic points are located half a cun bilateral to Du Mai from vertebrae T1 through L5. Classically, there are 17 pairs of points (34 points total) attributed to Hua Tuo. Within the last 2000 years, these points have extended both upward through the cervical spine and downward across the sacrum. The points in the cervical and sacrum are simply known as *jia* (lining) *ji* (spine).[3] The points lie along the interspinous transverse ligaments and muscles. Each point has its related posterior branch of the spinal nerve starting from below the vertebra and the accompanying artery and vein. It is understood that the stimulation of these points will treat problems of the organs and body parts that are located in the same general region. Their functions correspond roughly to those of the Bladder-associated Shu points.[4]

Main points according to Bob Damone[5]

Du 4, Du 3, Ren 4, Ren 3, Sp 6, Bl 23, Bl 52, Ki 3, St 36

EXPLANATION OF THE POINTS USED

Du 4: This point is called Ming Men (gate of vitality), with its location being exactly where the ministerial fire is commonly assumed to be (although that understanding has changed in different eras) It is precisely that ministerial fire that it can stir up, if necessary. Conversely, Du 4 also has the ability to discharge heat in the body that 'feels like fire'. The Classics of Difficulties quote that Ming Men is the residence of the Essence and stores semen in men. Du 4 further strengthens the Kidneys, but also influences Du Mai as the most important Yang meridian, which also runs around the genitals with its anterior course.

Du 3: Named 'Lumbar Yang gate', this point regulates the Lower Burner and is commonly used for seminal emission, impotence and other genital issues. It can also be used as a point on the Du Mai to strengthen Yang.

Ren 4: Its name 'Gate of the Original Qi' underlines the main function of this point: tonifying and strengthening. Ren 4 strengthens the original Qi and supports the Essence; it tonifies and strengthens the Kidneys and regulates the Lower Burner. It is located in the so-called lower Dantian (lower cinnabar field), a special centre of the deepest energies of the body, which extends from Ren 7 to Ren 4. The feeling of De-Qi should be directed towards the penis. The point strengthens the Bao, hence the genital system in men in general. It has a close relationship to the ancestral energy (pre-heaven).

Ren 3: The Front-Mu point of the Bladder and a crossing point of the Ren Mai with the Spleen, Liver and Kidney channels. It influences not only these three meridians but also the entire region of the lower abdomen. Ren 3 is preferred to Ren 4 in the case of fullness. It is especially popular in the treatment of abundance patterns, such as stagnation and accumulation of cold or heat. Its ability to evacuate dampness and heat makes it an important point for complaints of the genital region.

Sp 6: Meeting point of the three Yin channels of the leg. A very important and useful point for any kind of sexual dysfunction, including male infertility, as disharmonies in one of these three channels and organs are very likely to harm male fertility. In acupuncture manuals, it is ranked as one of the main points for treating sexual, urological and andrological diseases.

Bl 23: Back-Shu point of the Kidneys and, as such, an important point for the treatment of Kidney weakness in general, be it Kidney Qi vacuity, Kidney Essence deficiency, Kidney Yin or Kidney Yang deficiency.

Bl 52: Its name 'palace of Essence' or 'room of willpower' says a lot about its indication. In our context, it is used for its Kidney-tonifying effect as an alternative or supplement to BL 23 (both are at the same level). It supports the Essence and has the ability to strengthen Kidney Qi and Yang in order to strengthen sexual function and control the discharge of semen.

Ki 3: Used in any kind of Kidney weakness, like Bl 23. In addition, both Chong Mai and Ren Mai are rooted in the Kidneys, and patterns of disharmony in these two extraordinary meridians, which are so important for the male genital system, can be caused by Kidney weakness and treated with Ki 3.

St 36: This point tonifies Qi, nourishes Blood and Yin, strengthens the Stomach and Spleen and can clear dampness. As it stimulates Spleen and Stomach, it enhances the production of postnatal Qi which can be stored with prenatal Essence in the Kidneys. All these functions are essential for fertility.

TREATMENT PROTOCOLS ACCORDING TO THE PATTERNS

Kidney Yin vacuity
POINT SELECTION AND EXPLANATION

- **Lu 7–Ki 6** – open Ren Mai.[6]

- **Ki 3, Ki 6, Ki 9, Ren 4, Ren 12** – supplement Kidney Yin.

- **Bl 31, Bl 32** – local points to improve sperm quality.

- **Ki 2** – clears empty-heat (vacuity heat).

- **Pc 8, Ht 8, Liv 2** – purify empty-heat.[7]

- **St 36** – supports fluid.

- **Ki 11, Ki 12, Ren 3 and Ren 6** – tonify Kidney Qi in the Lower Burner.

- **Bl 23, Bl 52** – tonify Kidney Qi.[8]

- **Du 4** – activates Ming Men.

- **Sp 6** – focuses on the genital region.

- **Bl 15, Bl 43** – for excess nocturnal emissions with dreams.[9]

- **St 29, Sp 6** – increase Blood flow in the testicles (electroacupuncture (EA) 10 Hz joining same side 5–20 minutes).

Kidney Yang vacuity

POINT SELECTION AND EXPLANATION

- **SI 3–Bl 62** – open Du Mai.[10]

- **Ki 3, Ki 7, Ki 12** – supplement Kidney Qi and Kidney Yang.

- **Ki 2** – tonifies Kidney Yang.

- **St 29, Ren 8 with moxa** – help to warm the Lower Burner, help with impotence.

- **Bl 32, Bl 35, St 30, Ren 2 and Ren 4** – local points to promote Kidney Yang and help with sperm production.

- **Bl 23, Bl 52, Du 4** – warm and supplement and tonify Kidney Yang and Jing.[11] These three build the line of the Essence-tonifying points. Moxa!

- **Du 20** – raises the Yang.

- **Gb 25** – tonifies Kidneys as its Mu point.

- **Bl 30** – regulates genital function and sperm manufacture.[12]

- **Ki 14** – for leakage of sperm.[13]

- **Ren 6** – treats Qi, Yang and Jing.[14]

- **St 29, Sp 6** – increase Blood flow in the testicles (EA 10 Hz joining same side 5–20 minutes).[15]

Kidney Essence vacuity

POINT SELECTION AND EXPLANATION

- **Ki 12** – as confluence point of Chong Mai and Kidney channel. The Chong Mai is the channel to connect inherited and acquired constitution. EA on Ki 12 bilaterally with 10 Hz.[16]

- **Ren 2** – warms Yang and supplements Kidney.

- Ginger moxibustion on **Ren 3, Ren 4, Du 4**.

- **Ki 3 and Ki 6** – tonify the Kidney.

- **Bl 24 with Ren 4** – strengthen Qi of the Kidney Yang.

- **Sp 6 and Sp 8, St 36** – nourish and reinforce the acquired Essence.

- **St 27** – benefits the Essence and helps the Kidneys.

- **Bl 23, Bl 52 and Ki 7** – circulate and transport Kidney Qi.[17]

Spleen vacuity
POINT SELECTION AND EXPLANATION[18]

- **Sp 6** – strengthens Spleen, spreads Liver-Qi and benefits the Kidneys.

- **Sp 8** – Xi-cleft-point, circulates the Blood, regulates the Essence chamber.

- **St 30** – regulates Qi in abdomen, regulates the tendons.

- **St 36** – benefits Stomach and Spleen, tonifies Qi and Blood.

- **Ki 3** – tonifies the Kidney (Yin, Yang and Jing).

- **Liv 1, Liv 3** – move Qi.

- **Ren 6** – Lower Sea of Qi point, tonifies Qi and Yang.

- **Ren 17** – Lower and Upper Sea of Qi points.

- **Bl 20, Bl 21** – Back-Shu points of Stomach and Spleen.

- **Bl 17** – Influential point of Blood.

- **St 37, St 39, Bl 11** – Sea of Blood points that affect the amount and flow of Blood.

Blood stasis
POINT SELECTION AND EXPLANATION

- **Sp 4–Pc 6** – open Chong Mai as the Sea of Blood vessel.

- **Bl 31, Bl 32, Bl 35, St 29, St 30, Ren 1, Ren 2, Ren 3** – local points to invigorate Qi and Blood in the genital region, ease pain.

- **Liv 1, Liv 3, Liv 5, Liv 6** – move Qi and Blood in the genitals.

- **Liv 4, Ki 11** – move Qi (or treat swelling or pain) in the genitals.

- **Bl 17, Sp 10** – invigorate Blood.

- **St 29 with moxa** – warms the Lower Jiao, moves Blood and Qi in the Lower Burner.

- **Sp 6, Sp 8** – move Qi in the Lower Burner and in the genitals.[19]

- **St 29 and Sp 6** – with EA to increase the Blood flow of the testicles.[20]

- Bleed the following points with a lancet to dissolve stasis: **Sp 6, Sp 10, Liv 5, Bl 32, Ren 4 and Bl 17.**[21]

Liver Qi stagnation
POINT SELECTION AND EXPLANATION

- **Liv 10** – regulates the flow of Liver Qi and removes Blood stasis.

- **Ren 2** – the crossing point of the Ren channel and the Liver channel.

- **Ki 12, Ren 3, Liv 5, Liv 3, Sp 6, Ki 1** – a point combination that was found to be successful treating infertility due to aspermia.[22]

- **Pc 5, Pc 6** – calm the spirit and transform phlegm, mist heart orifices, regulate Qi.

- **Liv 8, Liv 14** – He-Sea and Front-Mu point of Liver channel to promote free Qi flow.

- **Ren 17** – Upper Sea of Qi point, regulates Qi and suppresses rebellious Qi.

- **Ren 1 and Ren 2** – increase the circulation of Qi and Blood in the genitals.[23]

- **St 30 and Bl 31** – remove stagnation in the Lower Burner.[24]

Cold in the Liver Channel[25]
POINT SELECTION AND EXPLANATION

- **St 29** – warms the Lower Burner and supports the genital region.

- **St 27** – strengthens Kidneys and tonifies Essence.

- **Ren 4** – warms and regulates the Essence chamber (room of sperm).

- **Ren 8** – warms the Yang, warms and harmonizes Intestines. Caution: moxa only!

- **St 36** – dispels pathogens.

- **Du 4** – benefits Essence and nourishes Yuan Qi.

- **Ki 2** – regulates the Lower Burner.

- **Liv 3, Liv 8, Liv 11** – regulate the Liver channel and the Lower Burner.

- **Bl 18** – Back-Shu point of the Liver.

- **Bl 23** – Back-Shu point of the Kidney to increase Qi and Yang.

- **Moxa** on all of these points recommended.

Damp-heat in the Lower Burner
POINT SELECTION AND EXPLANATION

- **GB 41, TH 5** – clear damp-heat in Lower Jiao via opening Dai Mai.[26]

- **GB 27** – clears damp-heat from Lower Jiao and Liver channel; also used as point on the Dai Mai.

- **St 28, St 30, Bl 28, Ren 3** – local points to remove damp-heat from the genitals.

- **Bl 35 and Ren 1** – clears damp-heat and treats impotence.

- **Bl 27, Bl 28** – clears genital discharge.

- **Liv 1, Liv 3, Liv 5, Liv 8, Ki 8, Ki 10** – eliminates damp-heat in the genitals, helps with itching and swelling.

- **St 28, Sp 9, Ren 9** – drain dampness from the Lower Burner.

- **Liv 2, LI 11, Ki 2** – clear heat and itching in the genital region.

- **Sp 6, Sp 7** – drain dampness.

- **Ki 3, Ki 7, Ren 4** – supplement Kidney Qi.[27]

- **Du 3** – clears damp and gently boosts Kidney Yang.[28]

Phlegm
POINT SELECTION AND EXPLANATION

- **St 40, Ren 9, Sp 9** – classical point combination to remove dampness and phlegm.[29]

- **St 36, Sp 3, Sp 8** – tonify Spleen to remove phlegm.[30]

- **Ren 3** – assists in the transforming function of Qi, regulates the room of sperm.

- **Ki 13** – circulates fluids and solves running piglet syndrome.

- **Liv 5** – important point for any genital problem, spreads Liver Qi.

Protocol if you do not get the pattern

Ren 4, Bl 23, Bl 32, Bl 35, St 36, Sp 6, Liv 3.

ACUPUNCTURE POINTS FOR MALE ON DAY OF SPERM DONATION[31]

We can only influence vitality and motility with this acupuncture sperm-booster, not the other parameters!

- **Ren 4** (deep needling!), **Ki 3, Ki 6, Lu 7** – reinforce Kidney Qi.

- **Ren 4 and Ren 6** with moxa (if cold), **Du 20** – fortify Yang.

- **St 29 and Sp 6** with EA (2 or 10 Hz, 5–10 minutes same side together) – regulate Blood flow to the testicles.

- **Sp 10, Liv 5, PC6** – reinforce and regulate Qi and Blood supply.

- **Liv 3, LI 4** – free flow of Qi.

- **Gb 41, TH 5** – clear damp-heat in Lower Jiao if necessary.

CHAPTER 16

Treatment Options from the Chinese Medicine 'Bag of Tricks' – Herbs

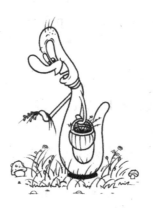

When looking for the ideal prescription for your patient, think your way through the diagram below. This special style of creating a herbal formula to treat male fertility issues is taught by Simon Becker, whom I truly admire for his unique didactics.

In Chapter 14, we sorted out the signs and symptoms to get the right pattern discrimination. Every pattern has its own guiding formula, often far more than one classic prescription, so you can choose the one that best suits your patient.

But now comes the very special unicorn power that gives the classical prescription you choose the important glitter, the two-step twist that makes you a prescriber 2.0.

The abnormalities in the semen analysis can also be categorized into patterns that can be considered just as much as the signs and symptoms of the patient, when defining a pattern. Finally, the classic prescription chosen and special medicinals are added, either according to the pattern or – more integrative – to the pathologies in the semen analysis.

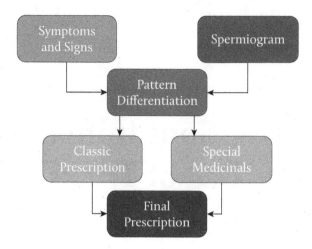

In this chapter, we will go through this special prescriptive style step by step, starting with the particular guiding formula for every pattern mentioned in Chapter 13.

GUIDING FORMULAS ACCORDING TO PATTERNS

Remember when I introduced myself as being kind of a curator of a gallery that collects the best pictures and brings them together in one place for people to look at and learn from? That is exactly how the presentation of the guiding formulas works. I combed through different sources, and here I can present my findings. As always, ask three doctors, get three diagnoses. It is the same with the perfect guiding formula for a pattern. With some patterns, the various authors are surprisingly concordant and in some not at all. It is up to you, as a prescriber, to choose the best one for your individual patient; these are just suggestions. It is only you who knows your patient, never a textbook! (Note: Next to the formula's name are the names of the authors using them in their books. Those books are listed in the Notes and Further Reading sections.)

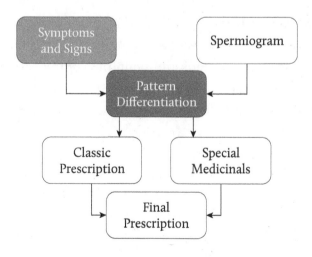

Kidney Yin deficiency

Basically, it comes down to four commonly suggested formulas for the herbal treatment of that pattern (see those *underlined*), or a combination of them.

Zuo Gui Wan (Restore the Left (Kidney) Pill) (Lin, Franconi, Weixin, Becker)

Shu Di Huang *Rx. Rehmanniae Preparata*
Shan Yao *Rx. Dioscoreae*
Gou Qi Zi *Fr. Lycii*
Shan Zhu Yu *Fr. Cornii*
Chuan Niu Xi *Rx. Cyathulae*
Tu Si Zi *Sm. Cuscutae*
Lu Jiao Jiao *Colla Cervi Cornus*
Gui Ban Jiao *Colla Plastrum Testudinis*

This formula nourishes Yin, tonifies the Kidneys without overheating or overloading and supplements Jing.

Liu Wei Di Huang Wan (Six-Ingredient Pill with Rehmannia) (Lin, Franconi, Weixin)

Shu Di Huang *Rx. Rehmanniae Preparata*
Shan Zhu Yu *Fr. Corni*
Shan Yao *Rx. Dioscoreae*
Fu Ling *Poria*
Mu Dan Pi *Cx. Moutan*
Ze Xie *Rhiz. Alismatis*

Nourishes Kidney Yin and also Liver Yin, clears empty-heat a little.

Wu Zi Yan Zong Wan (Five Ancestors Pill) (Glover, Franconi)

Gou Qi Zi *Fr. Lycii*	18 g
Fu Pen Zi *Fr. Rubi*	15 g
Che Qian Zi *Sm. Plantaginis*	15 g
Tu Si Zi *Sm. Cuscutae*	18 g
Wu Wei Zi *Fr. Schisandrae*	6 g

This formula is a brilliant all-in-one sperm-boosting composition. It supports Qi, Yin, Yang and Jing, secures Essence, eliminates damp-heat and heat in the Liver. *Fu Pen Zi* overall increases testosterone levels; *Gou Qi Zi* and *Tu Si Zi* improve sperm motility.

Zuo Gui Yin (Restore the Left (Kidney) Decoction) (Weixin, Glover)

Shu Di Huang Rx. Rehmanniae Preparata	12 g
Shan Yao Rx. Dioscoreae	12 g
Gou Qi Zi Fr. Lycii	12 g
Fu Ling Poria	12 g
Zhi Gan Cao Rx. Glycyrrhizae Preparata	3 g

This formula tonifies the Kidney and nourishes Yin. *Zuo Gui Yin* is less potent than *Zuo Gui Wan* and is used for milder and moderate cases of Kidney Yin deficiency. To further nourish Kidney Yin: *Gui Ban*, *Nu Zhen Zi*. To nourish Blood: *He Shou Wu*, *Bai Shao*, *Gou Qi Zi*.

Modification: *Wu Zi Yan Zong Wan* + *Zuo Gui Yin* (Damone, Dou)

Gou Qi Zi Fr. Lycii	15 g
Fu Pen Zi Fr. Rubi	15 g
Che Qian Zi Sm. Plantaginis	20 g
Tu Si Zi Sm. Cuscutae	15 g
Wu Wei Zi Fr. Schisandrae	10 g
Shu Di Huang Rx. Rehmanniae Preparata	10 g
Shan Yao Rx. Dioscoreae	10 g
Shan Zhu Yu Fr. Corni	10 g
Fu Ling Poria	10 g
Zhi Gan Cao Rx. Glycyrrhizae Prep	3 g

If there is a lot of empty-heat presenting, *Zhi Bai Di Huang Wan* (Phellodendron and Rehmannia Pill) is suggested (Lyttleton, Lin, Damone, Focks):

Zhi Mu Rx. Anemarrhenae
Huang Bai Cx. Phellodendri
Shu Di Huang Rx. Rehmanniae Preparata
Shan Zhu Yu Fr. Corni
Shan Yao Rx. Dioscoreae
Fu Ling Poria
Mu Dan Pi Cx. Moutan
Ze Xie Rhiz. Alismatis

Clears excess heat from the Lower Burner and nourishes Kidney Yin. Bob Damone adds *Che Qian Zi*, *Cang Zhu*, *Bi Xie* and *Tu Fu Ling* if there is also damp-heat in the Lower Burner.

Ye Ha Sheng Jing Tang (Maciocia)

Mu Dan Pi *Cx Moutan*
Di Gu Pi *Cx Lycii*
Chi Shao *Rx. Paeoniae Rubra*
Bai Shao *Rx. Paenoniae Alba*
Shan Zhu Yu *Fr. Corni*
Lian Qiao *Fr. Forsythiae*
Xia Ku Cao *Spica Prunellae*
Chai Hu *Rx. Bupleuri*
Dan Zhu Ye *Hb. Lophateri*
Fu Ling *Poria*
Sheng Di Huang *Rx Rehmanniae*
Xuan Shen *Rx Scrophulariae*
Mai Men Dong *Rx Ophiopogonis*
Zhe Bei Mu *Blb. Fritillariae Thunbergii*
Dan Shen *Rx. Slaviae Miltiorrhizae*
Gou Qi Zi *Fr. Lycii*
Yin Yang Huo *Hb. Epimedii*
Mu Li *Concha Ostrae*

Addendum: Becker's hitlist of Yin-deficiency medicinals

- **Nu Zhen Zi** *Fr. Ligustri Lucidi*

- **Huang Jing** *Rhiz. Polygonati*

- **Yu Zhu** *Rhiz. Polygonati Odorati*

- **Sang Shen** *Fr. Mori Fructus*

Kidney Yang deficiency

With this pattern, there are two formulas suggested by most of the authors (see those <u>underlined</u>), However, various other recommendations for prescriptions exist from various authors.

<u>*You Gui Wan*</u> (Restore the Right (Kidney) Pill) (Lin, Becker, Franconi)

Shu Di Huang *Rx. Rehmanniae Preparata*
Shan Yao *Rhiz. Dioscorea*
Shan Zhu Yu *Fr. Corni*

Gou Qi Zi Fr. Lycii
Du Zhong Cx. Eucommiae
Tu Si Zi Sm. Cuscutae
Fu Zi Rx. Aconiti lat. prep
Rou Gui Cx. Cinnamomi
Lu Jiao Jiao Cornu Cervi gelat.

Warms and tonifies Kidney Yang, replenishes Essence and Blood and Ming Men fire. Franconi advises the addition of He Shou Wu.

Jin Gui Shen Qi Wan (Kidney Qi Pill) (Franconi)

Shu Di Huang Rx. Rehmanniae Preparata
Shan Zhu Yu Fr. Corni
Shan Yao Rx. Dioscoreae
Fu Zi Aconiti Rx lat. prep
Gui Zhi Ram. Cinnamomi
Fu Ling Poria
Mu Dan Pi Cx. Moutan
Ze Xie Rhiz. Alismatis

Warms and tonifies the Kidneys, especially Kidney Yang. It is combined with other formulas such as:

Modified *Jin Gui Shen Qi Wan* + *Wu Zi Yan Zong Wan* (Dou, Zhi-Qiang)

Fu Zi Rx. Aconiti Lat. Prep	10 g
Rou Gui Cx. Cinnamomi	10 g
Shu Di Huang Rx. Rehmanniae Preparata	10 g
Shan Zhu Yu Fr. Corni	10 g
Shan Yao Rx. Dioscoreae	10 g
Tu Si Zi Sm. Cuscutae	10 g
Rou Cong Rong Hb. Cistanches	10 g
Xian Mao Rhiz. Curculiginis	10 g
Yin Yang Huo Hb. Epimedii	10 g
Wu Wei Zi Fr. Schisandrae	10 g
Gou Qi Zi Fr. Lycii	15 g

This combination strengthens the Kidneys, warms Yang and nourishes Essence. It strengthens the Yin in Yang. As quoted by the famous Zhang Jing-yue, 'If Yang is supported by Yin, his creation and transformation is endless'. The authors Zhi-Qiang, Li-Yun and Li suggest the same combination but add Fu Pen Zi Fr. Rubi 15 g for more Essence astringency.

Modified *You Gui Wan + Wu Zi Yan Zong Wan* (Damone)

Fu Zi Aconiti Rx. Aconiti Lateralis Preparata	6 g
Rou Gui Cx. Cinnamomi	6 g
Shu Di Huang Rx. Rehmanniae Preparata	10 g
Shan Zhu Yu Fr. Corni	12 g
Shan Yao Rx. Dioscoreae	12 g
Lu Jiao Jiao Cervi Cornu gelat	6 g
Du Zhong Cx. Eucommiae	15 g
Gou Qi Zi Fr. Lycii	15 g
Dang Gui Rx. Angelicae Sinensis	12 g
Wu Wei Zi Fr. Schisandrae	10 g
Fu Pen Zi Fr. Rubi	10 g
Tu Si Zi Sm. Cuscutae	15 g
Rou Cong Rong Hb Cistanches	10 g
Xian Mao Rhiz. Curculiginis	10 g
Yin Yang Huo Hb. Epimedii	12 g

Following the principle of never to forget to also nourish Kidney Yin when tonifying Kidney Yang, this formula consists of a lot of Yang tonics but also herbs to nourish Yin and Blood and to secure the Essence (*Wu Wei Zi*, *Fu Pen Zi*).

Da Tu Si Zi Wan (Major Cuscuta Pill) (Lin)

Tu Si Zi Sm. Cuscutae
Nu Zhen Zi Fr. Ligustri Lucidi
Gou Qi Zi Fr. Lycii
He Shou Wu Rx. Polygoni Multiflori
Shu Di Huang Rx. Rehmanniae Preparata
Shan Zhu Yu Fr. Corni
Han Lian Cao Hb. Ecliptae Prostratae
Sang Shen Fr. Mori Albae
Bu Gu Zhi Fr. Psoralae Corylifoliae
Rou Cong Rong Hb. Cistanches

It warms and reinforces Kidney Yang, warms Ming Men fire and includes a lot of astringent herbs to secure Kidneys and Jing and prevent abnormal leakage (e.g. seminal emission).

Zan Yu Dan (Special Pill to Aid Fertility) (Glover, Lin)

Shu Di Huang Rx. Rehmanniae Preparata	24 g
Bai Zhu Rhiz. Atractylodes Macrocephalae	24 g
Dang Gui Rx. Angelicae Sinensis	18 g
Gou Qi Zi Fr. Lycii	18 g
Du Zhong Cx. Eucommiae	12 g
Xian Mao Rhiz. Curculiginis	12 g
Shan Zhu Yu Fr. Corni	12 g
Yin Yang Huo Hb. Epimedii	12 g
Rou Cong Rong Hb. Cistanches	12 g
Jiu Cai Zi Sm. Allii Tuberosi	12 g
She Chuan Zi Sm. Cnidii Monneri	6 g
(Zhi) Fu Zi Rx. Aconiti Lat. Prep	6 g
Rou Gui Cx. Cinnamomi	6 g

Commonly used for Kidney Yuan Qi, Essence and Yang vacuity with infertility.

Wu Zi Yan Zong Wan (Five Ancestors Pill) (Maciocia)

Gou Qi Zi Fr. Lycii	18 g
Fu Pen Zi Fr. Rubi	15 g
Che Qian Zi Sm. Plantaginis	15 g
Tu Si Zi Sm. Cuscutae	18 g
Wu Wei Zi Fr. Schisandrae	6 g

This formula is a brilliant all-in-one sperm-boosting composition. It supports Yin, Qi, Yang and Jing, secures Essence, eliminates damp-heat and heat in the Liver. *Fu Pen Zi* overall increases testosterone levels; *Gou Qi Zi* and *Tu Si Zi* improve sperm motility.

You Gui Yin (Restore the Right Kidney Decoction) (Weixin, Glover)

Shu Di Huang Rx. Rehmanniae Preparata	15 g
Shan Yao Rhiz. Dioscorea	6 g
Shan Zhu Yu Fr. Corni	3 g
Gou Qi Zi Fr. Lycii	6 g
Du Zhong Cx. Eucommiae	6 g
Fu Zi Rx. Aconiti Lat. Prep.	3 g
Rou Gui Cx. Cinnamomi	3 g

This formula warms the Kidneys and replenishes the Essence. To tonify Kidney Yang even more, Glover adds *Tu Si Zi* (*Semen Cuscutae Chinesis*) 6 g and *Ba Ji Tian* (*Radix Morindae Officinalis*) 6 g.

Er Xian Tang (Two Immortals Decoction) (Weixin)

Xian Mao *Rhiz. Curculiginis*
Yin Yang Huo *Hb. Epimedii*
Ba Ji Tian *Rx. Morindae Officinalis*
Huang Bai *Cx. Phellodendri*
Zhi Mu *Rhiz. Anemarrhenae*
Dang Gui *Rx. Angelicae Sinensis*

Replenishes Kidney Yin and Yang, tonifies Kidney Jing and also purges deficiency fire. Regulates the Chong and Ren which are very important channels for fertility.

Gui Ling Ji (Tortoise Age Placenta Pill) (Franconi)

Ba Ji Tian *Rx. Morindae Officinalis*
Bu Gu Zhi *Fr. Psoralae*
Chuan Shan Jia *Sq. Mantis*
Du Zhong *Cx. Eucommiae*
Ding Xiang *Fl. Caryophylli*
Zhi Gan Cao *Rx. Glycyrrhizae Preparata*
Gou Qi Zi *Fr. Lycii*
Huang Qi *Rx. Astragali*
Lu Jiao *C. Cervi*
Huai Niu Xi *Rx. Achyranthis Bidentatae*
Ren Shen *Rx. Ginseng*
Rou Cong Rong *Hb. Cistanches*
Sha Ren *Fr. Amomi*
Shu Di Huang *Rx. Rehmanniae Preparata*
Suo Yang *Hb. Cynomorii*
Tian Men Dong *T. Asparagus*
Tu Si Zi *Sm. Cuscutae*
Ye Ju Hua *Fl. Crysanthemi Indici*
Yin Yang Huo *Hb. Epimedii*
Da Qing Yan Halitum

Used for Kidney Yang vacuity reaching all the organs. General Qi, Blood and Yang vacuity.

Pi Shen Shuan Bu Wan (Focks)

Dang Sheng Rx. Codonopsis	24 g
Ba Ji Tian Rx. Morindae Officinalis	9 g
Shan Yao Rhiz. Dioscoreae	12 g
Tu Si Zi Sm. Cuscutae	9 g
Shan Zhu Yu Fr. Corni	9 g
Sha Ren Fr. Amomi	6 g
Chen Pi Peric. Citri Reticulatae	4.5 g
Rou Dou Kou Sm. Myristicae	9 g
Bu Gu Zhi Fr. Psoralae	9 g
Wu Wei Zi Fr. Schisandrae	6 g
Lian Zi Sm Nelumbinis	12 g

If there is Kidney Yang deficiency accompanied by Spleen Yang-deficiency symptoms, such as thin stools and diarrhoea in the morning, use this one in combination with another Kidney Yang formula.

Addendum: Becker's hitlist of Yang-deficiency medicinals

- **Fu Pen Zi** Fr. Rubii
- **Tu Si Zi** Sm. Cuscutae
- **Du Zhong** Cx. Eucommiae
- **Xu Duan** Rx. Dipsaci
- **Yin Yang Huo** Hb. Epimedii
- **Ba Ji Tian** Rx. Morindae Officinalis
- **Xian Mao** Rhiz. Curculiginis
- **Huang Qi** Rx. Astragali
- **Lu Rong** Cornu Cervi Pantotrichum

Kidney Essence deficiency

Wu Zi Yan Zong Wan (Five Ancestors Pill) (Lin, Franconi, Glover)

Gou Qi Zi Fr. Lycii	18 g

Fu Pen Zi Fr. Rubi	15 g
Che Qian Zi Sm. Plantaginis	15 g
Tu Si Zi Sm. Cuscutae	18 g
Wu Wei Zi Fr. Schisandrae	6 g

This formula is a brilliant all-in-one sperm-boosting composition. It supports Kidney Yin, Kidney Yang and Jing, secures Essence, eliminates damp-heat and heat in the Liver. It tonifies the Kidneys and replenishes Essence. It can be used in most fertility patients as it warms but does not overheat, nourishes but is not overloading. *Fu Pen Zi* moreover increases testosterone levels. *Gou Qi Zi* and *Tu Si Zi* improve sperm motility (Glover).

Qi Zi Er Xian Wan (Seven Seed Two Immortals Pill) (Becker)

Gou Qi Zi Fr. Lycii
Fu Pen Zi Fr. Rubi
Che Qian Zi Sm. Plantaginis
Tu Si Zi Sm. Cuscutae
Wu Wei Zi Fr. Schisandrae
Xian Mao Rhiz. Curculiginis
Jiu Cai Zi Sm. Allii Tuberosi
Shen Zi Fr. Mori Albae
Dang Shen Rx. Codonopsis Pilosulae

In his original text, Becker refers to Huang Jing-juan *et al.* who do recommend that the formula should be prepared as a paste and that 10 g of that paste should be taken three times a day. The formula is based on *Wu Zi Yan Zong Wan* and therefore also focuses on warming Yang, replenishing Essence and supplementing the Kidneys as well as strengthening the Spleen and nourishing the Liver. It follows the principle of 'seeking Yang within Yin' and 'seeking Yin within Yang'. As its medicinals are level and harmonious, supplementing and not drying the formula is perfect for long-term use (Becker).

Bu Shen Yi Jing Fang (Supplement the Kidneys Benefit the Jing Formula) (Lyttleton)

He Shou Wu Rx. Polygonati Multiflori	15 g
Shu Di Huang Rx. Rehmanniae Preparata	15 g
Bai Shao Rx. Peoniae Alba	15 g
Gou Qi Zi Fr. Lycii	15 g
Shan Yao Rx. Dioscorea Oppositae	15 g
Shan Zhu Yu Fr. Corni	15 g
Nu Zhen Zi Fr. Ligustri Lucidi	15 g

Mu Dan Pi *Cx. Moutan*	15 g
Dang Shen *Rx. Codonopsis Pilosulae*	15 g
Huang Qi *Rx. Astragali*	15 g
Fu Pen Zi *Fr. Rubi*	15 g
Tu Si Zi *Sm. Cuscutae*	15 g
Yin Yang Huo *Hb. Epimedii*	15 g
Rou Cong Rong *Hb. Cistanches*	15 g
Ba Ji Tian *Rx. Morindae Officinalis*	12 g
Suo Yang *Hb. Cynamorii*	12 g
Dan Shen *Rx. Salviae Miltiorrhizae*	12 g
Lu Jiao Jiao *Cornu Cervi Parvum*	12 g
(**Gui Ban Jiao** *Gelat. PlastrumTestudinis*)	

This formula is a variation of *Bu Shen Sheng Jing Tang* (Supplement the Kidneys Engender Essence Decoction). It broadly addresses all the factors at play in Kidney-related male infertility. It includes Yang-tonifying herbs as well as Yin-supplementing ones. Bai Shao and He Shou Wu nourish the Blood, with He Shou Wu having a well-known effect on increasing semen quantity. Also there are three Qi tonics in there and Mu Dan Pi to clear heat. So it is a male fertility all-rounder when it comes to vacuity patterns as a cause.

Qi Bao Mei Sun (Ren) Wan (Seven-Treasure Special Pill for Beautiful Whiskers) (Lyttleton at HS)

He Shou Wu *Rx. Polygonati Multiflori*	15 g (300 g)
Gou Qi Zi *Fr. Lycii*	15 g (150 g)
Tu Si Zi *Sm. Cuscutae*	15 g (150 g)
Nu Zhen Zi *Fr. Ligustri Lucidi*	15 g*
Fu Ling *Poria*	15 g (150 g)
Dang Gui *Rx. Angelicae Sinensis*	15 g (150 g)
Bu Gu Zhi *Fr. Psoralae*	15 g (120 g)

* Anna Lin uses *Niu Xi Rx Achyratnis* 150 g instead.

Nourishes the Kidney and Liver Yin, replenishes the Kidney Essence, tonifies the Qi and nourishes the Blood. Processing *He Shou Wu* with *Hei Zhi Ma* (*Sm. Sesami Nigrum*) strengthens its Yin-nourishing properties. Anna Lin also recommends this formula. Her dosages are those in brackets above. Note: the ingredients are powdered and made into pills with one pill taken morning and evening per day which explains the dosage.

Nan Xing Bu Shen Fang (Men's Tonify Kidney Pill) (Franconi)

Bai Shao Rx. Peoniae Alba
Che Qian Zi Sm. Plantaginis
Fu Zi Rx. Aconiti Lat. Prep.
Fu Ling Poria
Rou Gui Cx. Cinnamomi
Shan Yao Rx. Dioscorea Oppositae
Shan Zhu Yu Fr. Corni
Shu Di Huang Rx. Rehmanniae Preparata
Wu Wei Zi Fr. Schisandrae
Ze Xie Rhiz. Alismatis

Gui Shen Wan (Restore the Kidneys Pill) (Weixin)

Shu Di Huang Rx. Rehmanniae Preparata
Shan Yao Rx. Dioscorea Oppositae
Shan Zhu Yu Fr. Corni
Fu Ling Poria
Gou Qi Zi Fr. Lyci
Du Zhong Cx. Eucommiae
Tu Si Zi Sm. Cuscutae
Dang Gui Rx. Angelicae Sinensis

Zuo Jia You Gui Wan ('Counterfeit' Restore the Right Kidney Pill) (Becker)

Shu Di Huang Rx. Rehmanniae Preparata
Shan Yao Rx. Dioscoreae
Shan Zhu Yu Fr. Corni
Gou Qi Zi Fr. Lycii
Chuan Niu Xi Rx. Cyathulae
Tu Si Zi Sm. Cuscutae
Lu Jiao Jiao Cornu Colla Cervi
Du Zhong Cx. Eucommiae
Fu Zi Rx. Aconiti Lat. Prep.
Rou Gui Cx. Cinnamomi
Gui Ban Jiao Colla Plastri Testudinis

Becker adds *Chuan Niu Xi* (*Rx. Cyathulae*) and *Gui Ban Jiao* (*Colla Plastri Testudinis*) to the classical formula. That's what makes it 'counterfeit'. *Gui Ban Jiao* focuses on Yin and Blood nourishment, whereas *Chuan Niu Xi* not only invigorates and regulates Blood but is also a guiding herb to the urogenital region.

Yi Jing Si Yu Tang (Boost Essence Birthing Success Decoction) (Becker)

Yin Yang Huo *Herba Epimedii*	30 g
Shu Di Huang *Radix Rehmanniae Preparata*	30 g
Shan Zhu Yu *Fructus Corni Officinalis*	15 g
Shan Yao *Radix Dioscoreae Oppositae*	15 g
Dan Shen *Radix Salviae Miltiorrhizae*	15 g
Dang Gui *Radix Angelicae Sinensis*	15 g
Tu Si Zi *Semen Cuscutae*	15 g
Gou Qi Zi *Fructus Lycii Chinensis*	15 g
Fu Pen Zi *Fructus Rubi*	15 g
Xian Mao *Rhiz. Curculiginis Orchioidis*	15 g
Hu Zhang *Rhiz. Polygoni Cuspidati*	15 g
Huang Bai *Cortex Phellodendri*	6 g

With this formula's herbs, Kidney Yin and Yang are supplemented simultaneously; in addition, it uses heat-clearing and toxin-resolving medicinals. *Dang Gui* and *Dan Shen* supplement and nourish the Blood, so as to make Blood exuberant and full and Essence sufficient. Both herbs also have the function of quickening the Blood and transforming stasis, and thus can promote the metabolism of the organism and reproductive organs. *Hu Zhang* and *Huang Bai* clear heat, resolve toxins and dry dampness, as well moving stasis and freeing stagnation. According to the author of the formula, Chen Jing-Rong, male sterility should not merely be attributed to either Kidney vacuity patterns or to Kidney repletion patterns. Rather, a combination of vacuity and repletion is often seen (Becker).

Addendum: Becker's hitlist of Kidney medicinals:

- **Di Huang** *Rx. Rehmanniae*

- **Tu Si Zi** *Sm. Cuscutae*

- **Nu Zhen Zi** *Fr. Ligustri Lucidi*

- **Huang Jing** *Rhiz. Polygonati*

- **Wu Wei Zi** *Fr. Schisandrae*

- **Gou Qi Zi** *Fr. Lycii*

- **Yin Yang Huo** *Hb. Epimedii*

- **Ba Ji Tian** Rx. Morindae Officinalis

- **Xian Mao** Rhiz. Curculiginis

Spleen vacuity (Qi and Blood deficiency)

The selection of a guiding formula for this pattern depends on whether Blood or Qi is more depleted and moreover on the state of the Middle Burner (Spleen and Stomach). Therefore, there are various formulas offered and hardly any consensus on one guiding formula.

FOR QI VACUITY IN THE MIDDLE BURNER (SPLEEN AND STOMACH VACUITY)

Bu Zhong Yi Qi Tang (Tonify the Middle and Augment the Qi Decoction) (Lin)

Huang Qi Rx. Astragali
Ren Shen Rx. Ginseng
Bai Zhu Rhiz. Atractylodes Macrocephalae
Zhi Gan Cao Rx. Glycyrrhizae Prep
Dang Gui Rx. Angelicae Sinensis
Chen Pi Pericap. Citri Reticulatae
Sheng Ma Rhiz. Cimicifugae
Chai Hu Rx. Bupleuri

Clearly tonifies the Middle Burner, benefits the Qi and raises sunken Qi. This formula's approach is to supplement post-heaven Essence to enhance fertility. As a side-effect, *Bu Zhong Yi Qi Tang* protects sperm from AsAb as shown in in vitro studies.

If Spleen vacuity has turned into Yang vacuity, add *Fu Zi Li Zhong Wan* (Lin) to the above formula:

Ren Shen Rx. Ginseng
Bai Zhu Rhiz. Atractylodis Macrocephalae
Gan Jiang Rhiz. Zinigiberis
Zhi Gan Cao Rx Glycyrrhizae Prep.
Fu Zi Rx. Aconiti Prep.
Rou Gui Cx. Cinnamomi

It warms Yang, dispels cold, tonifies Qi and strengthens the Spleen to aid the herbs in *Bu Zhong Yi Qi Tang*.

IF QI AND BLOOD ARE EQUALLY DIMINISHED

Modified *Ba Zhen Sheng Jing Tang* (Eight Treasures Decoction to Promote Jing) (Dou, Zhi-Qiang, Franconi)

Huang Qi Rx. Astragali	15 g
Dang Shen Rx. Codonopsis	10 g
Bai Zhu Rhiz. Atractylodes Macrocephalae	10 g
Gan Cao Rx. Glycyrrhizae	3 g
Dang Gui Rx. Angelica Sinensis	10 g
Bai Shao Rx. Paeoniae Alba	10 g
Ejiao Asini Corii Collla	10 g
Shu di Huang Rx. Rehmanniae Preparata	15 g
Gou Qi Zi Fr. Lycii	15 g
Fu Ling Poria	10 g
Huang Jing Rhiz. Polygonati	15 g
Tu Si Zi Sm. Cuscutae	15 g
Zi He Che Placenta Hominis	15 g

With its Qi-tonifying and Blood-nourishing components, it supplements both substances equally. *Tu Si Zi, Gou Qi Zi, He Shou Wu* and *Zi He Che* fortify the Kidneys and hence help producing sperm. Human placenta is frequently substituted by pig or cattle placenta. Be careful that *Dang Gui* in this high dosage often leads to bloating in Western people with our modern lifestyle gut issues. This side-effect could be prevented by adding *Sha Ren*.

Anna Lin recommends this formula too but uses the well-known classic prescription *Ba Zhen Tang* without any modification.

She further offers as an alternative:

Shi Quan Da Bu Tang (Perfect Major Supplementation Decoction) (Lin)

Huang Qi Rx. Astragali
Ren Shen Rx. Ginseng
Rou Gui Cx. Cinnamomi
Bai Zhu Rhiz. Atractylodis Macrocephalae
Dang Gui Rx. Angelicea Sinensis
Shu Di Huang Rx. Rehmanniae Preparata
Bai Shao Rx. Paeoniae Alba
Chuan Xiong Rhiz. Ligustici Wallichii
Fu Ling Poria
Zhi Gan Cao Rx. Glycyrrhizae Prep.

Replenishes Yang and warms and tonifies Qi and Blood.

Bob Damone combines the above with modified *Yu Lin Zhu* (Unicorn-Rearing Pill) in cases of dual vacuity of Spleen and Kidney Qi and insufficiency of Heart and Liver Blood as the added herbs more focus on supplementing the Kidneys.

Huang Qi Rx. Astragali	30 g
Ren Shen Rx. Ginseng	15 g
Rou Gui Cx. Cinnamomi	6 g
Chao Bai Zhu Rhiz. Atractylodis Macrocephalae frictum	15 g
Dang Gui Rx. Angelica Sinensis	12 g
Shu Di Huang Rx Rehmanniae Preparata	12 g
Bai Shao Rx. Peoniae Alba	12 g
Chuan Xiong Rhiz. Ligustici Wallicii	10 g
Fu Ling Poria	12 g
Zhi Gan Cao Rx Glycyrrhizae praep.	3 g

Added *Yu Lin Zhu* medication:

Tu Si Zi Sm. Cuscutae	15 g
Gou Qi Zi Fr. Lycii	15 g
Shan Yao Rhiz. Dioscorae Opp.	15 g
Shan Zhu Yu Fr. Corni	12 g
Du Zhong Cx. Eucommiae	15 g
Lu Jiao Jiao Cervi Cornus Gelatinum	10 g
Hua Jiao Peric. Zanthoxyli	3 g

Focks also suggests a modification of *Yu Lin Zhu* that includes *Ba Ji Tian (Rx. Morindae)* 9 g and *Tao Ren (Sm. Persicae)* 15 g.

IF QI VACUITY IS PREDOMINANT

Liu Jun Zi Tang (Six Gentlemen Decoction) (Lin)

Ren Shen Rx. Ginseng	10 g
Bai Zhu Rhiz. Atractylodes Macrocephalae	10 g
Fu Ling Poria	10 g
Zhi Gan Cao Rx. Glycyrrhizae Prep.	3 g
Chen Pi Pericap. Citri Reticulatae	10 g
Ban Xia Rhiz. Pinelliae Ternatae	10 g

This well-known classical prescription is commonly used for Spleen and Stomach Qi deficiency accompanied by dampness and phlegm. If this formula is modified by adding *Sha Ren*, *Mu Xiang* and *Sheng Jiang*, it becomes a formula named *Xiang Sha Liu Jun Zi Tang*, which is recommended by Weixin if you also want to address cold.

Liu Jun Zi Tang can also be used combined with *Wu Zi Yan Zhong Wan*, according to Anna Lin:

Gou Qi Zi Fr. Lycii
Fu Pen Zi Fr. Rubi
Che Qian Zi Sm. Plantaginis
Tu Si Zi Sm. Cuscutae
Wu Wei Zi Fr. Schisandrae

Alternatively, following Zhi-Qiang and Li-Yun, a variation of *Wu Zi Yan Zhong Wan* named *Shi Zi Tang* is used together with *Liu Jun Zi Tang*. Dou recommends the same combination of formulas if both Spleen and Kidney are deficient.

Shi Zi Tang (Ten Semen Decoction)

Tu Si Zi Sm. Cuscutae	15 g
Sang Shen Zi Fr. Mori	15 g
Gou Qi Zi Fr. Lycii	15 g
Nu Zhen Zi Fr. Ligustri Lucidi	15 g
Bu Gu Zhi Fr. Psoralae	15 g
She Chuang Zi Fr. Cnidii	15 g
Fu Pen Zi Fr. Rubi	10 g
Jin Ying Zi Fr. Rosae Laevigatae	10 g
Wu Wei Zi Fr. Schisandrae Chinensis	10 g
Che Qian Zi Sm. Plantaginis	20 g

It tonifies Yin as well as Yang, is drying as well as moistening. Combined with *Liu Jun Zi Tang*, it strengthens Spleen and Kidney, tonifies Qi, nourishes Blood and refills Kidney Essence.

IF BLOOD VACUITY IS MORE DOMINANT IN THIS PATTERN

Gui Pi Tang (Restore the Spleen Decoction) (Lin)

Ren Shen Rx. Ginseng
Huang Qi Rx. Astragali
Bai Zhu Rhiz. Atractylodes Macrocephalae
Fu Ling Poria

Suan Zao Ren Sm. Ziziphi Spinosae
Long Yan Rou Arillus Longan
Zhi Gan Cao Rx. Glycyrrhizae Prep.
Mu Xiang Rx. Saussurae
Dang Gui Rx. Angelicea Sinensis
Zhi Yuan Zhi Rx. Polygalae Prep.
Sheng Jiang Rx. Zingiberis Recens
Da Zao Fr. Jujubae

Being a well-known classical formula for the treatment of Spleen Qi deficiency and Heart Blood deficiency, it targets the problem of this pattern.

A variation of the above is *Ren Shen Gui Pi Wan*, which is recommended by Franconi:

Ren Shen Rx. Ginseng
Huang Qi Rx. Astragali
Bai Zhu Rhiz. Atractylodes Macrocephalae
Fu Ling Poria
Shan Yao Rhiz. Dioscorae
Xiang Fu Rhiz. Cyperi
Sha Ren Fr. Amomi
Chen Pi Pericarp. Citri Reticulatae
Zhi Yuan Zhi Rx. Polygalae
Dang Gui Rx. Angelicae Sinensis
Suan Zao Ren Sm. Ziziphi Spinosae

Often it is prescribed for chronically overworked men with intellectual exhaustion as both *Chen Pi* and especially *Xiang Fu* treat Liver Qi stagnation perfectly.

Liver Qi depression

Obviously, this is the pattern with the greatest agreement on how to treat it. The formula is:

Xiao Yao San (Free and Easy Wanderer Powder) (Lyttleton)

Chai Hu Rx. Bupleuri		9 g
Bai Shao Rx. Paeoniae Alba		12 g
Dang Gui Rx. Angelicae Sinensis		9 g
Bai Zhu Rhiz. Atractylodis Mac.		9 g
Fu Ling Poria		15 g
Sheng Jiang Rhiz. Zingiberis		3 g

Bo He *Hb. Menthae*	3 g
Gan Cao *Rx. Glycyrrhizae Uralensis*	3 g

It is the most commonly prescribed formula in the Western world, as it resolves Liver Qi stagnation but also nourishes Blood. If there are signs of heat, make it *Jia Wei Xiao Yao San* by adding *Zhi Zi* and *Mu Dan Pi*, which will help clear heat.

Si Ni San Jia Jian (modified Frigid Extremities Powder) (Becker)

Chai Hu *Rx. Bupleuri*	9 g
Bai Shao *Rx. Paeoniae Alba*	10 g
Mu Xiang *Rx. Aucklandiae*	9 g
Chen Pi *Peric. Citri Reticulatae*	6 g
Gan Cao *Rx. Glycyrrhizae*	6 g

Becker prefers *Chen Pi* over the classically used *Zhi Shi* due to its warm nature and because it also strengthens and benefits the Spleen. *Mu Xiang* is added to have another Qi-regulating herb in the formula. Anna Lin also uses this formula, but in its classic version.

Chai Hu Shu Gan Tang (Bupleurum Powder to Spread the Liver) (Lin)

Chai Hu *Rx. Bupleuri*
Bai Shao *Rx. Paeoniae Alba*
Zhi Ke *Fr. Aurantii*
Chuan Xiong *Rhiz. Ligustici Wallichii*
Xiang Fu *Rhiz. Cyperi*
Gan Cao *Rx. Glycyrrhizae*

To help to decide whether to use *Chai Hu Shu Gan San* rather than *Xiao Yao San*, there are two main points to consider: Liver is constrained with Qi stagnation, leading to Blood stasis and a wiry but not weak pulse!

Unnamed formula (Lin)

Chai Hu *Rx. Bupleuri*
Tai Wu Yao *Rx. Linderae Strychnifoliae*
Ju He *Sm. Citri Aurantii*
Chen Xiang *Lign. Aquilariae Agallochae*
Xiang Fu *Rhiz. Cyperi Rotundi*
Bai Shao *Rx. Paeoniae Albae*
Dang Gui *Rx. Angelicae Sinensis*

Yin Yang Huo *Hb. Epimedii*
Xian Mao *Rhiz. Curculiginis Orchoidis*
Gan Cao *Rx. Glycyrrhizae*

With the first five herbs coming from the category of Qi-regulating herbs, the focus of this formula is clear. But it also contains two Blood-tonifying herbs as well as two Yang tonics. Yang tonics are known to increase the ATP production in the mitochondria; for sperm cells, that means that motility increases.

If Liver Qi stagnation comes along with Kidney deficiency (for explanation see the section above: Kidney Yin deficiency), Maciocia recommends:

Zhi Bai Di Huang Wan (Phellodendron and Rehmannia Pill)

Zhi Mu *Rx. Anemarrhenae*
Huang Bai *Cx. Phellodendri*
Shu Di Huang *Rx. Rehmanniae Preparata*
Shan Zhu Yu *Fr. Corni*
Shan Yao *Rx. Dioscoreae*
Fu Ling *Poria*
Mu Dan Pi *Cx. Moutan*
Ze Xie *Rhiz. Alismatis*

Another option would be to use:

Modified Kai Yu Zhong Yu Tang (Opening Stagnation and Growing Jade Decoction) (Focks)

Chai Hu *Rx. Bupleuri*	9 g
Bai Shao *Rx. Paeoniae Alba*	15 g
Dang Gui *Rx. Angelicae Sinensis*	12 g
Bai Zhu *Rhiz. Atractylodis Mac.*	9 g
Fu Ling *Poria*	12 g
Xiang Fu *Rhiz. Cyperi Rotundi*	9 g
Ju He *Sm. Citri Aurantii*	9 g
Tian Hua Fen *Rx. Trichosantis*	12 g
Tao Ren *Sm. Persicae*	9 g
Wang Bu Liu Xing *Sm. Vaccariae*	15 g

This formula is a variation of *Xiao Yao San*. It is commonly used for infertility due to Liver disorders as it nourishes the Blood, tonifies the Spleen, soothes the Liver and clears Liver heat. The modification Focks offers adds *Ju He* as a Qi regulator, *Tao Ren* as a

Blood-regulating and invigorating herb as well as *Wang Bu Liu Xing*. The latter is a guiding herb to the testicles as well.

Yue Ju Wan (Escape Restraint Pill) (Glover)

Cang Zhu *Rhiz. Atractylodis Lanceae*	6 g
Chuan Xiong *Rx Ligustici Chuanxiong*	6 g
Xiang Fu *Rhiz. Cyperi Rotundi*	6 g
Zhi Zi *Fr. Gardeniae Jasminoidis*	6 g
Shen Qu *Massa Fermenta Medicinalis*	6 g

This formula regulates Qi and releases all types of stagnation (Qi, Blood, phlegm, fire, food and dampness). Possible modifications to intensify the Qi-moving aspect of the formula would be *Chai Hu* and *Chuan Lian Zi*.

Jia Wei Shao Yao Gan Cao Tang (Extended Peony and Licorice Decoction)

Bai Shao *Rx. Paeoniae Albae*	18 g
Zhi Gan Cao *mix-fried Rx. Glycyrrhizae Uralensis*	18 g
Tu Si Zi *Semen Cuscutae Chinesis*	15 g
He Huan Pi *Cx. Albizziae Julibrissinis*	15 g
Mai Ya *Fructus Germinatus Hordei Vulgaris*	15 g
Gou Qi Zi *Fuctus Lycii Chinensis*	10 g
Dang Gui *Rx. Angelicae Sinensis*	10 g
Yin Yang Huo *Hb. Epimedii*	10 g

This expanded formula, compared with the classic one that only consists of *Bai Shao* and *Gan Cao*, could be used as an add-on to other prescriptions of this section. The twist about it is that in a case series study it turned out that *Jia Wei Shao Yao Tang* increases testosterone levels up to normal and treats hyperprolactinemia in men by normalizing this parameter as well. This could not only be useful in impotence as in the study, but also for male-factor infertility.[1]

Blood stasis

Surprisingly consensual are the suggestions for the best formula to treat Blood stasis. It comes down to *Xue Fu Zhu Yu Tang*, which is recommended by almost every author, amended by various single named formulas from different authors.

Xue Fu Zhu Yu Tang (Decoction for Removing Blood Stasis in the Chest) (Lyttleton)

Dang Gui Rx. Angelicae Sinensis	12 g
Sheng Di Huang Rx. Rehmanniae Glutinosae	9 g
Chi Shao Rx. Paeoniae Rubrae	6 g
Chuan Xiong Rx. Ligustici Chuanxiong	6 g
Tao Ren Sm. Persicae	12 g
Hong Hua Fl. Carthami	9 g
Chai Hu Rx. Bupleuri	3 g
Zhi Ke Fr. Citri seu Ponciri	6 g
Chuan Niu Xi Rx. Cyathulae	9 g
Jie Geng Rx. Platycodi Grandiflori	6 g
Gan Cao Rx. Glycyrrhiazae	3 g

Another very well-known formula that invigorates Blood but also dispels Blood stasis, spreads Liver Qi and unblocks the channels. Most modern texts replace *Niu Xi* (*Rx. Achyranthis Bidentatae*) with *Chuan Niu Xi* (as in our formula above). According to Bensky as well as Chen, *Chuan Niu Xi* is stronger in activating Blood circulation, whereas *Huai Niu Xi* is stronger in tonifying the Liver and Kidney. That explanation makes it obvious why for the Blood stasis pattern *Chuan Niu Xi* should be preferred.

Zhi-Qiang modifies the formula by adding *Chuan Shan Jia* (*Sq. Mantis*), *Lu Lu Tong* (*Fr. Liquidambaris*), *Dan Shen* (*Rx. Salviae*) and *Wang Bu Liu Xing* (*Sm. Vaccariae*) for even more focus on solving Blood stasis. Additionally, *Lu Lu Tong* and *Wang Bu Liu Xing* work as guiding herbs to the testis.

Damone's modification includes *Lu Lu Tong* (*Fr. Liquidambaris*), *Dan Shen* (*Rx. Salviae*), *Wang Bu Liu Xing* (*Sm. Vaccariae*) as well as *San Leng* (*Rhiz. Sparganii*) and *E Zhu* (*Rhiz. Curcumae*). The last two not only invigorate Blood but also break Blood stasis.

Maciocia uses *Ge Xia Zhu Yu Tang* (Drive out Blood Stasis Below the Diaphragm Decoction) for Blood stasis and Qi stagnation:

Dang Gui Rx. Angelicae Sinensis	9 g
Chuan Xiong Rx. Ligustici Chuanxiong	6 g
Tao Ren Sm. Persicae	9 g
Mu Dan Pi Cx. Moutan	6 g
Chi Shao Rx. Paeoniae Rubrae	6 g
Wu Yao Rx. Linderae Strychnifoliae	6–12 g
Yan Hu Suo Rhiz. Corydalis	3 g
Gan Cao Rx. Glycyrrhizae	9 g
Xiang Fu Rhiz. Cyperi Rotundi	4.5 g

Hong Hua Fl. Carthami	9 g
Zhi Ke Fr. Citri seu Ponciri	4.5 g

This prescription invigorates the Blood, dispels Blood stasis and moves Qi and therefore stops pain. Commonly used for masses below the diaphragm and bearing-down sensation when lying down.

Simon Becker goes for *Shao Fu Zhu Yu Tang* as an alternative to *Xue Fu Zhu Yu Tang*, as does Glover:

Xiao Hui Xiang Fr. Foeniculi	2 g
Gan Jiang Rhiz. Zingiberis	1 g
Yan Hu Suo Rhiz. Corydalis	4 g
Mo Yao Myrrha	4 g
Dang Gui Rx. Angelicae sinensis	11 g
Chuan Xiong Rhiz. Chuanxiong	4 g
Rou Gui Cx. Cinnamomi	4 g
Chi Shao Rx. Paeoniae Rubra	4 g
Pu Huang Pollen Typhae	11 g
Wu Ling Zhi Faeces Trogopterori	7 g

This famous formula by Wangxinren states in the original text:

[T]his formula has a seemingly magical effect on planting seeds and therefore indicates its use for fertility problems especially when there is cold as an additional factor. Xiao Hui Xiang, Gan jiang, and Rou Gui are all acrid and warm or hot medicinals. Xiao Hui Xiang and Rou Gui enter the Lower Burner. This first group of medicinals hence not only warms the Lower Burner. Because of the acrid medicinals, it also moves qi and disperses cold. Thereby, it supports the movement of blood.[2]

Dou offers an unnamed prescription:

Chai Hu Rx. Bupleuri	10 g
Zhi Ke Fr. Citri seu Ponciri	10 g
Niu Xi Rx. Cyathulae	10 g
Tao Ren Sm. Persicae	10 g
Hong Hua Fl. Carthami	10 g
Chi Shao Rx. Paeoniae Rubrae	10 g
Dang Gui Rx. Angelicae Sinensis	10 g
Lu Lu Tong Fr. Liquidambaris	15 g
Dan Shen Rx. Salviae Milt.	20 g
Wang Bu Liu Xing Sm. Vaccariae	20 g
Chuan Shan Jia Sq. Mantis	15 g

This one really goes against Blood stasis by containing eight herbs from the category 'invigorate blood'. It might be necessary to add some Blood tonics for some patients.

Anna Lin offers two other options:

Tao Hong Si Wu Tang (Four Substances Decoction with Safflower and Peach Pit) (Lin)

Tao Ren *Semen Persicae*
Hong Hua *Flos Carthami*
Dang Gui *Radix Angelicae Sinensis*
Chuan Xiong *Rhizoma Chuanxiong*
Bai Shao *Radix Paeoniae Alba*
Shu Di Huang *Radix Rehmanniae Preparata*

This classical formula tonifies and invigorates the Blood, regulates Blood circulation and breaks up Blood stagnation.

Jiu Gui Shen Qi Wan modified (Kidney Pill)

Shu Di Huang *Rx. Rehmanniae Preparata*
Shan Zhu Yu *Fr. Corni*
Shan Yao *Rx. Dioscoreae*
Fu Zi *Rx. Aconiti Lat. Prep*
Gui Zhi *Ram. Cinnamomi*
Fu Ling *Poria*
Mu Dan Pi *Cx. Moutan*
Ze Xie *Rhiz. Alismatis*
+
Chuan Shan Jia *Sq. Mantis*
Wang Bu Liu Xing *Sm. Vaccariae*
Lu Lu Tong *Fr. Liquidambaris*
Niu Xi *Rx. Achyranthis Bidentatae*

This modification uses the warming and tonifying Kidney Yang effect of the basic formula and then adds strong Blood-moving herbs. On top of that it includes two guiding herbs, *Lu Lu Tong* to address the Lower Burner and *Wang Bu Liu Xing* to target the testicles directly.

Jill Glover suggests:

Ju He Wan (Tangerine Seed Pill) (Glover)

Ju He Sm. Citri Reticulatae	30 g
Chuan Lian Zi Fr. Meliae Toosendan	30 g
Yan Hu Suo Rhiz. Corydalis Yanhusuo	15 g
Mu Xiang Rx. Auklandiae Lappae	15 g
Tao Ren Sm. Persicae	30 g
Rou Gui Cx. Cinnamoni Cassiae	15 g
Mu Tong Caulis Mutong	15 g
Hou Po Cx. Magnoliae Officinalis	15 g
Zhi Shi Fr. Immaturus Citri Aurantii	15 g
Hai Zao Sargassum	30 g
Kun Bu Thallus Algae	30 g
Hai Dai Herba Laminaria Japonica	30 g

This formula is commonly used in Chinese Medicine andrology as its Western indications are hernia, orchitis, hydrocele and varicocele. It promotes the movement of Qi, softens hardness and dissipates nodules. As this formula traditionally is a Qi-regulating one, adding *San Leng* and *E Zhu* might be useful to focus more on solving Blood stasis.

Addendum: Becker's hitlist of stasis medicinals

- *Dan Shen* Rx. et Rhiz. Salviae Miltiorrhizae
- *E Zhu* Rhiz. Curcumae
- *San Leng* Rhiz. Sparganii
- *Mu Li* Conchae Ostrea
- *San Qi* Rx. et Rhiz. Notoginseng
- *Lu Lu Tong* Fr. Liquidambaris

Cold in the Liver

Not all authors describe this pattern, so the selection of prescriptions used is limited but quite coherent. To me, the pattern is relevant as a lot of male fertility patients do watersports and hence are prone to cold entering the Liver channel.

Nuan Gan Jian (Liver-Warming Brew) (Damone)

Rou Gui Cx. Cinnamomi	6 g

Xiao Hui Xiang Fr. Foeniculi	10 g
Wu Yao Rx. Linderae	10 g
Dang Gui Rx. Angelicae Sinensis	10 g
Fu Ling Poria	12 g
Sheng Jiang Rhiz. Zingiberis Recens	3 slices
Gou Qi Zi Fr. Lycii	15 g
Hu Lu Ba Sm. Trigonellae	10 g
Ba Ji Tian Rx. Morindae Officinalis	15 g

This formula warms the Liver and Kidneys, promotes Qi movement and dispels cold. It is used for lower abdominal pain that is sharp, localized and aggravated by the local application of cold and a swelling distention and pain of the scrotum.

Anna Lin uses the classical formula which excludes *Hu Lu Ba* and *Ba Ji Tian* but includes *Chen Xiang* (*Lign. Aquilariae Agallochae*).

Focks recommends a modification of:

Wen Jing Tang (Warm the Mensis (Collaterals) Decoction) (Focks)

Wu Zhu Yu Fr. Evodiae	3–6 g
Dang Gui Rx. Angelicae Sinensis	6–9 g
Bai Shao Rx. Paeoniae Albae	6 g
Chuan Xiong Rhiz. Ligustici Chuanxiong	6 g
Dang Shen Rx. Codonopsis	9 g
Gui Zhi Ram. Cinnamomi	6 g
E Jiao Colla Corii Asini	6–9 g
Ban Xia Rhiz. Pinelliae	6 g
Mu Dan Pi Cx. Moutan	6 g
Pao Jiang Rhiz. Zingiberis Prep.	6 g
Wu Yao Rx. Linderae	6–9 g
Xiao Hui Xiang Fr. Foeniculi	6 g
Li Zhi He Sm. Litchi	9–12 g

Commonly used for cold in the uterus, in our case it eliminates cold in the room of sperm. Additionally, it eliminates cold from Chong Mai and Ren Mai that is accompanied by Blood stasis. Interestingly, Dr Huang Huang describes the function of *Wen Jing Tang* as nourishing the Blood and enriching the Yin; to him it is first a moistening formula and second a warming formula. A good idea would be to combine the two formulas above to make *Nuan Gan Wen Jing Tang*.

Nuan Gan Wen Jing Tang (Warm the Liver and Jing Decoction)

Xiao Hui Xiang Fr. Foeniculi	15 g
Zi Shi Ying Amethystum	15 g
Ju He Sm. Citri	10 g
Li Zhi He Sm. Litchi	10 g
Fu Ling Poria	10 g
Jiu Cai Zi Sm. Allii Tuberosi	10 g
Rou Gui Cx. Cinnamomi	10 g
Ba Ji Tian Rx. Morindae Officinalis	6 g
Yin Yang Huo Hb. Epimedii	6 g
Wang Bu Liu Xing Sm. Vaccariae	6 g
Shen Jin Cao Hb. Lycopodii	12 g

Dang Gui Si Ni Tang (Dang Gui Decoction for Frigid Extremities) (Lin)

Dang Gui Rx. Angelicae Sinensis
Gui Zhi Ram. Cinnamomi
Bai Shao Rx. Paeoniae Albae
Mu Tong Caulis Akebiae Mutong
Xi Xin Hb. Cum Rad. Asari
Da Zao Fr. Ziziphi Jujubae
Zhi Gan Cao Rx. Glycyrrhizae Prep.

Warms the channels and disperses cold, nourishes the Blood and unblocks the Blood vessels.

Tian Tai Wu Yao San (Top Quality Lindera Powder) (Lin)

Xiao Hui Xiang Fr. Foeniculi
Wu Yao Rx. Linderae
Mu Xiang Rx. Saussureae
Qing Pi Peric. Citri Ret. Viridis
Gao Liang Jiang Rhiz. Alipinae Officinari
Bing Lang Sm. Arecae Catechu
Chuan Lian Zi Fr. Meliae Toosendanis
Ba Dou Sm. Crotonis

This formula is also commonly used in Chinese Medicine andrology for swollen scrotum, hernia and pain referring to the testis. It promotes Qi movement and spreads Liver Qi but also scatters cold and alleviates pain. If there is severe aversion to cold, add *Wu Zhu*

Yu (*Fructus Evodiae*) 6 g to warm the Liver channel. If there is severe pain in the testicles, add *Li Zhi He* (*Semen Litchi*) 10 g to regulate the circulation of Qi in the Liver channel and relieve the pain.

Damp-heat

Three main formulas are suggested for treatment by almost every author. Number one is:

Long Dan Xie Gan Tang

Long Dan Cao Rx. Gentianae	6 g
Huang Qin Rx. Scutellariae	9 g
Zhi Zi Fr. Gardeniae	9 g
Mu Tong Cl. Akebiae	9 g
Che Qian Zi Sm. Plantaginis	9 g
Ze Xie Rh. Alismatis	9 g
Chai Hu Rx. Bupleuri	9 g
Sheng Di Huang Rx. Rehmanniae	12 g
Dang Gui Rx. Angelicae sinensis	9 g
Gan Cao Rx. Glycyrrhizae	3 g

The first three herbs purge the Liver of the pathogenic fire, whereas *Mu Tong* and *Che Qian Zi* remove damp-heat. All the drugs of that prescription together not only purge and remove but also replenish and nourish, purging the Liver from excess, removing damp-heat from the middle Jiao. Focks recommends adding *Tao Ren*, *Hong Hua* and *Wang Bu Liu Xing*.

Bi Xie Fen Qing Yin (Dioscorea Separating the Clear Decoction) (Lyttleton)

Bi Xie Rhiz. Dioscorea	12 g
Yi Zhi Ren Fr. Alipinae Oxyphyllae	9 g
Wu Yao Rx. Linderae Strychnifoliae	9 g
Shi Chang Pu Rhiz. Acori Graminei	9 g

Bi Xie drains damp from the urogenital system and *Shi Chang Pu* opens orifices to facilitate this draining. *Yi Zhi Ren* and *Wu Yao* warm the Bladder and Kidney to facilitate efficient excretion of fluids. Lyttleton recommends using *Long Bi Xie Fen Qing Qin* if damp-heat is in the Lower Burner but *Long Dan Xie Gan Tang* if it is more in the genitals. Note that *Bi Xie* and *Bei Xi* are the same herb (the name is written differently in various books).

Bi Xie Shen Shi Tang (Dioscorea Decoction to Leach out Dampness) (Franconi)

Yi Yi Ren Sm. Coicis
Hua Shi Talcum
Bi Xie Rhiz. Dioscorea
Fu Ling Poria
Huang Bai Cx. Phellodendri
Mu Dan Pi Cx. Moutan
Ze Xie Rhiz. Alismatis
Tong Cao Tetrapanacis Medullae

If heat prevails more than dampness, this formula is superior to *Bi Xie Fen Qing Yin*. The formula is used to eliminate toxins, cool the Blood, clear heat, invigorate the Blood, resolve dampness in the Lower Jiao and disperse swelling. *Bi Xie Sheng Shi Wan* promotes natural urination.

Damone suggests a combination of the two formulas above, as do Dou and Zi-Qiang.

Bi Shen Shi Tang with *Long Dan Xie Gan Tang*

Long Dan Cao Radix et Rhizoma Gentianae	10 g
Huang Bai Cx. Phellodendri	10 g
Huang Qin Rx. Scutellariae	10 g
Zhi Zi Fr. Gardeniae	10 g
Mu Dan Pi Cx. Moutan	10 g
Ze Xie Rhiz. Alismatis Rhizoma	10 g
Bi Xie Rhiz. Dioscoreae Septemlobae	15 g
Yi Yi Ren Sm. Coicis	20 g
Fu Ling Poria	10 g
Tong Cao Med. Tetrapanacis	10 g
Che Qian Zi Sm. Plantaginis	12 g
Dang Gui Rx. Angelicae Sinensis	10 g
Sheng Di Rx. Rehmanniae	15 g

Weixin also offers some alternative prescriptions:

Wu Wei Xiao Du Yin (Five Ingredient Decoction to Eliminate Toxins) (Weixin)

Jin Yin Hua Fl. Lonicerae	9–25 g
Pu Gong Ying Hb. Taraxaci	3–30 g
Zi Hua Di Ding Hb. Violae	3–30 g
Ye Ju Hua Fl. Crysanthemi Indici	3–20 g

Tian Kui Zi Rx. Semiaquilegiae   3–15 g
Wine

In the formula, *Jin Yin Hua*, *Pu Gong Yin*, *Zi Hua Di Ding* and *Ju Hua* are used to clear heat and resolve toxins. The drugs together clear heat and resolve toxins, cool the Blood and disperse swelling. It reduces external carbuncles and furuncles if they show up as a sign of heat and toxins.

Zhi Bai Di Huang Wan (Weixin)

Zhi Mu Rx. Anemarrhenae
Huang Bai Cx. Phellodendri
Shu Di Huang Rx. Rehmanniae Preparata
Shan Zhu Yu Fr. Corni
Shan Yao Rx. Dioscoreae
Fu Ling Poria
Mu Dan Pi Cx. Moutan
Ze Xie Rhiz. Alismatis

Anna Lin's alternative suggestions are:

San Miao Wan (Three Marvel Pill) (Lin)

Huang Bai Cx. Phellodendri   12 g
Jin Cang Zhu Rhiz. Atractylodes soaked   18 g
Chuan Niu Xi Rx. Cyathulae   6 g
Sheng Jiang Rh. Zingiberis Recens   3 g

The formula clears heat and dries dampness. It is especially recommended for damp-heat in the Lower Jiao.

San Ren Tang (Three Seed Decoction) (Lin)

Xing Ren Sm. Pruni Armeniacae
Bai Dou Kou Fr. Amomi
Hou Po Cx. Magnoliae Off.
Ban Xia Rhiz. Pinelliae
Dan Zhu Ye Hb. Lophateri Gracilis
Yi Yi Ren Sm. Coicis
Tong Cao Med. Tetrapanacis Papyriferi
Hua Shi Talcum

With three herbs that transform dampness and the last three herbs to promote urination to clear dampness and heat, this classical formula fits perfectly if there is more dampness than heat accompanied by a weak Spleen Qi.

Huo Jinglun offers an unnamed prescription in his book *Acupuncture and Moxibustion Therapy in Gynecology and Obstretics*:[3]

Shu Di Huang *Rx. Rehmanniae Preparata*
He Shou Wu *Rx. Polygonati*
Lian Qiao *Fl. Lonicerae*
Qu Mai *Hb. Dianthi*
Che Qian Zi *Sm. Plantaginis*
Bi Xie *Rhiz. Dioscoreae Sept.*
Huang Bai *Cx. Phellodendri*
Mu Tong *Cl. Akebiae*
Hua Shi *Talcum*
Gan Cao *Rx. Glycyrrhizae*

Containing of a lot of dampness-draining but also heat-clearing herbs, the special thing about that formula is that, with *Shu Di Huang* and *He Shou Wu*, nourishing the Blood is considered. That makes this prescription very clearing but not drying.

Hong Teng Bai Jiang Wan (*Sargentodoxae Patrinae* Compound) (Glover)

Dang Gui *Radix Angelicae Sinensis*	9 g
Chi Shao *Radix Paeoniae Rubra*	9 g
Bai Shao *Radix Paeoniae Lactiflorae*	9 g
Hong Teng *Caulis Sargentodoxae*	15 g
Bai Jiang Cao *Herba cum Radice Patrinae*	15 g
Shan Zha *Fructus Crataegi*	12 g
Yan Hu Suo *Rhizoma Corydalis Yanhusuo*	9 g
Chai Hu *Radix Bupleuri*	6 g
Chen Pi *Pericarpium Citri Reticulate*	6 g
Mu Xiang *Radix Auklandiae Lappae*	6 g
Yi Yi Ren *Semen Coicis Lachryma-jobi*	15 g
Sang Ji Sheng *Ramulus Mori Albae*	12 g

Used for damp-heat accumulation and toxins. *Dang Gui*, *Bai Shao* and *Chi Shao* nourish and regulate the Blood. *Mu Xiang* and *Chen Pi* regulate the Spleen and Stomach Qi while *Chai Hu* moves the Liver Qi. *Hong Teng* and *Bai Jiang Cao* are herbs used to detoxify and disperse stagnant Blood and reduce inflammation. *Yan Hu Suo* and *Shan Zha* also move the

Blood. *Yi Yi Ren* clears damp. *Sang Ji Sheng* clears damp and at the same time supplements Liver and Kidney (Lyttleton).

Addendum: Becker's hitlist of damp-heat medicinals

- **Bai Jiang Cao** Hb. Patriniae
- **Tu Fu Ling** Rhiz. Smilacis Glabrae
- **Pu Gong Ying** Hb. Taraxaci
- **Hong Teng** Cl. Sargentodoxae
- **Bi Xie** Rhiz. Dioscoreae Septemlobae
- **Che Qian Zi** Sm. Plantaginis
- **Huang Bai** Cx. Phellodendri

Damp-phlegm

The most commonly suggested formula is *Cang Fu Dao Tan Tang*; all the others are mentioned only by one author.

Cang Fu Dao Tan Tang (*Atractylodes-Poria* Phlegm Dissipating Decoction)

Cang Zhu Rh. Atractylodis	12 g
Bai Zhu Rh. Atractylodis Macrocephalae	12 g
Xiang Fu Rh. Cyperi	12 g
Chen Pi Peric. Citri Reticulatae	10 g
Ban Xia Rh. Pinelliae	10 g
Zhi Shi Fr. Aurantii immaturus	10 g
Fu Ling Poria	12 g
Ze Xie Rhiz. Alismatis	12 g
Che Qian Zi Sm. Plantaginis	15 g
Lu Lu Tong Fr. Liquidambaris	6 g
Zhe Bei Mu Blb. Fritillariae Thunbergii	12 g
Zhi Gan Cao Rx. Glycyrrhizae Prep.	3 g

It promotes the flow of Qi, removes dampness and resolves phlegm. Men with a damp-phlegm pattern often present as adipose, showing a Tai-Yin body type. For them, the formula might need to be expanded with Spleen Qi-tonifying herbs such as *Huang Qi* or

Ren Shen. Not only is *Lu Lu Tong* a Blood-moving herb but it also works as a GPS herb for the testicles.

Dou modifies the prescription, adding *Dan Nan Xing* (*Arisaema cum Bile*) and *Chen Pi* (*Pericarp. Citri*) as well *as Chuan Shan Jia* (*Sq. Mantis*) but removes *Zhe Bei Mu* and *Gan Cao*.

Lin combines *Cang Fu Dao Tan Tang* with:

Ping Wei San (Calm the Stomach Powder)

Cang Zhu *Rhiz. Atractylodes*
Hou Po *Cx. Magnoliae*
Chen Pi *Peric. Citri*
Zhi Gan Cao *Rx. Glycyrrhizae Uralensis*

It is an ancient Chinese herbal medicine that eliminates dampness in the digestive tract and supports Stomach comfort to make it more suitable for patients with a weak Middle Burner.

or: *Er Chen Tang* (Decoction of Two Old Drugs)

Ban Xia *Rhiz. Pinelliae*
Chen Pi *Peric. Citri Ret.*
Fu Ling *Poria*
Sheng Jiang *Rhiz. Zingiberis Recens*
Zhi Gan Cao *Rx. Glycyrrhizae Uralensis Prep.*

This classical formula dries dampness, transforms phlegm, regulates Qi and harmonizes the Middle Burner.

Becker suggests a combination of *Er Chen Tang*, *Wu Ling San* and *Shen Ling Bai Zhu San* (note that several herbs in that combination of three overlap).

Wu Ling San (Five Ingredient Formula with Poria)

Ze Xie *Rhiz. Alismatis*
Fu Ling *Poria*
Zhu Ling *Polyporus*
Bai Zhu *Rhiz. Atractylodes Mac.*
Gui Zhi *Ram. Cinammomi*

Another well-known prescription with potential diuresis-inducing and Kidney-protective and warming activities. It may increase the removal of excess fluid, prevent the retention of water, maintain healthy water metabolism by promoting diuresis and protect Kidney function.

Shen Ling Bai Zhu San (Ginseng and Atractylodes Formula)

Ren Shen Rx. Ginseng
Bai Zhu Rhiz. Atractylodes Mac.
Fu Ling Poria
Zhi Gan Cao Rx. Glycyrrhizae Uralensis Prep.
Shan Yao Rhiz. Dioscoreae
Bai Bian Dou Sm. Lablab Album
Lian Zi Sm. Nelumbinis
Yi Yi Ren Sm. Coicis
Sha Ren Fr. Amomi

Used for dampness due to Spleen Qi deficiency, it is a classical Spleen tonic appropriate for long-term use. Shen Ling Bai Zhu San may also be helpful to support a healthy weight. Giovanni Maciocia has his own preferred formula for damp-phlegm:

Fang Ji Huang Qi Tang

Huang Qi Rx. Astragali
Bai Zhu Rhiz. Atractylodes Mac.
Zhi Gan Cao Rx. Glycyrrhizae Uralensis Prep.
Sheng Jiang Rhiz. Zingiberis Recens
Da Zao Fr. Jujubae
Dan Shen Rx. Salviae Mil.
Yin Chen Hao Hb. Artemisiae
Ze Xie Rhiz. Alismatis
Fu Ling Poria
Yin Yang Huo Hb. Epimedii
Gou Qi Zi Fr. Lycii
He Shou Wu Rhiz. Polygonati

This classical prescription supplements Qi and forces diuresis. It is commonly used for chronic issues that accompany oedema of the lower part of the body, with a soft but tensionless muscular aspect. *Fang Ji* (*Rx. Stephaniae Tetrandae*) is removed in Maciocia's version although it would match the pattern perfectly. A possible explanation might be that when *Radix Stephania Tetrandra* was misused with *Aristolochia* species (*Guan Fang Ji*), acute or chronic nephropathy caused by aristolochic acid occurred, causing a huge scandal. Maybe he eliminated the herb for safety reasons, which is not necessary when ensuring *Han Fang Ji* (*Rx. Stephaniae Tetrandae*) is used.

Damone also suggests using *Bi Xie Fen Qing Yin*:

Bi Xie Fen Qing Yin (Dioscorea Separating the Clear Decoction)

Chuan Bi Xie Rhiz. Dioscorea Hypoglaucae	9 g
Yi Zhi Ren Fr. Alipinae Oxyphyllae	9 g
Wu Yao Rx. Linderae Strychnifoliae	9 g
Shi Chang Pu Rhiz. Acori Graminei	9 g

Or alternatively Liu Jun Zi Tang:

Liu Jun Zi Tang

Ren Shen Rx. Ginseng	10 g
Bai Zhu Rhiz. Atractylodes Macrocephalae	10 g
Fu Ling Poria	10 g
Zhi Gan Cao Rx. Glycyrrhizae Prep.	3 g
Chen Pi Pericap. Citri Reticulatae	10 g
Ban Xia Rhiz. Pinelliae Ternatae	10 g

Addendum: Becker's hitlist of Spleen damp-phlegm medicinals

- **Cang Zhu** Rhiz. Atractylodis
- **Ban Xia** Rhiz. Pinelliae
- **Chen Pi** Peric. Citri Reticulatae
- **Kun Bu** Thallus Eckloniae
- **Hai Zao** Sargassum
- **Zhe Bei Mu** Blb. Fritillariae Thunbergii

PRESCRIPTIONS ACCORDING TO SPERMIOGRAM

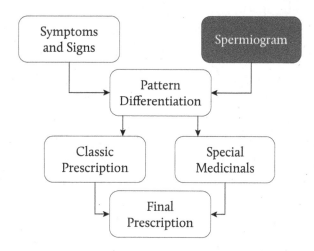

Note: Use the suggested formulas of this section in addition to the selected pattern-based formulas from above. Combine them or prescribe them alternately.

SPERM PATHOLOGIES

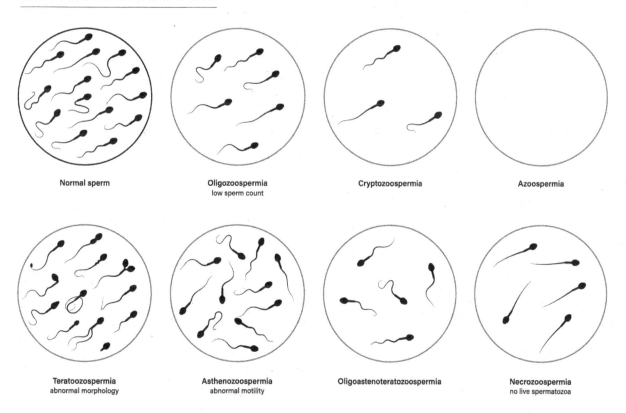

Oligospermia (Jing Shao)

In Chinese Medicine, oligospermia can be found in the category Jing shao (scantly seminal flow), Jing Qing (thin semen) or Xu Lao (consumption).

It is basically a Kidney Essence insufficiency problem, either constitutional or acquired. But it may also be due to a lack of transformation where the Spleen as the source of the post-heaven Essence is weak. In most cases, the decrease in sperm count is caused by deficiency of both the Spleen and the Kidney.

The treatment of oligospermia and – in extreme cases – azoospermia must focus on warming Yang to transform Qi and enriching the Kidneys to replenish the Essence; likewise, to strengthen the Spleen and to support movement to fill and nourish the Kidney Essence.

Oligospermia

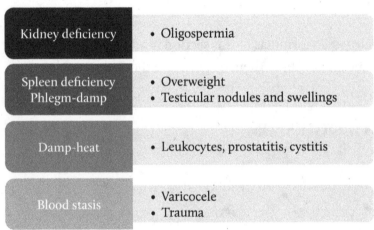

Kidney deficiency	• Oligospermia
Spleen deficiency Phlegm-damp	• Overweight • Testicular nodules and swellings
Damp-heat	• Leukocytes, prostatitis, cystitis
Blood stasis	• Varicocele • Trauma

Concerning pattern discrimination, most likely there are Kidney patterns, dampness and phlegm, damp-heat in the Lower Burner and stasis of Blood.

The suggested prescriptions are in addition to those from the basic patterns. They could be either used as alternatives or in combination.

Kidney patterns

KIDNEY ESSENCE DEFICIENCY

Sheng Jing Tang modified (Decoction for Engendering Semen) (Tiandong)

Fu Pen Zi Fr. Rubi	15 g
Tu Si Zi Sm. Cuscutae	15 g
Gou Qi Zi Fr. Lycii	15 g
Wu Wei Zi Fr. Schisandrae	10 g
Che Qian Zi Sm. Plantaginis	10 g
Dang Gui Rx. Angelicae Sinensis	15 g

Shu Di Huang Rx. Rehmanniae Prep.	20 g
Chi Shao Rx. Paeoniae Rubrae	10 g
Dang Shen Rx. Codonopsis	15 g
Bai Zhu Rhiz. Atractylodes Mac.	10 g
Fu Ling Poria	10 g
Xu Duan Rx. Dipsaci	15 g
Yin Yang Huo Hb. Epimedii	10 g
Gan Cao Rx. Glycyrrhizae	3 g

This formula reinforces the Kidney to generate Essence as well as replenishing both the Qi and Blood. In a nutshell, it is a pre- and post-heaven reinforcing prescription. It is a compound of *Wu Zi Yan Zong Wan*, *Si Wu Tang* and *Si Jun Zi Tang* with modifications.

It is the most commonly used formula for the treatment of oligospermia. Tiandong explains that in clinical practice most patients of this type cannot be identified in Chinese Medicine patterns for lack of apparent symptoms.

Anna Lin also suggests this formula for the treatment of combined Kidney and Spleen deficiency but uses *Huang Qi* instead of *Bai Zhu*, excludes *Chi Shao* and *Poria* but adds *Sang Shen* and *Chen Pi*.

Qi Zi Er Xian Wan (Becker)

Xian Mao Rhiz. Curculiginis
Yin Yang Huo Hb. Epimedii
Tu Si Zi Sm. Cuscutae
Gou Qi Zi Fr. Lycii
Fu Pen Zi Fr. Rubii
Jiu Cai Zi Sm. Alii Tuberosi
Sang Shen Fr. Mori
Wu Wei Zi Fr. Schisandrae
Che Qian Zi Sm. Plantaginis
Dang Shen Rx. Codonopsis

A good basic prescription composed from Essence-tonifying herbs and Yang tonics. By adding *Che Qian Zi* it also clears dampness from the Lower Burner.

Qiang Jing Jian (Clavey)

Yin Yang Huo Hb. Epimedii Herba	15 g
Rou Cong Rong Hb. Cistanches	12 g
He Shou Wu Rx. Polygoni Multiflori	15 g
Huang Jing Rhiz. Polygonati	15 g

Xu Duan Rx. Dipsaci	12 g
Gou Qi Zi Fr. Lycii	15 g
Shu Di Huang Rx. Rehmanniae Prep.	15 g
Lu Jiao Cornu Cervi Gelatinum	15 g
Tu Si Zi Sm. Cuscutae	12 g
Fu Ling Poria	12 g
Ze Xie Rhiz. Alismatis	12 g

If there is a tendency to Yin deficiency, this formula is the one Steve Clavey would go with. Once again, this formula is not only nourishing but also discharges dampness.

Jin Shi Yie Hua Sheng Jing Tang (Jin's Decoction for Replenishing Essence and Sperma Liquefication) (Weixin)

Mu Dan Pi Cx. Moutan	9 g
Di Gu Pi Cx. Lycii	9 g
Bai Shao Rx. Paeoniae Albae	9 g
Shu Di Huang Rx. Rehmanniae Prep.	9 g
Mai Men Dong Rx. Ophiopogonis	9 g
Xuan Shen Rx. Scrophulariae	9 g
He Shou Wu Rx. Polygoni Multiflori	15 g
Sang Shen Fr. Mori	15 g
Gou Qi Zi Fr. Lycii	15 g
Shan Zhu Yu Fr. Corni	9 g
Yin Yang Huo Hb. Epimedii	15 g
Fu Ling Poria	9 g
Dan Zhu Ye Hb. Lophateri	9 g
Mu Li Concha Ostrae	30 g
Dan Shen Rx. Salviae Milit.	30 g
Lian Qiao Fl. Forsythiae	12 g
Jin Yin Hua Fl. Lonicerae	18 g

A very useable formula that not only contains nourishing and tonifying herbs for the Liver, Blood and Kidney but also includes heat-clearing and Blood-cooling herbs. *Mu Li* soothes the Liver and checks exuberance of Yang, astringes and arrests discharge.

Anna Lin uses a variation of this formula with the addition of *Chi Shao* and *Zhe Bei Mu* for Essence vacuity with Yin deficiency.

Other formulas suggested by various authors are:

- *Ju Jing Tang*, modified (Decoction to Support Jing) (Franconi)

- *Yu Jing Tang* (Zi-Qiang)

- *Tu Si Zi Tang* (Zi-Qiang)

In the case of Kidney Essence deficiency with more Kidney Yang vacuity Anna Lin uses a combination of *Wu Zi Yan Zong Wan* and:

Shi Zi Wan

Sang Shen Zi *Fr. Mori Albi*
Fu Zi *Rx. Aconiti Prep.*
Jiu Cai Zi *Sm. Alii Tuberosi*
Hu Lu Ba *Sm. Trigonellae Foeni-greaci*
She Chuang Zi *Sm. Cnidii Monnieri*
Dang Gui *Rx. Angelicae Sin.*
Xu Duan *Rx. Dipsaci*
Dang Shen *Rx. Codonopsis*
Ba Ji Tian *Rx. Morindae*
Lu Jiao Jiao *Colli Cornu Cervi*

DEFICIENCY OF QI AND BLOOD/SPLEEN DEFICIENCY

Bu Jing Fang (Zi-Qiang)

Huang Jing *Rhiz. Polygonati*	20 g
Shan Yao *Rhiz. Dioscorae*	20 g
Dang Shen *Rx. Codonopsis*	20 g
Zhi Huang Qi *Rx. Astragali*	20 g
Xu Duan *Rx. Dipsaci*	20 g
Wu Wei Zi *Fr. Schisandrae*	10 g
Fu Pen Zi *Fr. Rubi*	10 g
Tu Si Zi *Sm. Cuscutae*	10 g
Che Qian Zi *Sm. Plantaginis*	10 g
Dang Gui *Rx. Angelicae Sinensis*	10 g
Fu Ling *Poria*	10 g

Indicated when there is oligospermia due to Essence deficiency and Spleen vacuity.

Jia Wei Bao Zhen Wan (Zi-Qiang)

Dang Shen *Rx. Codonopsis*	24 g
Huang Qi *Rx. Astragali*	24 g
Sang Ji Sheng *Hb. Taxilli*	15 g

Tu Si Zi Sm. Cuscutae	15 g
Fu Pen Zi Fr. Rubi	24 g
Yin Yang Huo Hb. Epimedii	24 g
Du Zhong Cx. Eucommiae	9 g

This formula is used for oligospermia due to Kidney and Spleen weakness.
Other formulas:

- *Shen Jing Tang* (Lin)

- *He Che Zhong Zi Wan* (Pill of Dried Human Placenta for Pregnancy) (Weixin)

- *Shi Quan Da Bu Wan* (All-Inclusive Great Tonifying Pill) (Clavey)

SPLEEN DEFICIENCY WITH PHLEGM-DAMP

Chu Shi Hua Tan Huo Zi Tang (Remove Damp Transform Phlegm and Obtain Progeny Decoction) (Clavey)

Chao Cang Zhu Rhiz. Atractylodes dry-fried	15 g
Yi Yi Ren Sm. Coicis	15 g
Ze Xie Rhiz. Alismatis	15 g
Che Qian Zi Sm. Plantaginis	10 g
Ban Xia Rhiz. Pinelliae T.	10 g
Chen Pi Peric. Citri Retic.	7 g
Quan Gua Lou Fr. et Peric. Trichosanthis	9 g
Chao Huang Bai Cx. Phellodendri dry-fried	9 g
Long Dan Cao Rx. Gentianae Scabrae	10 g
Kun Bun Thallus Algae	6 g
Hai Zao Sargassum	6 g
Gan Cao Rx. Glycyrrhizae Uralensis	6 g

This formula is often used when there are signs of a phlegm blockage – for instance, if the vas deferens is obstructed from a biomedical perspective, leading to azoospermia. But it can also be used in cases of oligospermia due to phlegm blockage.

Fang Ji Huang Qi Tang Jia Wei (Lin)

Huang Qi Rx. Astragali
Han Fang Ji Rx. Stephaniae Tetrandae
Bai Zhu Rhiz. Atractylodis Mac.
Zhi Gan Cao Rx. Glycyrrhizae Uralensis Prep.
Sheng Jiang Rhiz. Zingiberis Recens

Da Zao *Fr. Zizyphi Jujubae*
Dan Shen *Rx. Salviae Miltiorrhizae*
Yin Chen *Hb. Artemisiae Capillaris*
Ze Xie *Rhiz. Alismatis*
Fu Ling *Poria*
Gou Qi Zi *Fr. Lycii*
He Shou Wu *Rx. Polygoni Multiflori*

DAMP-HEAT

Qing Jing Jian (Clear the Jing Decoction) (Clavey)

Bie Xie *Rhiz. Dioscoreae*	15 g
Tu Si Zi *Sm. Cuscutae*	15 g
Che Qian Zi *Sm. Plantaginis*	15 g
Huang Bai *Cx. Phellodendri*	10 g
Zhi Mu *Rx. Anemarrhenae Asphodeloidis*	10 g
Chai Hu *Rx. Bupleuri*	10 g
Zhi Da Huang *Rx. et Rhizoma Rhei Prep.*	10 g
Hong Teng *Cl. Sargentodoxae Cuneatae*	15 g
Dan Shen *Rx. Salviae Miltiorrhizae*	15 g
Mu Dan Pi *Cx. Moutan Radicis*	10 g
Bai Hua She She Cao *Hb. Oldenlandiae Diffusae*	15 g
Wang Bu Liu Xing *Sm. Vaccariae*	10 g

BLOOD STASIS

Tong Jing Jian (Fee Jing Decoction) (Clavey)

Dan Shen *Rx. et Rh. Salviae Militorrhizae*	15 g
E Zhu *Rhiz. Curcumae*	15 g
Chuan Niu Xi *Rx. Cyathulae*	15 g
Dang Gui *Rx. Angelicae Sinensis*	10 g
Chuan Xiong *Rhiz. Chuanxiong*	10 g
Chai Hu *Rx. Bupleuri*	10 g
Huang Qi *Rx. Astragali*	30 g
Mu Li *Concha Ostrea*	30 g

The first five herbs remove Blood stagnation, with the *Niu Xi* drawing the effect downwards. *Chai Hu* frees Qi flow in the Liver channel and prolongs sperm activity. *Huang Qi* benefits Qi and livens the flow of Blood without damaging the correct (zheng) Qi. *Mu Li* softens hard lumps and helps eliminate old stagnant Blood. According to Steve Clavey, Blood stasis has a lot to do with varicocele. If there is such a venal formation, there is certainly Blood stasis. Even without it, there might be Blood stasis causing oligo- or azoospermia. Generally, Blood-moving herbs should be added to most of the formulas as Blood stasis has a huge negative impact on spermatogenesis. Chronic illnesses tend to be accompanied by Blood stasis as they enter the Luo vessels causing it. *Mu Li* and *E Zhu* are the major workers in this formula as they break Blood; *Huang Qi* is almost as important as it moves Blood by enhancing Qi circulation. If there is pain in the testicles, *Qing Pi* and *Yan Hu Suo* should be added.

There are rare cases where the pattern causing oligospermia is cold and damp in the Lower Burner. Only Anna Lin lists it, so the recommendation is by her:

Shao Fu Zhu Yu Tang He Si Ling Tang Jia Jian

Xiao Hui Xiang Fr. Foeniculi	6 g
Pao Jiang Rhiz. Zingiberis	10 g
Dang Gui Rx. Angelicae Sinensis	10 g
Rou Gui Cx. Cinnamomi	6 g
Chi Shao Rx. Paeoniae Radix	10 g
Long Yan Rou Arillus Euphoriae Longanae	10 g
Bai Shao Rx. Paeoniae Albae	13 g
Ze Xie Rhiz. Alismatis	10 g
Fu Ling Poria	10 g
Bie Xie Rhiz. Dioscorae	10 g
Niu Xi Rx. Achyrantihis Bidentatae	10 g

Azoospermia (Wu Jing)

The main cause of no sperm in the ejaculate from a Chinese Medicine perspective is Kidney Qi and Yin vacuity. Sometimes this vacuity is complicated by the 'duo infernale' – Qi stagnation and Blood stasis. Some sources add damp-heat as a possible pattern.

Modern books divide the pattern causing azoospermia according to Western Medicine into azoospermia due to obstruction and non-obstructive azoospermia. The obstructive type is secondary to Blood, phlegm or heat that blocks the sperm channel, whereas the non-obstructive azoospermia is secondary to Kidney and Liver patterns (Franconi). In any case, azoospermia is a serious condition and, as with the Western prognosis, not easy to treat successfully.

KIDNEY YANG DEFICIENCY

Huang Qi Zeng Jing Wan (Astragalus Supplement Jing Pill) (Clavey)

Fu Zi Rx. Aconiti Carmichaeli Prep.	90 g
Jiu Cai Zi Sm. Allii Tuberosi	60 g
Yin Yang Huo Hb. Epimedii	100 g
Tu Si Zi Sm. Cuscutae	60 g
Lu Rong Cornu Cervi Parvum	60 g
Rou Cong Bai Blb. Allii Fistulosi	60 g
Gou Qi Zi Fr. Lycii Chinensis	60 g
Shi Hu Hb. Dendrobii	15 g
Fu Pen Zi Fr. Rubi	60 g
Huai Niu Xi Rx. Achyranthis Bidentatae	30 g

Modified *Bu Tian Yu Ling Dan* (Tonify Heaven, Raise Boy Pill) (Franconi)

Rou Gui Cx. Cinnamomi	10 g
Tu Si Zi Sm. Cuscutae	10 g
Rou Cong Rong Hb. Cistanches	10 g
Shu Di Huang Rx. Rehmanniae Prep.	20 g
Gou Qi Zi Fr. Lycii	10 g
Mu Dan Pi Cx. Moutan	10 g
Dang Shen Rx. Codonopsis	15 g
Bai Zhu Rhiz. Atractylodes Mac.	10 g
Ze Xie Rhiz. Alismatis	10 g
Che Qian Zi Sm Plantaginis	10 g
Shan Zhu Yu Fr. Corni	10 g
Wu Wei Zi Fr. Schisandrae	6 g
Fu Ling Poria	10 g

KIDNEY YIN DEFICIENCY

Zi Yin Sheng Jing Fu Yu Tang (Nourish Yin Produce Jing and Double Fertility Decoction) (Clavey)

Shu Di Huang Rx. Rehmanniae Prep.	15 g
Shan Zhu Yu Fr. Corni Officinalis	12 g
Shan Yao Rx. Dioscoreae Oppositae	12 g
Mu Dan Pi Cx. Moutan Radicis	10 g
Ze Xie Rhiz. Alismatis	10 g
Fu Ling Poria	10 g

Chao Huang Bai dry-fried *Cortex Phellodendri*	9 g
Tu Si Zi Sm. Cuscutae	12 g
Rou Cong Bai Blb. Allii Fistulosi	12 g
Gou Qi Zi Fr. Lycii Chinensis	12 g
Nu Zhen Zi Fr. Ligustri Lucidi	12 g
He Shou Wu Rx. Polygoni Multiflori	12 g

Modified *Shen Sui Yu Lin Dan* (Elixier to Promote the Production of Sperm) (Franconi)

Rou Cong Rong Hb. Cistanches	10 g
Tu Si Zi Sm. Cuscutae	10 g
Shu Di Huang Rx. Rehmanniae Prep.	20 g
Gou Qi Zi Fr. Lycii	10 g
Shan Zhu Yu Fr. Corni	10 g
Dang Shen Rx. Codonopsis	15 g
Bai Zhu Rhiz. Atractylodes Mac.	10 g
He Shou Wu Rx. Polygoni Multif.	10 g
Shan Yao Rx. Dioscorae Opp.	15 g
Shen Qu Massa Fermentata	10 g
Mai Ya Fr. Hordei Vulg.	10 g

QI BLOCKAGE AND BLOOD STAGNATION IN AZOOSPERMIA

Fu Jing Zi Tang (Double Sperm Decoction) (Clavey)

Chai Hu Rx. Bupleuri	9 g
Chao Ju He Sm. Citri Reticulatae dry-fried	9 g
Li Zhe He Sm. Litchi Chinensis	10 g
Zao Jiao Ci Spina Gleditsiae Sinensis	10 g
Lu Lu Tong Fr. Liquidambaris Taiwanianae	12 g
Chao Tao Ren Sm. Persicae dry-fried	12 g
Hong Hua Fl. Carthami Tinctorii	12 g
Chi Shao Rx. Paeoniae Rubrae	6 g
Sheng Huang Qi Fresh Radix Astragali	15 g
Chen Pi Peric. Citris Reticulatae	6 g
Tu Si Zi Sm. Cuscutae	15 g
Niu Xi Rx. Achyranthis Bidentatae	9 g

Modified *Xie Fu Zhu Yu Tang* (Decoction to Eliminate Stasis in the House of Blood) (Franconi)

Tao Ren Sm. Pruni Persicae	10 g
Hong Hua Fl. Carthami	10 g
Dan Shen Rx. Salviae Miltiorrhizae	10 g
E Zhu Rhiz. Curcumae	10 g
Niu Xi Rx. Cyathulae	10 g
Dang Gui Wei Rx. Angelicae Sinensis	10 g
Chai Hu Rx. Bupleuri	6 g
Zhi Ke Fr. Citri Aurantii	6 g
Chuan Xiong Rx. Ligustrici Wallichii	10 g
Shu Di Huang Rx. Rehmanniae Glut	15 g
Fu Ling Poria	10 g
Bai Zhu Rhiz. Atractylodes Mac.	10 g
Shen Qu Massa Fermentata	6 g
Gan Cao Rx. Glycyrrhizae	6 g

PHLEGM-DAMP OCCLUSION

Chu Shi Hua Tan Huo Zi Tang (Remove Damp Transform Phlegm and Obtain Progeny Decoction) (Clavey)

Chao Cang Zhu Rhiz. Atractylodis dry-fried	15 g
Yi Yi Ren Sm. Coicis Lachryma-jobi	15 g
Ze Xie Rhiz. Alismatis	15 g
Che Qian Zi Sm. Plantaginis	10 g
Ban Xia Rhiz. Pinelliae Ternatae	10 g
Chen Pi Peric. Citri Reticulatae	7 g
Quan Gua Lou Fr. et Peric. Trichosanthis	9 g
Chao Huang Bai Cortex Phellodendri dry-fried	9 g
Long Dan Cao Rx. Gentianae Scabrae	10 g
Kun Bu Thallus Algae	6 g
Hai Zao Sargassum	6 g
Gan Cao Rx. Glycyrrhizae Uralensis	6 g

Ju He Wan (Focks)

Chao Ju He Sm. Citri Reticulatae	9 g
Chao Chuan Lian Zi Fr. Toosendan	9 g
Hai Zao Sargassum	9 g
Kun Bu Thallus Eckloniae	9 g

Tao Ren *Sm. Persicae*	9 g
Hou Po *Cx. Magnoliae Off.*	3 g
Mu Xiang *Rx. Aucklandiae*	3 g
Yan Hu Suo *Rhiz. Corydalis*	3 g
Zhi Shi *Fr. Aurantii Immaturus*	3 g
Rou Gui *Cx. Cinnamomi*	3 g

DAMP-HEAT AND STASIS BLOCK THE CHANNEL

Wu Shen Tang (Five-Miracle Decoction) (Franconi)

Che Qian Zi *Sm. Plantaginis*	10 g
Sheng Yi Ren *Sm. Coicis Lachryma*	15 g
Yin Hua *Fl. Lonicerae*	10 g
Tu Fu Ling *Rhiz. Smilacis Glabrae*	10 g
Gan Cao *Rhiz. Glycyrrhizae Uralensis*	6 g
Chuan Niu Xi *Rx. Cyathulae*	15 g
Yi Mu Cao *Hb. Leonuri*	10 g
Bei Mu *Blb. Fritillariae*	12 g
Xuan Shen *Rx. Scophulariae*	15 g
Shi Chang Pu *Rhiz. Acori Gram.*	6 g

Sheng Jing Zan Yu Wan modified (Pill for Spermatogeny and Supporting Fertility) (Weixin)

Yin Yang Huo *Hb. Epimedii*
Shi Hu *Hb. Dendrobii*
Xian Mao *Rhiz. Curculiginis*
Gou Qi Zi *Fr. Lycii*
Huang Bai *Cx. Phellodendri*
Zhi Mu *Rhiz. Anemarrhenae*
Long Dan Cao *Rx. Gentianae*
Ju Hua *Fl. Chrysanthemi*

Asthenospermia

There is no equivalent of this type of infertility in Chinese Medicine literature, and it may fall into the category of jing leng (精冷 seminal cold). According to Anna Lin and some others, sperm motility mainly depends on Kidney Yang. If Kidney Yang is diminished – due to different causes – motility problems result. Bear in mind that every movement in general depends on Yang, and the same is true for sperm cells. Certainly, there can be a vacuity of

Kidney Yang and Kidney Yin, even leading to vacuity fire with all its symptoms, but still the underlying problem will be the Kidney Yang vacuity. A sperm chamber that isn't heated properly will not create moveable sperm cells. Dampness and heat are other causes for sperm motility issues, as both directly harm and damage sperm cells.

Asthenospermia

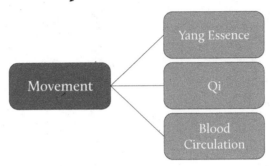

KIDNEY ESSENCE VACUITY

Qiang Jing Tang (Sperm-Fortifying Decoction) (Tiandong)

Gou Qi Zi Fr. Lycii	10 g
Tu Si Zi Sm. Cuscutae	10 g
Che Qian Zi Sm. Plantaginis	10 g
Fu Pen Zi Fr. Rubi	10 g
Wu Wei Zi Fr. Schisandrae	10 g
Jiu Cai Zi Sm. Allii Tuberosi	10 g
Sha Yuan Zi Sm. Astragali Complanati	10 g
Sang Shen Fr. Mori	10 g
Wu Yao Rx. Linderae	10 g
Chen Xiang Lign. Aquilariae Resinatum	3 g
Xi Xin Hb. Asari	2 g
Huai Niu Xi Rx. Achyranthis Bid.	15 g
Xu Duan Rx. Dipsaci	10 g
Zi He Che Placenta Hominis	5 g
Ba Ji Tian Rx. Morindae Officinalis	10 g
Rou Cong Rong Hb. Cistanches	10 g
Tao Ren Sm. Persicae	6 g
Wu Gong Scolopendra	1 piece

KIDNEY YANG VACUITY

Fu Ming Sheng Huo Dan (Support Life and Produce Fire Pill) (Clavey)

Fu Zi Rx. Aconiti Prep.	6 g
Rou Gui Cx. Cinnamomi Cassiae	6 g
Lu Rong Cornu Cervi Parvum	6 g
Ren Shen Rx. Ginseng	9 g
Ba Ji Tian Rx. Morindae Off.	9 g
Shan Zhu Yu Fr. Corni Off.	9 g
Wu Wei Zi Fr. Schisandrae	9 g
Shu Di Huang Rx. Rehmanniae Glut.	18 g
Huang Qi Rx. Astragali	15 g
Bai Zhu Rhiz. Atractylodes Mac.	15 g
Rou Cong Rong Hb. Cistanches	15 g
Du Zhong Cx. Eucommiae	15 g
Long Gu Os Draconis	15 g
Shou Zao Ren Sm. Ziziphae Spin, baked	15 g
Yin Yang Huo Hb. Epimedii	15 g

Guiding Formula (Lin)

Shu Di Huang Rx. Rehmanniae Prep.	10 g
Shan Yao Rx. Rhiz. Dioscorae	30 g
Gou Qi Zi Fr. Lycii	15 g
Tu Si Zi Sm. Cuscutae	30 g
Nu Zhen Zi Fr. Ligustri Lucidi	20 g
Han Lian Cao Hb. Ecliptae	15 g
Wu Wei Zi Fr. Schisandrae	6 g
Sang Ji Sheng Hb. Taxilli	15 g
Lu Jiao Jiao Cornu Cervi Gelatinum	12 g
Yin Yang Huo Hb. Epimedii	15 g
Suo Yang Hb. Cynomorii	12 g
Ba Ji Tian Rx. Morindae	10 g
Sha Ren Fr. Amomi	6 g
Gan Cao Rx. Glycyrrhizae Uralensis	2 g

Wen Shen Yi Jing Wan (Luo Yuan-Kai)

Pao Tian Xiong Tuber Aconiti Laterale Tianxiong	180 g
Shu Di Huang Rx. Rehmanniae Prep.	18 g
Tu Si Zi Sm. Cuscutae	480 g

Lu Jiao Shuang *Cornu Cervi Degelatinatum*	120 g
Bai Zhu *Rhiz. Atractylodes Mac.*	480 g
Rou Gui *Cx. Cinnamomi*	30 g

Processed into honey pills, take 6 g twice a day. Used for low motility caused by Kidney Yang vacuity and Ming Men fire burning low.

YIN VACUITY

Er Xian Tang (Lin)

Xian Mao *Rhiz. Curguliginis*	6 g
Yin Yang Huo *Hb. Epimedii*	6 g
Ba Ji Tian *Hb. Ecliptae*	6 g
Dang Gui *Rx. Angelicae Sinensis*	6 g
Zhi Mu *Rhiz. Anemarrhenae*	10 g
Huang Bai *Cx. Phellodendri*	10 g

Zi Yin Zhong Zi Wan (Nourish Yin to Enhance Fertility Pill) (Clavey)

Zhi Mu *Rx. Anemarrhenae*	9 g
Huang Bai *Cx. Phellodendri*	9 g
Tian Men Dong *Tuber Asparagi Cochinchinensis*	9 g
Mai Men Dong *Tuber Ophiopogonis Japonici*	9 g
Sang Shen Zi *Fr. Mori Albae*	9 g
Gou Qi Zi *Fr. Lycii Chinensis*	9 g
Tu Si Zi *Sm. Cuscutae*	9 g
Wu Wei Zi *Fr. Schisandrae Chinensis*	9 g
Shu Di Huang *Rx. Rehmanniae Prep.*	12 g
Huang Jing *Rhiz. Polygonati*	12 g
He Shou Wu *Rx. Polygoni Multiflori*	12 g
Fu Ling *Poria*	12 g
Bai Zi Ren *Sm. Biotae Orientalis*	12 g
Shan Yao *Rx. Dioscoreae Oppositae*	12 g
Chuan Niu Xi *Rx. Cyathulae*	12 g

QI AND BLOOD DEFICIENCY

Yu Lin Zhu (Filial Progeny Pill) (Zhang Jing-Yue)

Ba Zhen Tang (Eight Treasure Decoction)
+

Tu Si Zi *Sm. Cuscutae*

Du Zhong Cx. Eucommiae Ulmoidis
Lu Jiao Shuang Cornu Cervi Gelatinum
Chuan Jiao Peric. Zanthoxyli Bungeani
Gou Qi Zi Fr. Lycii Chinensis
Lu Jiao Jiao Colla Cornu Cervi
Shan Yao Rx. Dioscoreae Oppositae
Shan Zhu Yu Fr. Corni Officinalis
Ba Ji Tian Rx. Morindae Officinalis
Walnut flesh

Zi Ni Zu Jing Tang (Self-Made Spermia-Strengthening Decoction) (Weixin)

Tu Si Zi Sm. Cuscutae	12 g
Gou Qi Zi Fr. Lycii	10 g
Sang Shen Fr. Mori	12 g
Fu Pen Zi Fr. Rubi	12 g
Che Qian Zi Sm. Plantaginis	12 g
Wu Wei Zi Fr. Schisandra	12 g
Xian Mao Rhiz. Curculiginis	15 g
Yin Yang Huo Hb. Epimedii	15 g
Huang Qi Rx. Astragali	30 g
Shu Di Huang Rx. Rehmannia Prep.	30 g
Chuan Xiong Rx. Ligustri	12 g
Xu Duan Rx. Dipsaci	18 g
Dang Gui Rx. Angelicae Sinensis	15 g
Dang Sheng Rx. Codonopsis	30 g
E Jiao Colla Cori Asini	
Shan Yao Rhiz. Dioscorae	

DAMP-HEAT BLOCKS THE LOWER BURNER

Bi Yu San (Jasper Powder) (Franconi)

Hua Shi Talcum	36 g
Gan Cao Rx. Glycyrrhizhae	6–30 g
Qing Dai Indigo Pulverata Levis	4.5–9 g

This formula is used for summer heat and dampness with Liver and Gallbladder heat as well as Urinary Bladder damp-heat. It clears heat, relieves toxicity and promotes urination. It eliminates summer heat, tonifies Qi and moreover cools the Blood.

Zini Qing Re Hua Shi Tang (Self-Made Decoction for Removing Heat and Eliminating Damp) (Weixin)

Fu Ling *Poria*	15 g
Qi Ye Yi Zhi Hua *Hb. Paris Polyphyllae*	9 g
Huang Qin *Rx. Scutellariae*	9 g
Huang Lian *Rhiz. Coptidis*	3 g
Huang Bai *Cx. Phellodendri*	6 g
Che Qian Zi *Sm. Plantaginis*	15 g
Sheng di Huang *Rx. Rehmanniae Glutinosae*	12 g
Mu Dan Pi *Cx. Moutan*	9 g
Yin Yang Huo *Hb. Epimedii*	12 g
Ba Ji Tian *Rx. Morindae*	9 g
Tu Si Zi *Sem. Cuscutae*	9 g
Chen Pi *Peric. Citri Ret.*	9 g
Gan Cao *Rx. Glycyrrhizae*	6 g

The first herbs in the formula all clear heat and remove toxins, promote diuresis and purge fire. The Yang tonics within the prescription invigorate the Kidney and replenish Essence to high-quality sperm. The prescription as a whole clears heat, eliminates damp, invigorates the Kidney, replenishes Essence, removes dead sperm and produces survival sperm (Weixin).

OBSTRUCTION OF THE COLLATERALS – BLOOD STASIS

Si Yu Tang (Zhi-Qiang)

Dang Shen *Rx. Codonopsis*	15 g
Bai Zhu *Rhiz. Atractylodes Mac.*	15 g
Fu Ling *Poria*	10 g
Dang Gui *Rx. Angelicae Sinensis*	10 g
Bai Shao *Rx. Paeoniae Albae*	10 g
Sheng Di Huang *Rx. Rehmannia Rec.*	10 g
Mu Dan Pi *Cx. Moutan*	10 g
Tu Si Zi *Sm. Cuscutae*	10 g
Rong Cong Rong *Hb. Cistanches*	10 g
Yin Yang Huo *Hb. Epimedii*	10 g
Zi He Che *Placenta Hominis*	10 g
Gan Cao *Rx. Glycyrrhizae*	6 g

This formula is indicated when there is low motility and a decreased number of living spermatozoa due to Spleen and Kidney vacuity and a blockage due to Blood stasis.

Qiang Jing Jian (Zhi-Qiang)

Shu Di Huang *Rx. Rehmanniae Prep.*	12 g
Shan Yao *Rhiz. Dioscorae Opp.*	12 g
Shan Zhu Yu *Fr. Corni*	12 g
Dang Gui *Rx. Angelicae Sinensis*	12 g
Gou Qi Zi *Fr. Lycii*	12 g
Zi He Che *Placenta Hominis*	15 g
Zhi Jiang Can *Bombyx Batryticatus* (fried)	15 g
Gan Di Long *Pheretima* (dried)	15 g
Rou Cong Rong *Hb. Cistanches*	10 g
Lu Kiao Pian *Cornu Cervi* (cut)	10 g

This prescription is ideal in case of sperm motility issues due to Spleen and Kidney vacuity with stagnation of the collateral vessels.

Shao Fu Zhu Yu Tang plus **Lu Lu Tong** (*Fr. Liquidambaris*), **Wang Bu Liu Xing** (*Sm. Vaccariae*) and **Dan Shen** (*Rx. Salviae Milt.*) (Focks)

Teratospermia

Chinese Medicine regards abnormal morphology to be primarily caused by weakness of the Spleen and Kidneys, with damp accumulating and slowing Blood circulation. In the West, excessive heat (either deficient or excess type, but most often the latter) is a primary factor in this pathology.[4] Therefore, resolving Blood stasis is one of the key factors when treating malformed spermatozoa. Hans-Joachim Stelting, for example, recommends using Blood-moving herbs such as *Dan Shen* (*Rx. Salviae Milt.*), *Ji Xue Teng* (*Caulis Spatholobi*), *To Ren* (*Sm. Persicae*) and *Niu Xi* (*Rx. Achyranthis*).[5]

Nevertheless, there is very little literature on the treatment of this sperm parameter available. Furthermore, it is definitely the most difficult parameter to treat.

Teratospermia (according to Clavey)

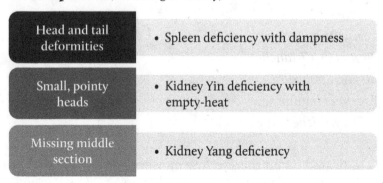

Head and tail deformities	• Spleen deficiency with dampness
Small, pointy heads	• Kidney Yin deficiency with empty-heat
Missing middle section	• Kidney Yang deficiency

SPLEEN DEFICIENCY WITH EXCESS DAMP CAUSING POOR MORPHOLOGY

Jian Pi Li Shi Zhi Ji Tang (Strengthen Spleen Clear Damp Treat Abnormality Decoction) (Clavey)

Cang Zhu Rhiz. Atractylodis		15 g
Ban Xia Rhiz. Pinelliae Ternatae		15 g
Xiang Fu Rhiz. Cyperi Rotundi		15 g
Fu Ling Scler. Poriae Cocos		30 g
Chen Pi Peric. Citri Reticulatae		10 g
Shen Qu Massa Fermentata		20 g
Chuan Xiong Rx. Ligustici Wallichii		5 g
Huang Qi Rx. Astragali		15 g
Yuan Zhi Rx. Polygalae Tenuifoliae		10 g

This type will have abnormalities primarily in the body and tail of the sperm.

Li Shi Yi Shen Tang (Focks)

Bie Xie Rhiz. Dioscorae		18 g
Yi Yi Ren Sm. Coicis		18 g
Tu Fu Ling Rhiz. Smilacis Glab.		18 g
Che Qian Zi Sm. Plantaginis		9 g
Shan Yao Rhiz. Dioscorae		9 g
Bai Zhu Rhiz. Atractylodes Mac.		9 g
He Tao Ren Sm. Juglandis		15 g
Niu Xi Rx. Achyranthis Bidentatae		15 g

This formula is suitable if the Spleen deficiency causes an accumulation of damp-heat in the Lower Burner as it clears heat, eliminates dampness but also replenishes Essence.

KIDNEY AND SPLEEN DEFICIENCY CAUSING POOR MORPHOLOGY

The name of that pattern by Steve Clavey does not match the prescription according to Simon Becker. He names that pattern 'Kidney Yin vacuity with empty-heat' in his article.[6]

Zi Yin Qing Re Zhi Ji San (Nourish Yin Cool Heat Treat Abnormality Powder) (Clavey)

Sheng Di Huang Rx. Rehmanniae Glutinosae		15 g
Shan Zhu Yu Fr. Corni Officinalis		15 g
Shan Yao Rx. Dioscoreae Oppositae		15 g
Tu Si Zi Sm. Cuscutae		15 g

Shui Niu Jiao Cornu Bubali	50 g
Gou Qi Zi Fr. Lycii Chinensis	12 g
Mu Dan Pi Cx. Moutan Radicis	10 g
Fu Ling Scl. Poriae Cocos	10 g
Yan Huang Bai Cx. Phellodendri, soaked in salt	9 g
Shan Zhi Zi Fr. Gardeniae Jasminoidis	5 g
Huang Qin Rx. Scutellariae Baicalensis	5 g
Xiang Fu Rhiz. Cyperi Rotundi	5 g
Ze Xie Rhiz. Alismatis	5 g

Powder finely and take 7.5 g before meals in the morning and evening with salt water. This pattern type will show abnormalities primarily of the head of the sperm in the sperm test, particularly small pointed heads and malformed heads. As the name of the formula suggests, it not only strengthens the Kidneys but also clears heat.

Da Bu Yin Wan (Great Tonify the Yin Pill) (Focks)

Shu Di Huang Rx. Rehmanniae Prep.	6–30 g
Su Jiu Gui Ban Pl. Testudinis (deep-fried)	6–30 g
Chao Huang Bai Cx. Phellodendri (deep-fried)	4–20 g
Jiu Chao Zhi Mu Rx. Anemarrhenae (wine-fried)	4–20 g
Zhu Ji Shui (pig spinal cord)	25–50 g
Feng Mel	

There is research showing that this prescription may have an ameliorative effect on mitochondrial dysfunction.

KIDNEY YANG DEFICIENCY AND BLOOD STAGNATION CAUSING POOR MORPHOLOGY

Wen Shen Hua Yu Zhi Ji Tang (Warm Kidneys Transform Stagnation Treat Abnormality Decoction) (Clavey)

Chao Bai Zhu Rhiz. Atractylodis Macrocephalae dry-fried	15 g
Ba Ji Tian Rx. Morindae Officinalis	15 g
Ren Shen Rx. Ginseng	10 g
Chao Du Zhong Eucommiae Ulmoidis dry-fried	15 g
Tu Si Zi Sm. Cuscutae	20 g
Chao Qian Shi Semen Euryales Ferox dry-fried	15 g
Rou Gui Cx. Cinnamomi Cassiae	5 g
Lu Jiao Shuang Cornu Cervi Gelatinum	10 g
Suo Yang Hb. Cynomorii Songarici	10 g
Hong Hua Fl. Carthami Tinctorii	5 g
Yan Hu Suo Rhiz. Corydalis Yanhusuo	10 g

This pattern type will have abnormalities primarily of the head of the sperm, particularly small pointed heads; and also sperm lacking a middle section. If there is additional Yin vacuity, herbs such as *Gou Qi Zi* (*Fr. Lycii*), *Wu Wei Zi* (*Fr. Schisandrae*) and *Nu Zhen Zi* (*Fr. Ligustri Lucici*) can be incorporated.

KIDNEY YIN AND YANG DEFICIENCY CAUSING POOR MORPHOLOGY

Shi Zi Er Xian Tang (Ten Seeds Two Immortals Decoction) (Clavey)

Tu Si Zi Sm. Cuscutae	10 g
Fu Pen Zi Fr. Rubi	10 g
Wu Wei Zi Fr. Schisandrae Chinensis	5 g
Che Qian Zi Sm. Plantaginis	10 g
Gou Qi Zi Fr. Lycii Chinensis	10 g
Nu Zhen Zi Fr. Ligustri Lucidi	15 g
Sha Yuan Ji Li Sm. Astragalai	10 g
Jiu Cai Zi Sm. Alii Tuberosi	10 g
She Chuang Zi Fr. Cnidii Monnieri	9 g
Sang Shen Zi Fr. Mori Albae	10 g
Xian Mao Rhiz. Curculiginis Orchioidis	15 g
Yin Yang Huo Hb. Epimedii	15 g

This pattern type will have low sperm count as well as high abnormality.

Zan Yu Dan Jia Jian (Special Pill to Enhance Fertility) (Clavey)

Shu Di Huang Rx. Rehmanniae Praeparata

Dung Gui Rx. Angelicae Sinensis

Du Zhong Cx. Eucommiae

Ba Ji Tian Rx. Morindae Officinalis

Rou Cong Rong Hb. Cistanches

Yin Yang Huo Hb. Epimedii

Rou Gui Cx. Cinnamomi

Bai Zhu Rhiz. Atractylodis Macrocephalae

Gou Qi Zi Fr. Lycii

Xian Mao Rhiz. Curculiginis

Shan Zhu Yu Fr. Corni

Jiu Zi Sm. Alii Tuberosii

Fu Zi Rx. Aconiti Lateralis Praeparata or *Ren Shen* Rx. Ginseng

Lu Rong Cornu Cervi Pantotrichum

Focks also lists this prescription but puts it in the category Kidney Yang vacuity or Kidney vacuity in general.

Liquefication problems

Reduced Viscosity: Etiology

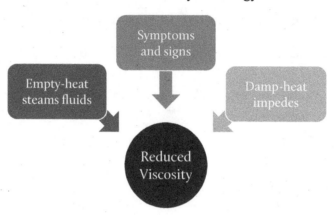

This is also a common cause of male infertility. The normal process of liquefication of the ejaculate from a Chinese Medicine perspective depends on Kidney Essence and Ming Men fire interacting by using the transformation power of Qi. According to its manifestation, liquefication problems may fall into the category of jing zhuo (seminal turbidity), jing re (seminal heat), jing han (seminal cold) and lin zhuo (strangury-turbidity) in Chinese Medicine. The main pathologic factors include downward flow of damp-heat, depletion and deficiency of Kidney Yin, insufficiency of Kidney Yang, accumulation of phlegm turbidity in the interior, and mutual mingling of phlegm and stasis.[7]

DAMP-HEAT POURING DOWNWARDS CAUSING POOR LIQUEFICATION

Cu Ye Hua Tang (Liquefaction-Promoting Decoction) (Tiandong)

Bi Xie *Rhiz. Dioscoreae Hypoglaucae*	15 g
Shi Chang Pu *Rhiz. Acori Tatarinowii*	10 g
Che Qian Zi *Sm. Plantaginis*	10 g
Lian Zi Xin *Plumula Nelumbinis*	5 g
Fu Ling *Poria*	15 g
Huang Bai *Cx. Phellodendri*	5 g
Long Dan Cao *Rx. Gentianae*	8 g
Tu Fu Ling *Rhiz. Smilacis Glabrae*	20 g
Huang Qin *Rx. Scutellariae*	10 g
Ku Shen *Rx. Sophorae Flavescentis*	10 g

Chi Shao Rx. Paeoniae Rubra	10 g
Bai Mao Gen Rhiz. Imperatae	10 g
Yi Mu Cao Hb. Leonuri	10 g
Qian Cao Rx. Rubiae Cordifoliae	10 g
Wu Yao Rx. Linderae	10 g
Yi Zhi Fr. Alpiniae Oxyphyllae	5 g

The formula of Liquefaction-Promoting Decoction is based on *Bixie Fen Qi*. This is a suitable formula for a case of chronic prostatitis, which should be treated on the principle of clearing away heat and removing dampness as well as promoting Blood circulation and resolving stasis according to the pattern identified.

Shui Zhi Ye Hua Tang

Shui Zhi Fen Hirudo	2 g
Zhi Mu Rhiz. Anemarrhenae	30 g
Huang Bai Cx. Phellodendri	10 g
Tian Men Dong Rx. Aspagari	15 g
Mai Men Dong Tuber Ophiopogonis Japonici	15 g
Sheng Di Huang Rx. Rehmanniae glut.	30 g
Xuan Shen Radix Scrophulariae Ningpoensis	15 g
Shi Hu Caulis Dendrobii	5 g
Mu Tong Caulis Akebiae	9 g
Gan Cao Rx. Glycyrrhizae	6 g

Long Dan Xie Gan Tang (Gentiana Longdancao Decoction to Drain the Liver) plus Zhi Bai Di Huang Tang (Anemarrhena, Phellodendron and Rehmannia Decoction) (Clavey, Weixin)

KIDNEY YIN VACUITY (WITH EMPTY-HEAT) CAUSING POOR LIQUEFACTION

Ye Hua Tang (Liquefaction Decoction) (Clavey)

Zhi Mu Rx. Anemarrhenae Asphodeloidis	9 g
Huang Bai Cx. Phellodendri	9 g
Bai Shao Rx. Paeoniae Lactiflorae	9 g
Chi Shao Rx. Paeoniae Rubrae	9 g
Mai Men Dong Tuber Ophiopogonis Japonici	9 g
Tian Hua Fen Rx. Trichosanthis	9 g
Dan Shen Rx. Salviae Miltiorrhizae	30 g
Gou Qi Zi Fr. Lycii Chinensis	15 g

Yin Yang Huo Hb. Epimedii	15 g
Sheng Di Huang Rx. Rehmanniae Prep.	12 g
Xuan Shen Rx. Scrophulariae Ningpoensis	9 g
Zhu Ye Hb. Lophatheri Gracilis	9 g
Che Qian Cao Gen Rx. Rubiae Cordifoliae	15 g

Yie Hua Tang (Decoction for Semen Liquefication) (Zi-Qiang)

Zhi Mu Rhiz. Anemarrhenae	15 g
Huang Bai Cx. Phellodendri	10 g
Sheng Di Huang Rx. Rehmanniae Prep.	15 g
Xian Mao Rhiz. Curculiginis	10 g
Che Qian Cao Hb. Plantaginis	10 g
Tian Hua Fen Rx. Trichosanthis	10 g
Nan Gua Zi Sm. Cucurbitae	10 g
Bai Shao Rx. Paeoniae Albae	10 g
Shu Di Huang Rx. Rehmanniae Prep.	15 g
Mai Men Dong Rx. Ophiopogonis	10 g
Xuan Shen Rx. Scrophulariae	10 g
Gou Qi Zi Fr. Lycii	10 g
Yin Yang Huo Hb. Epimedii	10 g
Dan Shen Rx. Salviae Milit.	15 g

Weixin uses the same formula but uses *Chi Shao* (*Rx. Paeoniae Rubrae*) and *Dan Zhu Ye* (*Hb. Lophatheri*) instead of *Nan Gua Zi* and *Xian Mao*.

Zhi Bai Di Huang Wan (Clavey)

KIDNEY YANG VACUITY CAUSING POOR LIQUEFACTION

Sheng Jing Tang (Produce Jing Decoction) (Clavey)

Yin Yang Huo Hb. Epimedii	15 g
Xu Duan Rx. Dipsaci	15 g
Shu Di Huang Rx. Rehmanniae Prep.	15 g
He Shou Wu Rx Polygoni Multiflori	15 g
Sang Shen Zi Fr. Mori Albae	15 g
Dang Shen Rx. Codonopsis Pilosulae	15 g
Huang Qi Rx. Astragali	18 g
Dang Gui Rx. Angelicae Sinensis	9 g
Fu Pen Zi Fr. Rubi	9 g

Weixin uses a modification of this formula adding *Tu Si Zi* (*Sm. Cuscutae*) 9 g, *Chen Pi* (*Peric. Citri Retic*) 9 g, *Che Qian Zi* (*Sm. Plantaginis*) 9 g, *Ba Ji Tian* (*Rx. Morindae*) 9 g, *Fu Zi* (*Rx. Aconiti Prep.*) 3–6 g, *Wu Yao* (*Rx. Linderae*) 6 g, *Xiao Hui Xiang* (*Fr. Foeniculi*) 6 g, *Wu Zhu Yu* (*Fr. Evodiae*) 9 g.

OTHER FORMULAS

- *Jin Gui Shen Qi Wan* plus *Wu Zi Yang Zong Wan* (Clavey)

Immuninfertility (*Jing Zi Mi Du Zeng Gao*)

The anti-sperm antibodies (AsAb) act like Velcro – sperm cells surrounded by antibodies attached to their plasma membrane become stuck to other sperm in the same condition, causing clumping and thus inability to move forward.

Most authors highlight the importance of using Blood-moving herbs as autoimmune diseases often belong to the category of Blood stasis. The combination of *Dan Shen* and *Huang Qi* is a Dui Yao pair commonly used in autoimmune pathologies for example. Another treatment strategy would be to tonify the Zheng Qi while expelling dampness, heat and Blood stasis as pathogens causing the autoimmune infertility.

Clinical research confirms that herbs for promoting Blood circulation and removing Blood stasis have some suppressive effects on substances that cause humeral and cellular immunity. Those drugs have curative effects in treating especially autoimmune diseases. Drugs for nourishing Yin and removing heat from Blood can supress immunological hyperfunction. Herbs for clearing heat and toxins can supress immunoreaction and increase the phagocytic function of the reticuloendothelial system. Drugs for expelling wind, removing damp and clearing cold diminish inflammation and suppress the release of allergic transmitters and regulate the permeability of Blood vessels.[8]

ALL-IN-ONE – USED FOR ANY PATTERN FORMULA

Xiao Kang Tang (Antibody-Resolving Decoction) (Tiandong)

Nu Zhen Zi Fr. Ligustri Lucidi	10 g
Mo Han Lian Herba Ecliptae	10 g
Sheng Di Huang Rx. Rehmanniae	10 g
Xuan Shen Rx. Scrophulariae	10 g
Pu Gong Ying Hb. Taraxaci	10 g
Jin Yin Hua Fl. Lonicerae	10 g
Chai Hu Rx. Bupleuri	10 g
Hu Zhang Rhiz. Polygoni Cuspidati	15 g
Dan Shen Rx. Salviae Miltiorrhizae	10 g

Chi Shao Rx. Paeoniae Rubra	10 g
Chuan Shan Jia Squama Manitis	5 g
Wang Bu Liu Xing Sm. Vaccariae	10 g
Tian Qi Mo Rad. Pulvis Notoginseng	1 g
Pu Huang Pollen Typhae	10 g
Hai Ma Hippocampus	1 piece
Dang Shen Radix Codonopsis	10 g

This formula enriches Yin, clears away heat, removes dampness, invigorates Blood circulation and resolves stasis.

BLOOD STASIS

Guiding formula (Lin)

Lu Lu Tong Fr. Liquidambaris	30 g
San Leng Rhiz. Sparganii	15 g
E Zhu Rhiz. Curcumae	15 g
Tao Ren Sm. Persicae	15 g
Hong Hua Fl. Carthami	10 g
Chi Shao Rx. Paeoniae Rubrae	10 g
Chuan Xiong Rhiz. Lugustri Chuanxiong	10 g
Niu Xi Rx. Achyranthis Bident.	30 g
Zhi Mu Rhiz. Anemarrhenae	10 g
Huang Bai Cx. Phellodendri	10 g
Gou Qi Zi Fr. Lycii	30 g
Fu Pen Zi Fr. Rubi	30 g
Mu Dan Pi Cx. Moutan	30 g

This prescription activates the Blood and transforms stasis, assisted by enriching Yin, boosting Essence and descending fire as necessary.

KIDNEY YANG DEFICIENCY IN ANTI-SPERM ANTIBODIES
Cold leads to seminal congelation.

Huang Shi Zeng Jing Wan (Mr Huang's Augment Jing Pill) (Huang Hai-Bo)

Zhi Fu Zi Rx. Aconiti Carmichaeli Prep.	90 g
Rou Gui Cx. Cinnamomi Cassiae	60 g
Jiu Cai Zi Sm. Alii Tuberosi	90 g
Yin Yang Huo Hb. Epimedii	90 g

Tu Si Zi Sm. Cuscutae	180 g
Lu Rong Cornu Cervi Parvum	90 g
Lu Jiao Jiao Colla Cornu Cervi	270 g
Bai Shao Rx. Paeoniae Lactiflorae	150 g
Ren Shen Rx. Ginseng	30 g

Powder finely, sieve and make pills with 'toffied' (cooked) honey, each pill 12 g. Take one pill morning, noon and night with wine.

Zi Ni Wen Ning Tang (Self-Made Decoction for Warming Agglutination) (Weixin)

Yin Yang Huo Hb. Epimedii	15 g
Ba Ji Tian Rx. Morindae	9 g
Tu Si Zi Sm. Cuscutae	9 g
Fu Zi Rx. Aconiti Prep.	6 g
Rou Gui Cx. Cinnamomi	6 g
Ren Shen Rx. Ginseng	3–6 g
Dang Gui Rx. Angelicae Sin.	9 g
Huang Qi Rx. Astragali	30 g
Bai Shao Rx. Paeoniae Albae	9 g
Xu Chang Qing Rx Cynanchi Paniculati	9 g
Gan Cao Rx. Glycyrrhizae Ural.	6 g

Xu Chang Qing is considered to process anti-immunological function.

KIDNEY YIN DEFICIENCY IN ANTI-SPERM ANTIBODIES
A lack of fluids and Yin leads to thickening.

Yi Shen Bu Jing San (Benefit Kidneys and Tonify Jing Powder) (Huang Hai-Bo)

Lu Rong Cornu Cervi Parvum	30 g
Yin Yang Huo Hb. Epimedii	120 g
Tu Si Zi Sm. Cuscutae	150 g
Lu Jiao Jiao Colla Cornu Cervi	80 g
Huang Jing Rhiz. Polygonati	180 g
Wu Wei Zi Fr. Schisandrae Chinensis	90 g
Nu Zhen Zi Fr. Ligustri Lucidi	90 g
Ren Shen Rx. Ginseng	60 g
Zi He Che Placenta Hominis	180 g

Powder finely, take three times per day with salt water. Avoid hot spicy foods.

Zi Ni Xiao Ning Tang (Self-Made Agglutination-Relieving Decoction) (Weixin)

Shu Di Huang Rx. Rehmanniae	12 g
Mai Men Dong Rx. Ophiopogonis	9 g
Xuan Shen Rx. Scophulariae	9 g
Bai Shao Rx. Paeoniae Albae	9 g
Nu Zhen Zi Fr. Ligustri Lucidi	12 g
Han Lian Cao Hb. Ecliptae	12 g
Gui Ban Plastrum Testudinis	30 g
Bie Jia Carapax Trionycis	30 g
Chi Shao Rx. Paeoniae Rubrae	9 g
Mu Dan Pi Cx. Moutan	9 g
Dan Shen Rx. Salvia Milt.	30 g
Xu Chang Qing Rx. Cynanchi Paniculati	9 g
Gan Cao Rx. Glycyrrhizae Ural.	6 g

Drugs aiming at nourishing Yin and cooling Blood can inhibit hyperimmunological function and counteract against pathological changes. Drugs that activate the circulation of Blood and remove Blood stasis not only have anti-inflammatory effects but also lower capillary permeability and inhibit cellular immunity.

LIVER CHANNEL DAMP-HEAT IN ANTI-SPERM ANTIBODIES
Dampness and heat bind the sperm.

Qing Re Chu Shi Xiao Ning Tang (Cool Heat Eliminate Damp and Dissolve Coagulation Decoction) (Huang Hai-Bo)

Long Dan Cao Rx. Gentianae Scabrae	12 g
Ku Shen Rx. Sophorae Flavescentis	9 g
Chao Huang Bai Cortex Phellodendri dry-fried	6 g
Dan Zhu Ye Hb. Lopthatheri Gracili	9 g
Ze Xie Rhiz. Alismatis	9 g
Mu Dan Pi Cx. Moutan Radicis	6 g
Han Fang Ji Rx. Stephaniae Tetrandae	9 g
Cang Zhu Rhiz. Atractylodis	9 g
Chi Fu Ling Scl. Poriae Cocos Rubrae	9 g

Zi Ni Chu Ning Tang (Self-Made Decoction for Removing Agglutination) (Weixin)

Long Dan Cao Rx. Gentianae	9 g
Huang Lian Rhiz. Coptidis	3 g
Huang Qin Rx. Scuttellariae	9 g
Da Huang Rx. et Rhiz. Rei	3 g
Shu Di Huang Rx. Rehmanniae Prep.	12 g
Mu Dan Pi Cx. Moutan	9 g
Dang Gui Rx. Angelicae Sin.	15 g
Lian Qiao Fr. Forsythiae	12 g
Pu Gong Ying Hb. Taraxaci	18 g
Bai Hua She She Cao Hb. Hedyotis	15 g
Gan Cao Rx. Glycyrrhizzae	6 g

The above drugs play their roles through cAMP and cGMP level regulation, therefore an anti-autoimmune effect is achieved.

LIVER QI BLOCKAGE IN ANTI-SPERM ANTIBODIES

The free flow of Liver Qi is obstructed, leading to agglutination.

Si Ni San (Frigid Extremities Powder) with additions (*Huang Hai-Bo*)

Chai Hu Rx. Bupleuri	90 g
Bai Shao Rx. Paeoniae Lactiflorae	100 g
Zhi Xiang Fu Rhiz. Cyperi Rotundi	90 g
Mu Xiang Rx. Saussureae seu Vladimirae	90 g
Chen Pi Peric. Citri Reticulatae	60 g
Gan Cao Rx. Glycyrrhizae Uralensis	60 g

Powder finely and sieve; take 9–12 g twice a day.

SPECIAL MEDICINALS

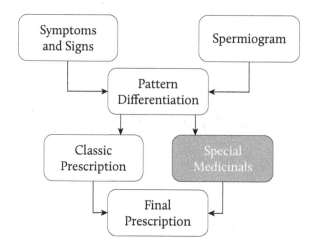

Guiding medicinals

- **Lu Lu Tong** Fr. Liquidambaris

- **Wang Bu Liu Xing** Sm. Vaccariae

Both of the above are guiding medicinals to the testicles. *Lu Lu Tong* is more often used if there is additional need of a Blood-moving herb in the prescription, whereas *Wang Bu Liu Xing* can be seen as useable in any case as it is a very mild herb.

- **Niu Xi** Rx. Achyranthis

- **Chuan Niu Xi** Rx. Cyathulae

Both of these Blood-moving herbs work as guiding medicinals that bring the effect of a prescription down to the Lower Burner.

Mycoplasma infection

- **Bai Bu** Rx. Stemonae

- **She Chuang Zi** Fr. Cnidii

Prolactinemia

- **Mai Ya** Fr. Hordei Vulgaris germ.

- **Chai Hu** Rx. Bupleuri

Special medicinals for anti-sperm antibodies

- **Huang Qi** Rx. Astragali
- **Zhi Mu** Rhiz. Anemarrhenae
- **Nu Zhen Zi** Fr. Ligustri Lucidi
- **Zhu Ling** Polyporus

Reduced viscosity

- **Bie Xie** Rhiz. Dioscoreae Septemlobae – if there is dampness hindering liquefication
- **Mai Ya** Fr. Hordei germ. – contains a lot of enzymes that help the often-missing plasminogen of the prostate secretion to liquefy semen
- **Zhi Ke** Fr. Auranti

Sperm movement

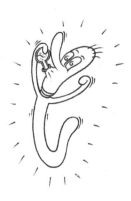

Tonifying Yang to improve motility is a well-known concept. From a modern perspective, it makes even more sense when knowing that Yang tonics increase ATP production in the mitochondria that are settled in the sperm's middle piece.

- **Tu Si Zi** Sm. Cuscutae
- **Xian Mao** Rhiz. Curculiginis
- **Ba ji Tian** Rx. Morindae

Also Qi tonics work well in motility treatments. Studies showed that Huang Qi, for example, could increase motility 1.5-fold.

- **Huang Qi** Rx. Astragali

When sperm's ability to move suffers from microtrauma, such as induced by mountain biking, Blood-moving herbs should be taken into account.

- *Niu Xi* Rx. Achyranthis

- *Lu Lu Tong* Fr. Liquidambaris

- *San Qi* Rx. Notoginseng

- *Dan Shen* Rx. Salviae

Damp-heat and toxins

- *Bai Jiang Cao* Hb. Patriniae

- *Tu Fu Ling* Rhiz. Smilacis Glabrae

- *Pu Gong Ying* Hb. Taraxaci

- *Hong Teng* Cl. Sargentodoxae

— CHAPTER 17 —

Evidence

(or: How Sexy Can Research Be?)

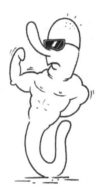

To have evidence that our empirically effective therapeutic interventions are also statistically relevant is of enormous importance. This is the tool to be able to get in touch with reproductive endocrinologists, gynaecologists, andrologists and all the different sub-groups you need and want to work with. But those specialists are used to talking in a scientific language and don't know what to do with terms like Qi and Jing. So you'll need to learn to speak 'scientific' at least a little, to be able to communicate with them.

This is a selection of research done in the field of acupuncture and herbs to give you some talking tools. As research is fast-moving and, fortunately, a lot of it is done in the Chinese Medicine field, this chapter would need to grow and to be updated constantly, which is not possible in a printed book. So please see this chapter as a 'teaser' and reach out to recent research presented at congresses or in published articles.

RESEARCH ON ACUPUNCTURE FOR MALE FERTILITY PROBLEMS

As with any indication, acupuncture studies are always quite difficult to design and their quality varies a lot. Concerning acupuncture and male infertility, there are some studies that stand out due to their high quality and some due to their interesting findings. This is kind of a 'best of' mixture of both categories, but the fact remains that much more research is needed in the acupuncture field.

SUMMARIES OF THE RESEARCH STUDIES

Acupuncture and OATS

A prospective, randomized, single-blind, placebo-controlled trial.

All male partners from infertile couples with sperm concentrations < 1 million sperm/ml who presented at the Division of Reproductive Endocrinology and Infertility, Department of Obstetrics and Gynaecology, University of Witten/Herdecke.

Patients were randomized to receive either acupuncture or placebo acupuncture twice weekly for 6 weeks (28/29).

Points used: *Zusanli* (St 36, bilateral), *Sanyinjiao* (Sp 6, bilateral), *Taixi* (Ki 3, bilateral), *Taichong* (Liv 3, bilateral), *Shenshu* (Bl 23, bilateral), *Ciliao* (Bl 32, bilateral), *Guilai* (St 29, bilateral), *Xuehai* (Sp 10, bilateral) and *Guanyuan* (Ren 4).

Result: A significantly higher percentage of motile sperm (World Health Organization categories A–C), but no effect on sperm concentration, was found after acupuncture compared with placebo acupuncture.

Source: Dieterle, S., Li, C., Greb, R., Bartzsch, F., Hatsmann, W. and Huang, D. (2009) 'A prospective randomized placebo-controlled study of the effect of acupuncture in infertile patients with severe oligoasthenozoospermia.' *Fertility and Sterility 92*, 4, 1340–1343.

Electroacupuncture (EA) and semen parameter

A total of 121 patients diagnosed with oligospermia, asthenospermia or oligoasthenospermia were randomized into four groups (three treatment groups, one control):

Points used: The TEAS (transcutaneous electric acupoint stimulation) groups were treated with 2Hz (n=31), 100Hz (n=31), or mock stimulation (n=29) at acupuncture points Bl 23, St 36, CV 1 and CV 4 for two months. The control group (n=30) was provided with lifestyle advice only.

Result: Best was the 2 Hz group which showed a significant change in total sperm count and motility, neutral α-glucosidase (NAG) and zinc levels as well as fructose levels.

Explanation: The upregulation of calcium and integrin-binding protein 1 (CIB1) and downregulation of cyclin-dependent kinase 1 b (CDK1) by TEAS may be associated with its positive effects on sperm motility and count.

Source: Yu, Y., Sha, S.-B., Zhang, B., Guan, Q. *et al.* (2019) 'Effects and mechanism of action of transcutaneous electrical acupuncture point stimulation in patients with abnormal semen parameters.' *Acupuncture in Medicine 37*, 1, 25–32.

Comparing effects of acupuncture and varicocelectomy on sperm parameters in infertile varicocele patients

Between January 2008 and May 2010, 30 men with primary infertility (one year of unprotected intercourse, healthy wife) and varicocele with normal hormone levels and abnormal semen analysis were randomized into two groups. Group 1 underwent subinguinal microscopic varicocelectomy, and Group 2 underwent acupuncture treatment twice a week for two months. Both groups were evaluated with semen analysis at six months after the treatment.

Results: Sperm concentration and motility improved significantly in both groups after the treatment. Increase in sperm concentration was higher in the acupuncture group compared to the varicocelectomy group (P=0.039). The average follow-up was 42 months, and pregnancy rates of 33% were observed in both groups.

Source: Kucuk, E.V., Bindayi, A., Boylu, U., Onol, F.F. and Gumus, E. (2016) 'Randomised clinical trial of comparing effects of acupuncture and varicocelectomy on sperm parameters in infertile varicocele patients.' *Andrologia 48*, 10, 1080–1085.

Quantitative evaluation of spermatozoa ultrastructure after acupuncture treatment for idiopathic male infertility

Twenty-eight patients received acupuncture twice a week over a period of five weeks; there were 12 men in the untreated control group (range: 25–46 years).

Points used: Primary points – Ren 4, UB 23 bilateral, Bl 32 bilateral, Liv 3 bilateral, Ki 3 bilateral; secondary points – St 36 bilateral, Sp 10 bilateral, Sp 6 bilateral, St 29 bilateral, Du 20.

Results: Quantitative analysis by transmission electron microscopy (TEM) showed a statistically significant improvement in acrosome position and shape, nuclear shape, axonemal pattern and shape, and accessory fibres of sperm organelles; and statistically significant increase after acupuncture in the percentage and number of sperm without ultrastructural defects in the total ejaculates.

Source: Pei, J., Strehler, E., Noss, U., Abt, M. *et al.* (2005) 'Quantitative evaluation of spermatozoa ultrastructure after acupuncture treatment for idiopathic male infertility.' *Fertility and Sterility 84*, 1, 141–147.

Effects of acupuncture and moxa treatment in patients with semen abnormalities

In a prospective, controlled and blind study, 19 patients aged 24–42 years, without children, with semen abnormalities in concentration, morphology and/or progressive motility without any apparent cause, were randomized into two groups. There was a study group that received acupuncture and moxa treatment at well-known therapeutic points that work for fertility issues and a control group. They received acupuncture and moxa at the indifferent points. Both groups received therapy for ten weeks. Semen analyses were performed before and after the treatment course.

Points used:

Points needled	
St 30	Ki 3
St 36	Ll 4
Sp 6	Sp 4
Liv 3	Pc 6

Points treated with moxa			
Bl 23	Ren 6	Ren 5	Ex-CA (Qimen)
Bl 52	Ren 4	Lu 9	Ex-CA 1 (Zigong)
Bl 22	Du 3	Bl 13	
Du 4	Bl 20	Bl 14	
Bl 32	Bl 21	Bl 15	

Results: The patients of the study group presented a significant increase in the percentage of normal-form sperm compared to the control group. The comparison of other pre- and post-treatment data (volume, concentration, progressive motility and number of round cells) did not show significant differences between the two groups.

Explanation: The authors' explanation for the acupuncture effect was that needling caused a vasodilatation in the testicles as well as in the epidymidis, which lowered the ROS.

Source: Gurfinkel, E., Cedenho, A.P., Yamamura, Y. and Srougi, M. (2003) 'Effects of acupuncture and moxa treatment in patients with semen abnormalities.' *Asian Journal of Andrology 5*, 4, 345–348.

Success of acupuncture treatment in patients with initially low sperm output is associated with a decrease in scrotal skin temperature

Question: To verify whether the influence of acupuncture treatment on sperm output in patients with low sperm density is associated with a decrease in scrotal temperature.

Study design: The experimental group included 39 men who were referred for acupuncture owing to low sperm output. The control group, which comprised 18 normal fertile men, was used to define a threshold (30.5°C) above which scrotal skin temperature was considered to be high. Scrotal skin temperature and sperm concentration were measured before and after acupuncture treatment.

Each patient in the experimental group underwent a course of 8–10 acupunctural treatments (two treatments a week).

Points used: Acupuncture points appropriate for the deficiency of the Kidneys (hormonal imbalance) and damp-heat syndromes (inflammation of the genital tract) were regarded as main points: Sp 6 (*Sanyinjiao*), Ren 4 (*GuanYuan*), Lu 7 (*Liegue*), Kl 6 (*Zhohai*) and ST 30 (*Qicong*) were used for both syndromes.

Four additional main points – Ki 3 (*Taixi*), Bl 23 (*Shenshu*), Ki 11 (*Henggu*) and Bl 52 (*Zhishi*) – were used only for the Kidney Yang deficiency syndrome (spermatogenic failure).

Five other main points – Sp 9 (*Yinlingquan*), Liv 5 (*Ligou*), Ll 11 (*Quchi*), St 28 (*Shuidao*) and Gb 41 (*Zuliqi*) – were used only for damp-heat in the genital system (inflammation of the genital tract).

Secondary points: Ll 4 (*Hegu*), St 36 (*Zusanli*), Sp 10 (*Xuehai*), Ht 7 (*Shenmen*), Bl 20 (*Pishu*), Pc 6 (*Neiguan*), Ren 1 (*Huiyin*), Ren 2 (*Qugu*), Ren 6 (*Qihai*), Du 4 (*Ming Men*), Du 20 (*Baihui*), Gb 20 (*Fengchi*), Liv 3 (*Taichong*), Ki 7 (*Fulu*) and Gb 27 (*Wushu*).

Specific combinations of main and secondary points were selected for each patient during treatment, according to the principles of traditional acupuncture.

No more than 12 points were punctured during any single session.

Results: 34 of the 39 participants in the experimental group initially had high scrotal skin temperature; the other five had normal values. The five patients with initially normal scrotal temperatures were not affected by the acupuncture treatment.

Following treatment, 17 of the 34 patients with hyperthermia, all of whom had genital tract inflammation, had normal scrotal skin temperature; in 15 of these 17 patients, sperm count was increased.

In the remaining 17 men with scrotal hyperthermia, neither scrotal skin temperature nor sperm concentration was affected by the treatment.

About 90% of the latter patients suffered from high gonadotropins or mixed etiological factors.

Source: Siterman, S., Eltes, F., Schechter, L., Maimon, Y., Lederman, H. and Bartoov, B. (2009) 'Success of acupuncture treatment in patients with initially low sperm output is associated with a decrease in scrotal skin temperature.' *Asian Journal of Andrology* 11, 2, 200–208.

Influence of acupuncture on idiopathic male infertility in assisted reproductive technology

The clinical effects of acupuncture on idiopathic male infertility in sperm parameter and on therapeutic results in assisted reproductive technology were investigated.

Study design: 22 unsuccessful intracytoplasmic sperm injection (ICSI) patients with idiopathic male infertility were treated with acupuncture twice weekly for eight weeks, followed by ICSI treatment again. Sperm concentration, motility, morphology, fertilization rates and embryo quality were observed.

Results: Quick sperm motility after acupuncture (18.3% +/– 9.6%) was significantly improved as compared with that before treatment (11.0% +/– 7.5%, P < 0.01).

The normal sperm ratio was increased after acupuncture (21.1% +/– 10.4% vs 16.2% +/– 8.2%, P < 0.05).

The fertilization rates after acupuncture (66.2%) were obviously higher than those before treatment (40.2%, P < 0.01).

There was no significant difference in sperm concentration and general sperm motility between before and after acupuncture.

Embryo quality after acupuncture was improved, but the difference between them was not significant (P > 0.05). Acupuncture can improve sperm quality and fertilization rates in assisted reproductive technology.

Source: Zhang, M., Huang, G., Lu, F., Paulus, W.E. and Sterzik, K. (2002) 'Influence of acupuncture on idiopathic male infertility in assisted reproductive technology.' *Journal of Huazhong University of Science and Technology: Medical Sciences* 22, 3, 228–230.

Finally, here are the results of two different systematic reviews on acupuncture for male fertility:

Article 1

THE EFFECTIVENESS AND SAFETY OF ACUPUNCTURE FOR POOR SEMEN QUALITY IN INFERTILE MALES: A SYSTEMATIC REVIEW AND META-ANALYSIS

Ui Min Jerng, Jun-Young Jo, Seunghoon Lee, Jin-Moo Lee and Ohmin Kwon

DOI: 10.4103/1008-682X.129130

In this systematic review and meta-analysis the researchers searched for randomized controlled trials (RCTs) that compared acupuncture, with or without additional treatment, against placebo, sham, no treatment or the same additional treatment. The outcomes they looked at were pregnancy rates (defined as a positive pregnancy test), sperm concentration and motility.

Results: Acupuncture increased sperm motility (the percentage of sperm moving with rapid progression) as well as sperm concentration. As these two results were heterogeneous among the included studies, the researchers end with the well-known words: 'Further large, well-designed RCTs are required.'

Citation: Jerng, U.M., Jo, J.Y., Lee, S., Lee, J.M. and Kwon, O. (2014) 'The effectiveness and safety of acupuncture for poor semen quality in infertile males: A systematic review and meta-analysis'. *Asian Journal of Andrology 16*, 6, 884–891.

Source: pubmed.ncbi.nlm.nih.gov

Article 2

EFFICACY AND SAFETY OF ACUPUNCTURE FOR THE TREATMENT OF OLIGOASTHENOZOOSPERMIA: A SYSTEMATIC REVIEW.

Fang You, Lianguo Ruan, Li Zeng and Yan Zhang

DOI:10.1111/and.13415

As oligoasthenospermia is a common factor causing male infertility, which is treated frequently with Chinese Medicine, this review tried to assess the evidence of acupuncture for this indication. They included 12 randomized controlled trials (RCTs) with 1088 participants. 'According to the narrative analysis, acupuncture or acupuncture combined with another intervention was effective in improving the semen quality based on the included studies.' But as the methodological quality of most studies included was low, again the researchers end with the sentence that full-scale RCTs are needed to be able to validate the effect of acupuncture in the therapy of oligoasthenospermia.

Citation: You, F., Ruan, L., Zeng, L. and Zhang, Y. (2019) 'Efficacy and safety of acupuncture for the treatment of oligoasthenozoospermia: A systematic review'. *Andrologia 52*, 1, e13415.

Source: pubmed.ncbi.nlm.nih.gov

RESEARCH HERBS AND PRESCRIPTIONS

A quick reminder

The hypothalamic-pituitary-gonadal (HPG) axis is a major positive- and negative-endocrine feedback system that regulates testis function. Hormone levels that are either too high or too low are detrimental to spermatogenesis.

Modern research has demonstrated that Kidney deficiency often manifests with the dysfunction and impaired structure of the HPG axis.

Experiments have shown that Kidney-supplementing formulas could repair the structure and restore the function of the HPG axis, bidirectionally regulate the hormone levels of follicle-stimulating hormone (FSH) and luteinizing hormone (LH), and eventually increase the level of testosterone (T) to improve the quality of semen.

Sources: Cen, Y.H., Zhao, F.L., Fan, R. and He, G.Z. (2014) 'Research progress in the reproductive-related kidney deficiency and kidney tonifying Chinese medicine mechanism.' *Medical Recapitulate 20*, 2226–2228.

Fenglei, Q., Fanhui, Z. and Weiquan, F. (2005) 'Effects of Chinese herbal preparation for invigorating kidney on function of hypothalamic-pituitary-gonad axis in rats.' *Chinese Journal of Sports Medicine 24*, 5, 571.

Enhancement of follicle-stimulating hormone levels, regulation of luteinizing hormone level[1]

Low levels of FSH imply hypospermatogenesis. Kidney-supplementing and replenishing herbal medicines heightened testicular function in spermatogenesis through upregulation of FSH:

- **Gou Qi Zi** (*Lycium Barbarum*): Could significantly raise FSH and LH levels.

- **Ren Shen** (*Ginsenoide*): Ginsenosides were able to stimulate cultured anterior pituitary cells to secrete FSH and LH in vitro.

Sources: Luo, Q., Li, Z., Huang, X., Yan, J., Zhang, S. and Cai, Y.Z. (2006) 'Lycium barbarum polysaccharides: Protective effects against heat-induced damage of rat testes and H2O2-induced DNA damage in mouse testicular cells and beneficial effect on sexual behavior and reproductive function of hemicastrated rats.' *Life Sciences 79*, 7, 613–621.

Li, X., Liu, S., Ma, X. and Xu, J. (1988) 'A study of the effect of ginsenosides on the secretion of gonadotropins.' *Journal of Norman Bethune University of Medical Sciences 14*, 293–295.

- **Liu Wei Di Huang Wan** significantly increased FSH and LH levels in Kidney Yin-deficient infertile men.

- **Wu Zi Yan Zong Wan** promotes the secretion of FSH and simultaneously reduces LH levels through a negative feedback pathway.

Sources: Ye, Z., Chen, D., Zhong, J., Zhang, Y. *et al.* (2013) 'Effect of Jiawei Wuzi Yanzong decoction on sperm quality and hormone level.' *World Chinese Medicine 8*, 626–629.

Xie, J., Wang, J., Chen, M. and Liu, H. (2011) 'Influence of Guilingji capsules on spermatogenesis and sexual hormones in oligospermatism rats.' *Journal of Guangzhou University of Traditional Chinese Medicine 2011*, 6, 621–623.

Reducing FSH levels, regulating LH levels[2]

Abnormally high FSH and LH levels suggest injured spermatogenesis in the testis. Kidney-supplementing and Essence-replenishing herbal medicines can repair the damaged histologic structure of the seminiferous epithelium and stimulate spermatogenesis by downregulating FSH levels:

- **Wu Wei Zi** (*Schisandra Chinensis*) reduced FSH and LH levels (in rats).

- **Jin Gui Shen Qi** was capable of decreasing FSH levels and increasing LH levels in model rats.

Sources: Zhang, Y., Shen, N., Qi, L., Chen, W., Dong, Z. and Zhao, D.H. (2013) 'Efficacy of Schizandra chinesis polysaccharide on cyclophosphamide induced dyszoospermia of rats and its effects on reproductive hormones.' *Chinese Journal of Integrated Traditional and Western Medicine 33*, 3, 361–364.

Ma, L., Jia, M., Nan, Y.Y., Liu, M.L., Wang, Z.R. and Ma, J. (2011) 'Effects of Jingui Shenqi pills on sperm quality and contents of hormones in adenine-induced infertility rats.' *Journal of Shandong University of Traditional Chinese Medicine 35*, 431–433.

Shu Di Huang *R. Rehmanniae Praeparatae*	24 g
Shan Zhu Yu *Fr. Corni Officinalis*	12 g
Shan Yao *R. Dioscorae Oppositae*	12 g
Fu Zi *R. Lateralis Aconiti Carmichaeli Praeparata*	3 g
Gui Zhi *Ram. Cinnamomi Cassiae*	3 g
Ze Xie *Rh. Alismatis Orientaiis*	9 g
Fu Ling *Sclerotium Poriae Cocos*	9 g
Mu Dan Pi *C. Moutan Radicis*	9 g

Regulating the HPG axis to raise testosterone levels

- **Rou Cong Rong** (*Cistanche Tub.*) significantly enhanced testosterone biosynthesis by increasing the expression of key steroidogenic enzymes.

Kidney-supplementing herbal medicines elevate testosterone levels via multiple targets and pathways.

Source: Jiang, Z., Wang, J., Li, X. and Zhang X. (2016) 'Echinacoside and Cistanche tubulosa (Schenk) R. wight ameliorate bisphenol A-induced testicular and sperm damage in rats through gonad axis regulated steroidogenic enzymes.' *Journal of Ethnopharmacology 193*, 321–328.

Regulating FSH and LH levels bidirectionally[3]

TCM regulates FSH and LH level bidirectionally, maintaining endocrine homeostasis.

- **Bu Shen Sheng Jing Pill** increased LH levels in Kidney Yang-deficient infertile men, and decreased FSH levels in Kidney Yin-deficient and Kidney Yin- and Yang-deficient men.

Source: Yue, G.P., Chen, Q. and Dai, N. (1996) 'Eighty-seven cases of male infertility treated by bushen shengjing pill in clinical observation and evaluation on its curative effect.' *Chinese Journal of Integrated Traditional and Western Medicine 16*, 8, 463–466.

BU SHEN SHENG JING PILL

Shan Zhu Fu *Fr. Corni Officinalis*	15 g
Tu Si Zi *Sm. Cuscutae*	15 g
Dang Shen *Rx. Codonopsis Pilosulae*	15 g
Wu Wie Zi *Fr. Schisandrae Chinensis*	15 g
Du Zhong *Cx. Eucommiae Ulmoidis*	15 g
He Shou Wu *Rx. Polygoni Multiflori*	15 g
Shu Di Huang *Rx. Rehmanniae Glutinosae Conquitae*	15 g
Xian Mao *Rhiz. Curculiginis Orchioidis*	10 g
Xian Ling Pi *Herba Epimedii*	10 g
Chao Bai Zhu stir-fried *Rhiz. Atractylodis Macrocephalae*	10 g

Boosting the function of Sertoli cells and Leydig cells[4]

A reduction in the number of Sertoli cells leads to a proportional decrease in the number of germ cells and Leydig cells, with detrimental effects on fertility.

Sertoli cells secrete androgen-binding protein under the regulation of FSH, while LH stimulates Leydig cells to synthesize testosterone. These two processes cooperate to maintain normal spermatogenesis.

- **Wu Zi Yan Zong Wan:** Previous studies have demonstrated that this could dramatically enhance the activity of Sertoli cells. WYP prominently elevated levels of serum inhibin B.

- **Liu Wei Di Huang Wan:** capable of stimulating Sertoli cells to proliferate.

Sources: Yang, A., Liu, B., Zhang, S., Xie, C. *et al.* (2010) 'Mechanism of Wuziyanzong pills in improvement of function of Sertoli cells in rats with insufficiency of kidney essence.' *Journal of Beijing University of Traditional Chinese Medicine 33*, 378–380.

Xu, Y.P., Liu, B.X., Zhang, X.P., Yang, C.W. and Wang, C.H. (2014) 'A Chinese herbal formula,

Wuzi Yanzong pill, improves spermatogenesis by modulating the secretory function of Sertoli cells.' *Chinese Journal of Integrative Medicine 20*, 3, 194–199.

Ke, M., Liu, B., Wang, C. and Pei, X. (2016) 'Study on the effects of Wuzi Yanzong pill on semen quality and its related mechanism.' *Chinese Journal of Andrology 30*, 30–33.

Wang, Q.Z., Wang, D.F., Liu, H.L., Feng, D.J., Wang, H.H. and Guo, Z.B. (2013) 'Effects of extracts from Liuwei dihuang Pill on the proliferation of mouse Sertoli cells.' *Lishizhen Medicine and Materia Medica Research 24*, 1363–1365.

- **Yang Jing capsule:** Could significantly upregulate testosterone synthesis in Leydig cells.

The capsule is composed of 11 traditional Chinese drugs: 13.3% *Yinyanghuo* (*Herba Epimedii Brevicornus*), 13.3% *Muli* (*Concha Ostreae* (calcined)), 13.3% *Wangbuliuxing* (*Semen Vaccariae Segetalis*), 10% *Huangqi* (*Radix Astragali Mongolici*), 10% *Danggui* (*Radix Angelicae Sinensis*), 6.7% *Huangjing* (*Rhizoma Polygonati Sibirici*), 6.7% *Shayuanzi* (*Semen Astragali Complanati*), 6.7% *Ziheche* (*Placenta Hominis*), 6.7% *Shudihuang* (*Radix Rehmanniae Preparata*), 6.7% *Lizhihe* (*Semen Litchi*) and 6.7% *Shuizhi* (*Hirudo*).

- *Icariin* (in **Yin Yang Huo**) significantly promotes the proliferation of Leydig cells and stimulates the proliferation of Sertoli cells.

Sources: Gu, Y., Zhang, X., Sun, D., Zhao, H. *et al.* (2015) 'The stimulative effect of Yangjing capsule on testosterone synthesis through Nur77 pathway in Leydig cells.' *Evidence-Based Complementary and Alternative Medicine 2015*, 408686.

Xu, Y., Wu, B. and Jiang, Y. (2013) 'Effect of icariin on the proliferation, apoptosis and testosterone synthesis of immature rat Leydig cells.' *Modern Journal of Integrated and Traditional Chinese and Western Medicine 22*, 2864–2866.

Nan, Y., Zhang, X., Yang, G., Xie, J. *et al.* (2014) 'Icariin stimulates the proliferation of rat Sertoli cells in an ERK1/2-dependent manner in vitro.' *Andrologia 46*, 12, 9–16.

Preventing oxidative stress[5]

Excessive reactive oxygen species (ROS) attack the membrane and DNA of sperm cells, leading to decreased fluidity and impeded permeability of the sperm plasma membrane. This causes a higher DFI, which would contribute to infertility.

Chinese Medicine has been demonstrated to scavenge ROS, improve the antioxidant capacity of the seminal plasma, lower sperm DFI, and protect the male reproductive system from the lesions induced by ROS.

- *Ba Ji Tian* (Morinda), *Tu Si Zi* (Cuscutae), *Gou Qi Zi* and *Wu Wei Zi* protect the sperm cell from oxidative stress.

- *Wu Zi Yan Zong Wan* improved the survival rate of Sertoli cells against oxidative stress.

- *Jin Gui Shen Qi Wan* protects from oxidative stress.

Sources: Yang, X., Ding, C.F., Zhang, Y.H., Yan, Z.Z. and Du, J. (2006) 'Extract from Cuscuta chinensis against the structure of human sperm membrane and the oxidative injury of function.' *Chinese Pharmaceutical Journal 41*, 515–518.

Shi, G.J., Zheng, J., Wu, J., Qiao, H.Q. *et al.* (2017) 'Beneficial effects of Lycium barbarum polysaccharide on spermatogenesis by improving antioxidant activity and inhibiting apoptosis in streptozotocin-induced diabetic male mice.' *Food and Function 8*, 3, 1215–1226.

Yu, H.Y., Chen, Z.Y., Sun, B., Liu, J. *et al.* (2014) 'Lignans from the fruit of Schisandra glaucescens with antioxidant and neuroprotective properties.' *Journal of Natural Products 77*, 6, 1311–1320.

Yin, J.L., Xu, Y. and Wu, B. (2013) 'Wuziyanzong compound relieves oxidative stress injury and inhibits the apoptosis of Sertoli cells.' *National Journal of Andrology 19*, 3, 257–261.

Li, W.L., Dai, Y., Xu, D. and Ji, Y.B. (2007) 'Effects of different polar fractions from Jinkuishenqiwan on testosterone and oxidative stress in rats with kidney-yang deficiency induced by hydrocortisone.' *Chinese Journal of New Drugs 16*, 1944–1946.

Supplementing trace elements[6]

Zinc and selenium are essential trace elements for testicular development and spermatogenesis. Zinc plays an important role in antioxidation, DNA repair mechanisms and maintaining genomic stability. Selenium is a critical component to shield membrane lipids from oxidation. It is also a constituent of the mitochondrial sheath of spermatozoa.

Manganese is also an essential trace element that acts as a potent trigger of sperm motility.

- *Yin Yang Huo* and *Xian Mao*: Kidney-supplementing herbal medicines such as Epimedium and Curculigo were rich in zinc and manganese.

- *Shu Di Huang* has high levels of selenium.

Sources: Yu, N.C. and Guan, J.H. (1997) 'Study on trace elements in 8 kidney-tonifying Chinese medicines and their clinical efficacy.' *ShiZhen Journal of Traditional Chinese Medicine Research 8*, 33–34.

Lin, S., Zhao, L., Dong, S. and An, D. (1989) 'Determination of selenium in ten kinds of traditional Chinese medicine by fluorescence spectrophotometry.' *Journal of China Pharmaceutical University 20*, 46–47.

Ameliorating the microcirculation of the testis

Spermatogenesis is a highly metabolic process that is susceptible to disruptions in the supply of nutrients and oxygen. Sufficient blood supply for the testis is a prerequisite for normal spermatogenesis.

Blood-quickening medicines ameliorated the microcirculation and metabolism of the testis and ensured an adequate nutrient supply for the testis. They also alleviated inflammatory effusion and inflammation and unblocked the vas deferens.

Source: Zhou, S.H. and Xie, J.X. (2007) 'The application of treating male diseases from the perspective of Blood stasis.' *Journal of New Chinese Medicine 39*, 97–98.

- **Bu Shen Huo Xue** could upregulate the protein expression of vascular endothelial growth factor (VEGF) to facilitate testicular microcirculation.

Bu Shen Huo Xue was composed of *Rehmanniae Radix Preparata, Radices Paeoniae Alba, Angelica Sinensis, Ligusticum Wallichii, Semen Cuscutae, Herba Epimedii, Rhizoma Anemarrhenae, Golden Cypress* and *Radix Bupleuri.*

Source: Dong, W., Jin, B., Sun, D., Cai, B. *et al.* (2018) 'Bushenhuoxue prescription facilitates testicular microcirculation in dyszoospermia mice via activating VEGF/VEGFR2 pathway.' *Chinese Journal of Andrology 32*, 30–35.

Improving semen quality and pregnancy rate[7]

Fructose and alpha-glucosidase are the major components of seminal plasma. Fructose is the energy source for sperm; it is metabolized into adenosine triphosphate (ATP) by glycolysis and is associated with sperm motility. Alpha-glucosidase can catalyze the degradation of the glycogen stores of sperm in the epididymis, supplying energy for the maturation and motion of sperm.

- **Jia Wei Wu Zi Yan Zong Wan** increased fructose levels in seminal plasma in infertile men with asthenozoospermia.

- **Sheng Jing** significantly increased the levels of seminal plasma alpha-glucosidase and fructose.

Western name	Chinese name
Antler gelatin	Lu Jiao Jiao
Epimedium	Yin Yang Huo
Curculigo	Xian Mao
Cherokee rosa	Jin Ying Zi
Schizandra	Wu Wei Zi
Loranthus	Sang Ji Sheng
Rehmannia	Shu Di Huang
Lycium	Gou Qi Huang
Cuscuta	Tu Si Zi
Dendrobium	Shi Hu
Morinda	Ba Ji Tian
Rubus	Fu Pen Zi
Achyranthes	Huai Niu Xi
Scripus	San Leng
Zedoaria	E Zhu

A randomized controlled study showed that both *Jiawei Wuzi Yanzong Decoction* and *Liuwei Dihuang Pill* treatments improved sperm vitality and motility in Kidney Yin-deficient infertile men.

A multi-centre study found that the *Qilin Pill* and the *WYP* could effectively improve seminal concentration and sperm motility in OATS patients, similiarily to the *Sheng Jing* prescription.

Qilin Pill: *Radix Polygoni Multiflori Praeparata cum Succo Glycines Sotae, Herba Ecliptae, Herba Epimedii, Semen Cuscutae, Herba Cynomorii, Radix Codonopsis, Radix Curcumae, Fructus Lycii, Fructus Rubi, Rhizoma Dioscoreae, Radix Et Rhizoma Salviae Miltiorrhizae, Radix Astragali, Radix Paeoniae Alba, Pericarpium Citri Reticulatae Viride, Fructus Mori.*

Sources: Ye, Z., Chen, D., Zhong, J., Zhang, Y. *et al.* (2013) 'Effect of Jiawei Wuzi Yanzong decoction on sperm quality and hormone level.' *World Chinese Medicine 8*, 626–629.

Shang, X.J., Guo, J., Chen, L., Deng, C.H. *et al.* (2011) 'Qilin pills for oligoasthenospermia: A multi-centered clinical trial.' *National Journal of Andrology 17*, 12, 1139–1142.

- *Sheng Jing* prescription treatment improved normal sperm morphology and acrosin activity, reducing sperm DFI.

- Meta-analysis indicated that Chinese Medicine and Chinese–Western combined therapy significantly enhanced the pregnancy rate.

Sources: Sun, Z.G., Lian, F., Jiang, K.P., Zhang, J.W. *et al.* (2012) 'Shengjing prescription improves semen parameters of oligoasthenozoospermia patients: Efficacy and mechanism.' *National Journal of Andrology 18*, 8, 764–767.

Au, C., Yeung, W. and Xu, F. (2015) 'Meta-analysis on TCM diagnosis and treatment of oligoasthenospermia.' *Chinese Archives of Traditional Chinese Medicine 33*, 2268–2273.

Zhou, J.F., Li, Q., Zhang, Q.H., Lin, R.W., Chen, Z.Q. and Xiang, S.T. (2015) 'Kidney-tonifying Chinese medicine for male infertility: A systematic review of randomized controlled trials.' *National Journal of Andrology 21*, 9, 833–840.

Alleviating inflammation[8]

Mycoplasma and chlamydia infections of the male genital tract are a common aetiology of male infertility, resulting in decreased sperm motility and increased abnormal sperm counts.

Inflammation leads to leukocyte infiltration into the seminal plasma, and the leukocytes release excessive ROS, which attack the plasma membrane and DNA of sperm.

- *Huang Bai*, *Huang Qin* and *Pu Gong Yi* could kill mycoplasma and chlamydia in experiments (rats).

- *Zhi Bai Di Huang Tang* could treat infection experimentally with ureoplasma by increasing the levels of IL-2 and TNF-α.

Source: Lu, F., He, Q., Zhang, B., Liu, Z. and Li, L. (2011) 'Effects of Zhibai Dihuang decoction on expression of IL-2, TNF-α in the testis of rats infected by ureaplasma urealyticum.' *China Journal of Traditional Chinese Medicine and Pharmacy 26*, 448–450.

Decreasing the level of anti-sperm antibodies[9]

Sperm is a specific antigen that causes the human body to generate anti-sperm antibodies (AsAb) when the immune system is exposed to it.

AsAb decrease sperm motility, impede sperm from undergoing capacitation and acrosome reactions, and interfere with sperm–oocyte recognition and fusion.

- *Zhi Bai Di Huang Tang* decoction treatment could remarkably reduce serum levels of AsAb in rats. While the concrete mechanism is obscure, Chinese Medicine may eliminate testicular immunological complexes and regulate the ratio of CD4/CD8 T cells to cure immune-induced infertility.

Sources: Li, X., Yu, X., Liu, J., Liao, X. and Miao, Y. (1997) 'An experimental study of the effect of Zhibai Dihuang decoction on immunological infertility.' *Traditional Chinese Drug Research and Clinical Pharmacology 8*, 83–85.

Wang, W., Huang, Z., Tang, M., Li, X. *et al.* (2001) 'A histological and immunohistochemical study on MianBu I & II treating immunological infertility of male mice.' *Chinese Journal of Histochemistry and Cytochemistry 10*, 81–85.

- *Yikang Tang* soothes the Liver, reinforces the Kidney, clears toxic heat and dampness, invigorates the blood and dispels Blood stasis.

Chai Hu Rx. Bupleuri	9 g
Sheng Di Huang Rx. Rehmanniae	10 g
Chuan Xiong Rhiz. Chuan Xiong	9 g
Bai Hua She She Cao Hb. Hedyotis Diffusae	12 g
Ban Zhi Lian Hb. Scutellariae Barbatae	10 g
Bai Dou Kou Fr. Amomi Rotundusg	9 g
Yin Yang Huo Hb. Epimedii	12 g
Sheng Huang Qi Rx. Astragali	20 g
Mu Dan Pi Cx. Moutan	9 g
Zhi Mu Rhiz. Anemarrhenae	9 g
Huang Bai Cx. Phellondri	9 g

Source: Sun, Z. and Bao, Y. (2006) 'TCM treatment of male immune infertility: A report of 100 cases.' *Journal of Traditional Chinese Medicine 26*, 36–38.

Modifying epigenetic markers[10]

- Epigenetics is the study of modification of gene expression without changing the DNA sequence, and epigenetic processes include DNA methylation, histone modification and chromatin remodelling.

- Normal H19 gene expression is crucial to spermatogenesis, and many patients with OATS had hypomethylation at the H19 locus.

Shengjing Formula treatment could improve sperm concentration, motility and clinical pregnancy rate by reducing the loss rate of the H19 imprinted gene.[11]

— CHAPTER 18 —

Low Level Laser Therapy (LLLT) and Mitochondrial Medicine in Male Reproductive Medicine

DR MICHAEL WEBER, MD

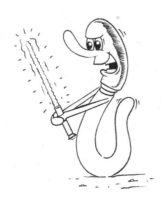

Disturbances of cellular and subcellular physiology are the root of male infertility. In particular, impairment of mitochondrial physiology by an excess of reactive oxygen species (ROS) will lead to measurable decrease of ATP production. Beside the targeted use of minerals and trace elements, the use of laser acupuncture and LLLT can improve the mitochondrial performance and enhance reproductive performance.

In this chapter you will learn about basic mitochondrial physiology, common disturbances and suggestions for a sucessful treatment. All known acupuncture points can be treated by laser irradiation with additional beneficial effects on cellular functions. The use of photobiomodulation is a promising tool for 'mitochondrial medicine' because most of the antenna pigments for the absorption of the photones are located within the mitochondrial membranes.

About 50% of infertility disorders are related to men. Poor semen quality is the main cause of infertility in men.[1] Cellular physiology, especially mitochondrial function, does play a crucial role in the pathology of male infertility (and degenerative diseases in general).

ROS and other oxidant radicals (such as NO and derivates) play a harmful role in male-factor infertility and human reproduction.

The male and female reproductive processes depend on the sufficient supply of cellular energy. In a healthy tissue, most of the energy production is generated by the powerhouses of our cells, by the mitochondria. 'Oxidative phosphorylation' (OxPhos) generates a vast amount of adenosine triphosphate (ATP). The five components of OxPhos are located within the inner mitochondrial membranes.

A mitochondrion (Greek: *mitos* = filament; *chondros* = grain) is a subcellular organelle enclosed by a double membrane with its own genome in the form of a circular DNA (mtDNA). Mitochondria occur in the cytosol of all body cells with the exception of mature erythrocytes. They were first described in 1865 as cell organelles in skeletal muscles. Each day the human body produces about 60 kg of ATP. Depending on the energy requirements of an organ, there are a few hundred to several thousand mitochondria in each cell. Most organs contain 500 to 2000 mitochondria per cell, and even oocytes contain around 100,000 mitochondria per cell. The mitochondrial genome is exclusively maternally inherited.

The most important functions of the mitochondria include: energy generation, regulation of the citrate cycle (Krebs cycle), beta-oxidation, regulation of apoptosis, synthesis of iron-sulphur clusters for the synthesis of respiratory chains, enzymes and the mitochondrial respiratory chain with oxidative phosphorylation.

In the mitochondrial respiratory chain, electrons are transferred to oxygen with the formation of water. The NADH from the citric acid cycle (generated by the oxidation of glucose and fatty acids) is the first complex of OxPhos. The electrons (e-) enter the electron transport chain via the electron carriers NADH and FADH2. FAD consists of adenosine diphosphate linked to riboflavin (vitamin B2). The other complexes of the mitochondrial respiratory chain are coenzyme Q10 (in its reduced form as ubiquinol) and the copper-dependent cytochrome C oxidase (CCO).

During the electron transfer, protons (H +) are transported from the mitochondrial matrix into the intermembrane space (between the outer and inner mitochondrial membrane). This creates an electrochemical proton gradient that is used at the end of OxPhos on the inner mitochondrial membrane to synthesize ATP from ADP and inorganic phosphate with the help of the magnesium-dependent ATP synthase. The conservation of the energy obtained here in the form of ATP is the actual step of the 'oxidative phosphorylation'. The newly synthesized ATP is transported by the adenine nucleotide translocase (ANT) in exchange for ADP for renewed ATP synthesis from the matrix into the cytosol.

From the very beginning, mitochondrial energy production is of utmost importance for sufficient male fertility. The early development of gonads has a higher energy requirement than ovaries.[2] The presence of many mitochondria in male germ cells highlights their importance in testicular metabolism. The germ cells' survival in the adult testis is dependent on carbohydrate metabolism, including glycolysis and mitochondrial oxidative phosphorylation.

During spermatogenesis, many changes in the energy metabolism of germ cells are involved, mainly due to the blood–testis barrier and changes to the surrounding medium.

Oxidative energy production is inevitably associated with the generation of ROS, excessive concentrations of which can lead to cellular pathology. The superoxide anion, the hydroxyl radical and the hypochlorite radical are some of the highest reactive radicals of oxygen. Within the cell membranes, the cytosol and the mitochondria, there are a number of defence systems to scavenge these ROS at an early stage. The superoxide dismutase (SOD) is one of the first-line molecules to detoxify the superoxide anion. Three different subtypes of SOD exist in the human cells, the copper- and zinc-dependent SOD are within the cytosol, the manganese containing one in the mitochondria.

If the ROS defence system of the cells is impaired, the oxygen radicals may interact with nitrite and form reactive nitrogen radicals. Reactive nitrogen species (RNS) is the name for highly reactive nitrogen compounds. They play an important role in a number of physiological but also pathophysiological processes. Analogous to the ROS that cause oxidative stress, reactive nitrogen species cause nitrosative stress. The reactive nitrogen species are responsible for some cell pathological phenomena that used to be attributed exclusively to the reactive oxygen species. Nitric oxide and its secondary product peroxynitrite (ONOO–) are counted among the reactive nitrogen species. Peroxynitrite anions arise from the recombination of nitrogen monoxide and superoxide radicals. NO blocks the CCO reversible whereas ONOO– leads to an irreversible block of CCO and thereby impaired ATP production.

Acquired secondary mitochondrial diseases can affect all organ systems, however, especially those with high oxygen and energy requirements. These include the brain, the sensory organs, the heart, the muscles and the reproductive organs. The mitochondria use over 90% of cellular oxygen for ATP synthesis. In addition to ATP production, there is also an amount of 0.5–5.0% of ROS, initially of the superoxide anion radical ($\cdot O_2-$).[3] In our organism, these compounds can react with other compounds (proteins, DNA) and cause severe damage and contribute to infertility. Several studies describe the constant increase of cellular injuries due to ROS during the ageing process. ROS can produce extensive protein damage and cytoskeletal modifications and inhibit cellular mechanisms as well as have adverse effects on lipid peroxidation. In healthy tissue, there is a balance between ROS and scavengers. ROS in excess may lead to severe impairment of cellular functions; however, ROS are necessary for several signalling functions in every organ, including male reproductive organs. ROS do have positive effects on sperm depending on the concentration and the nature of the ROS involved. They are necessary in regulating the hyperactivation and the ability of the spermatozoa to undergo acrosome reaction.[4]

In contrast to nuclear DNA, mitochondrial DNA (mtDNA) has significantly less effective repair mechanisms and is therefore much more susceptible to oxidative damage. Complex I (NADH dehydrogenase) and complex IV (CCO) are particularly affected by mutations caused by attack by free radicals, as these are predominantly encoded by the mtDNA.

Sperm production as well as the velocity of sperm movements depend on proper function of the mitochondrial ATP production. A pathological excess of ROS will ultimately lead to defective sperm function. Damaging of lipoproteins, cell and mitochondrial membranes by ROS frequently causes male infertility, due to abnormal flagella movement, failure to recognize the zona and inhibition of sperm–oocyte fusion. On the other hand, a temporary increased amount of superoxide anion (O_2-) is one of the first steps required by the spermatozoa for induction and development of hyperactivation and capacitation.

Male germ cells are enormously vulnerable to oxidative stress as the sperm membrane is rich in unsaturated fatty acids and lacks the capacity for DNA repair. Spermatozoa are principally susceptible to ROS-induced damage because their plasma membranes contain huge quantities of polyunsaturated fatty acids (PUFA) and their cytoplasm contains low concentrations of the scavenging enzymes.

Countless studies from all fields of medicine could prove that laser irradiation with red or near infrared light is a safe method for treatment and enhances mitochondrial performance and ATP production. Numerous studies confirm the positive influence of LLLT on the spermatozoa of various animals:[5] their motility and the content of ATP[6] increases,[7] cell life expectancy increases[8] and the probability of fertilization increases.

LLLT is a well-established medical treatment option in many fields of medicine including infertility. A huge number of scientific studies have shown that LLLT is beneficial in treating male infertility. LLLT can significantly improve the survival, motility and speed of movement of spermatozoa. Laser therapy of patients with prostatitis and vesiculitis can eliminate infiltrative-exudative changes, improve reproductive and copulatory functions. Local illumination of red (635 nm) and near infrared (808 or 904 nm) spectra can be combined with intravenous laser blood illumination (ILBI) of red (635 nm) spectra.

Improving sperm motility may increase the likelihood of natural conception or at least result in assisted/artificial reproductive technology (ART) techniques associated with a lower burden for the healthy female partner – for example, intrauterine insemination (IUI) instead of intracytoplasmatic sperm injection (ICSI).

Energy for flagellar movement is provided by mitochondria occurring as the mitochondrial sheath within the midpiece of the spermatozoon.[9] Stimulation of mitochondria, consequently, will result in increased sperm motility.[10]

Guilherme Henrique's research showed that LLLT increases the percentage of live sperm cells and sperm motility with more positive results. He practised radiation with the wavelength of 660 nm, 30 mw power and energy of 4 and 6 joules for 80–120 seconds.[11]

In a case study on a 32-year-old idiopathic infertile male patient with low number and quality of sperm (oligoasthenoteratozoospermia), according to 2010 WHO standards, the following laser acupuncture and LLLT treatment was performed: laser acupuncture treatment by laser pen with the following setting of: wavelength 810 nm (near infrared laser), output power 400 mW, Nogier B (584 Hz) frequency, each point 4 joules on average per acupuncture point. Treatment was performed on these points: Ll 4, Liv 3, Sp 6, Kid 3, Kid 6,

Sp 5, Ren 3, St 29, Du 4, St 36, Bl 23 and also auricular points: prostate gland, interferon, Kidney, Liver, Spleen and Shenmen in 15 sessions twice a week. In addition, super pulse laser with peak power 5 x 60 W = 300 W, impulse duration 200 ns, wavelength 904 nm, Nogier B frequency, 10 J was applied to the symphysis pubis, prostate gland and pelvic area. The treatment was done twice a week in 15 sessions.

The clinical outcome did show an increase of ejaculate volume from 1 ml to 4 ml, the motility of sperm increased from 20 to 43, together with normalizing of the sperm morphology.[12]

In conclusion, analysis of the scientific literature suggests that laser therapy should be used as much as possible in the complex treatment of men with infertility,[13] since the effectiveness of the method is good and often has no alternatives. For laser illumination, it is best to use LLLT red light (635/650 nm) and infrared (810/904 nm) for local illumination. Further research studies are suggested.

PBM positively affects sperm motility and velocity at doses of 4–6 J/cm in semen samples of asthenozoospermic patients. Applying LMqPCR on the same samples, no significant changes in the DNA fragmentation level after PBM could be detected.[14] Furthermore, the CD46 expression pattern confirmed the maintenance of acrosomal integrity after PBM. PBM therefore represents a promising future application for the improvement and success of ART.

Notes

CHAPTER 1

1   Purell, S. (2008) 'Erectile dysfunction and traditional oriental herbal medicinals.' *Sun Ten Newsletter*, Spring 2008.

CHAPTER 2

1   Van Blerkom, J. and Davis, P. (1995) 'Evolution of the sperm aster after microinjection of isolated human sperm centrosomes into meiotically mature human oocytes.' *Human Reproduction 10*, 8, 2179-2182. doi:10.1093/oxfordjournals.humrep.a136264.

2   Okabe, M. (2013) 'The cell biology of mammalian fertilization.' *Development 140*, 22, 4471-4479. doi:10.1242/dev.090613.

3   Parekattil, S.J., Esteves, S.C. and Agarwal, A. (eds) (2020) *Male Infertility: Contemporary Clinical Approaches, Andrology, ART and Antioxidants*. Cham: Springer.

4   Carlson, A.E., Westenbroek, R.E., Quill, T., Ren, D. *et al.* (2003) 'CatSper1 required for evoked Ca2+ entry and control of flagellar function in sperm.' *PNAS 100*, 25, 14864-14868. doi:10.1073/pnas.2536658100.

5   Armon, L. and Eisenbach, M. (2011) 'Behavioral mechanism during human sperm chemotaxis: Involvement of hyperactivation.' *PLOS ONE 6*, 12, e28359. doi:10.1371/journal.pone.0028359.

6   Parekattil, S.J., Esteves, S.C. and Agarwal, A. (eds) (2020) *Male Infertility: Contemporary Clinical Approaches, Andrology, ART and Antioxidants*. Cham: Springer.

7   Inoue, N., Ikawa, M., Isotani, A. and Okabe, M. (2005) 'The immunoglobulin superfamily protein Izumo is required for sperm to fuse with eggs.' *Nature 434*, 7030, 234-238. doi:10.1038/nature03362.

CHAPTER 3

1   Parekattil, S.J., Esteves, S.C. and Agarwal, A. (eds) (2020) *Male Infertility: Contemporary Clinical Approaches, Andrology, ART and Antioxidants*. Cham: Springer, Chapter 6.

2   Parekattil, S.J., Esteves, S.C. and Agarwal, A. (eds) (2020) *Male Infertility: Contemporary Clinical Approaches, Andrology, ART and Antioxidants*. Cham: Springer, Chapter 6.

3   Parekattil, S.J., Esteves, S.C. and Agarwal, A. (eds) (2020) *Male Infertility: Contemporary Clinical Approaches, Andrology, ART and Antioxidants*. Cham: Springer, Chapter 6.

4   Bezold, G., Lange, M. and Peter, R.U. (2001) 'Homozygous methylenetetrahydrofolate reductase C677T mutation and male infertility.' *New England Journal of Medicine 344*, 15, 1172-1173. doi:10.1056/NEJM200104123441517.

5   Motrich, R.D., Maccioni, M., Molina, R., Tissera, A. *et al.* (2005) 'Reduced semen quality in chronic prostatitis patients that have cellular autoimmune response to prostate antigens.' *Human Reproduction 20*, 9, 2567-2572. doi:10.1093/humrep/dei073.

6   Cho, C.L., Esteves, S.C. and Agarwal A. (2016) 'Novel insights into the pathophysiology of varicocele and its association with reactive oxygen species and sperm DNA fragmentation.' *Asian Journal of Andrology 18*, 2, 186-193. doi:10.4103/1008-682X.170441.

7   Parekattil, S.J., Esteves, S.C. and Agarwal, A. (eds) (2020) *Male Infertility: Contemporary Clinical Approaches, Andrology, ART and Antioxidants*. Cham: Springer, Chapter 6.

8   Agarwal, A., Virk, G., Ong, C. and du Plessis, S.S. (2014) 'Effect of oxidative stress on male reproduction.' *World Journal of Men's Health 32*, 1, 1–17. doi:10.5534/wjmh.2014.32.1.1.

9   Parekattil, S.J., Esteves, S.C. and Agarwal, A. (eds) (2020) *Male Infertility: Contemporary Clinical Approaches, Andrology, ART and Antioxidants.* Cham: Springer, Chapter 6.

10   Parekattil, S.J., Esteves, S.C. and Agarwal, A. (eds) (2020) *Male Infertility: Contemporary Clinical Approaches, Andrology, ART and Antioxidants.* Cham: Springer, Chapter 6.

11   Parekattil, S.J., Esteves, S.C. and Agarwal, A. (eds) (2020) *Male Infertility: Contemporary Clinical Approaches, Andrology, ART and Antioxidants.* Cham: Springer, Chapter 6.

12   Kandil, H., Agarwal, A., Saleh, R., Boitrelle, F. *et al.* (2021) 'Editorial commentary on draft of World Health Organization Sixth Edition Laboratory Manual for the Examination and Processing of Human Semen.' *World Journal of Men's Health 39*, 4, 577–580. doi:10.5534/wjmh.210074.

13   Majzoub, A. and Agarwal, A. (2018) 'Systematic review of antioxidant types and doses in male infertility: Benefits on semen parameters, advanced sperm function, assisted reproduction and live-birth rate.' *Arab Journal of Urology 16*, 1, 113–124. doi:10.1016/j.aju.2017.11.013.

14   Agarwal, A., Virk, G., Ong, C. and du Plessis, S.S. (2014) 'Effect of oxidative stress on male reproduction.' *World Journal of Men's Health 32*, 1, 1–17. doi:10.5534/wjmh.2014.32.1.1; Hamada, A., Esteves, S.C. and Agarwal, A. (2013) 'Insight into oxidative stress in varicocele-associated male infertility: Part 2.' *Nature Reviews: Urology 10*, 1, 26–37. doi:10.1038/nrurol.2012.198.

15   Parekattil, S.J., Esteves, S.C. and Agarwal, A. (eds) (2020) *Male Infertility: Contemporary Clinical Approaches, Andrology, ART and Antioxidants.* Cham: Springer, Chapter 6.

CHAPTER 4

1   Agarwal, A. and Said, T.M. (2005) 'Oxidative stress, DNA damage and apoptosis in male infertility: A clinical approach.' *BJU International 95*, 4, 503–507. doi:10.1111/j.1464-410x.2005.05328.x.

2   Agarwal, A. and Said, T.M. (2005) 'Oxidative stress, DNA damage and apoptosis in male infertility: A clinical approach.' *BJU International 95*, 4, 503–507. doi:10.1111/j.1464-410x.2005.05328.x.

3   Agarwal, A., Leisegang, K., Majzoub, A., Henkel, R. *et al.* (2021) 'Utility of antioxidants in the treatment of male infertility: Clinical guidelines based on a systematic review and analysis of evidence.' *World Journal of Men's Health 39*, 2, 233–290. doi:10.5534/wjmh.200196.

4   Ross, C., Morriss, A., Khairy, M., Khalaf, Y. *et al.* (2010) 'A systematic review of the effect of oral antioxidants on male infertility.' *Reproductive Biomedicine Online 20*, 6, 711–723. doi:10.1016/j.rbmo.2010.03.008; Salas-Huetos, A., Rosique-Esteban, N., Becerra-Tomás, N., Vizmanos, B., Bullo, M. and Salas-Salvado, J. (2018) 'Effect of nutrients and dietary supplements on sperm quality parameters: A systematic review and meta-analysis of randomized clinical trials.' *Advances in Nutrition 9*, 6, 833–848. doi:10.1093%2Fadvances%2Fnmy057.

5   Paciera, D. (2019) 'What actually are those "other ingredients" on a Thorne product label?' Take 5 Daily. www.thorne.com/take-5-daily/article/what-actually-are-those-other-ingredients-on-a-thorne-product-label#:~:text=Thorne's%20%E2%80%9CNo%20List%E2%80%9D%20includes%20artificial,%2C%20and%20nut%2Dderived%20ingredients.

6   Kaarouch, I., Bouamoud, N., Madkour, A., Louanjli, N. *et al.* (2018) 'Paternal age: Negative impact on sperm genome decays and IVF outcomes after 40 years.' *Molecular Reproduction and Development 85*, 3, 271–280. doi:10.1002/mrd.22963.

7   Agarwal, A., Leisegang, K., Majzoub, A., Henkel, R. *et al.* (2021) 'Utility of antioxidants in the treatment of male infertility: Clinical guidelines based on a systematic review and analysis of evidence.' *World Journal of Men's Health 39*, 2, 233–290. doi:10.5534/wjmh.200196.

8   Colagar, A.H., Marzony, E.T. and Chaichi, M.J. (2008) 'Zinc levels in seminal plasma are associated with sperm quality in fertile and infertile men.' *Nutrition Research 29*, 2, 82–88. doi:10.1016/j.nutres.2008.11.007.

9   Colagar, A.H., Marzony, E.T. and Chaichi, M.J. (2008) 'Zinc levels in seminal plasma are associated with sperm quality in fertile and infertile men.' *Nutrition Research 29*, 2, 82–88. doi:10.1016/j.nutres.2008.11.007.

10   Kerns, K., Zigo, M. and Sutovsky, P. (2018) 'Zinc: A necessary ion for mammalian sperm fertilization competency.' *International Journal of Molecular Sciences 19*, 12, 4097. doi:10.3390%2Fijms19124097.

11   Allouche-Fitoussi, D. and Breitbart, H. (2020) 'The role of zinc in male fertility.' *International Journal of Molecular Sciences 21*, 20, 7796. doi:10.3390/ijms21207796.

12 Higdon, J. (2019) 'Zinc.' Linus Pauling Institute, Micronutrient Information Center. https://lpi.oregon-state.edu/mic/minerals/zinc.

13 Higdon, J. (2015) 'Selenium.' Linus Pauling Institute, Micronutrient Information Center. https://lpi.oregonstate.edu/mic/minerals/selenium.

14 Hawkes, W.C., Alkan, Z. and Wong, K. (2009) 'Selenium supplementation does not affect testicular selenium status or semen quality in North American men.' *Journal of Andrology 30*, 5, 525–533. doi:10.2164/jandrol.108.006940.

15 Scott, R., MacPherson, A., Yates, R.W., Hussain, B. and Dixon, J. (1998) 'The effect of oral selenium supplementation on human sperm motility.' *British Journal of Urology 82*, 1, 76–80. doi:10.1046/j.1464-410x.1998.00683.x; Safarinejad, M.R. and Safarinejad, S. (2009) 'Efficacy of selenium and/or N-acetyl-cysteine for improving semen parameters in infertile men: A double-blind, placebo controlled, randomized study.' *Journal of Urology 181*, 2, 741–751. doi:10.1016/j.juro.2008.10.015.

16 Safarinejad, M.R. and Safarinejad, S. (2009) 'Efficacy of selenium and/or N-acetyl-cysteine for improving semen parameters in infertile men: A double-blind, placebo controlled, randomized study.' *Journal of Urology 181*, 2, 741–751. doi:10.1016/j.juro.2008.10.015.

17 Higdon, J. (2015) 'Selenium.' Linus Pauling Institute, Micronutrient Information Center. https://lpi.oregonstate.edu/mic/minerals/selenium.

18 Mantle, D. and Dybring, A. (2020) 'Bioavailability of coenzyme Q_{10}: An overview of the absorption process and subsequent metabolism.' *Antioxidants (Basel) 9*, 5, 386. doi:10.3390%2Fantiox9050386.

19 Durairajanayagam, D., Singh, D., Agarwal, A. and Henkel, R. (2021) 'Causes and consequences of sperm mitochondrial dysfunction.' *Andrologia 53*, 1, e13666. doi:10.1111/and.13666.

20 Safarinejad, M.R., Safarinejad, S., Shafiei, N. and Safarinejad, S. (2012) 'Effects of the reduced form of coenzyme Q10 (ubiquinol) on semen parameters in men with idiopathic infertility: A double-blind, placebo controlled, randomized study.' *Journal of Urology 188*, 2, 526–531. https://doi.org/10.1016/j.juro.2012.03.131.

21 Safarinejad, M.R. (2009) 'Efficacy of coenzyme Q10 on semen parameters, sperm function and reproductive hormones in infertile men.' *Journal of Urology 182*, 1, 237–248. doi:10.1016/j.juro.2009.02.121.

22 Mantle, D. and Dybring, A. (2020) 'Bioavailability of coenzyme Q_{10}: An overview of the absorption process and subsequent metabolism.' *Antioxidants (Basel) 9*, 5, 386. doi:10.3390%2Fantiox9050386.

23 Mantle, D. and Dybring, A. (2020) 'Bioavailability of coenzyme Q_{10}: An overview of the absorption process and subsequent metabolism.' *Antioxidants (Basel) 9*, 5, 386. doi:10.3390%2Fantiox9050386.

24 Mantle, D. and Dybring, A. (2020) 'Bioavailability of coenzyme Q_{10}: An overview of the absorption process and subsequent metabolism.' *Antioxidants (Basel) 9*, 5, 386. doi:10.3390%2Fantiox9050386.

25 Ratner, M. (2004–2021) 'NeoQ10 Coenzyme Q10 Supplement.' https://theralogix.com/products/neoq10-coenzyme-q10-supplement.

26 Safarinejad, M.R. and Safarinejad, S. (2009) 'Efficacy of selenium and/or N-acetyl-cysteine for improving semen parameters in infertile men: A double-blind, placebo controlled, randomized study.' *Journal of Urology 181*, 2, 741–751. doi:10.1016/j.juro.2008.10.015.

27 Haghighian, H., Haidari, F., Mohammadi-Asi, J. and Dadfar, M. (2015) 'Randomized, triple-blind, placebo-controlled clinical trial examining the effects of alpha-lipoic acid supplement on the spermatogram and seminal oxidative stress in infertile men.' *Fertility and Sterility 104*, 2, 318–324. doi:10.1016/j.fertnstert.2015.05.014.

28 Kessopoulou, E., Powers, H.J., Sharma, K.K., Pearson, M.J. *et al.* (1995) 'A double-blind randomized placebo cross-over controlled trial using the antioxidant vitamin E to treat reactive oxygen species associated male infertility.' *Fertility and Sterililty 64*, 4, 825–331. doi:10.1016/s0015-0282(16)57861-3.

29 Greco, E., Iacobelli, M., Rienzi, L., Ubaldi, F., Ferrero, S. and Tesarik, J. (2005) 'Reduction of the incidence of sperm DNA fragmentation by oral antioxidant treatment.' *Journal of Andrology 26*, 3, 349–353. doi:10.2164/jandrol.04146.

30 Ghanem, H., Shaeer, O. and El-Segini, A. (2010) 'Combination clomiphene citrate and antioxidant therapy for idiopathic male infertility: A randomized controlled trial.' *Fertility and Sterility 93*, 7, 2232–2235. doi:10.1016/j.fertnstert.2009.01.117; Suleiman, S.A., Ali, M.E., Zaki, Z.M., El-Malik, E.M. and Nasr, M.A. (1996) 'Lipid peroxidation and human sperm motility: Protective role of vitamin E.' *Journal of Andrology 17*, 5 530–537.

31 Higdon, J. (2018) 'Vitamin C.' Linus Pauling Institute, Micronutrient Information Center. https://lpi.oregonstate.edu/mic/vitamins/vitamin-C.

32 Higdon, J. (2015) 'Vitamin E.' Linus Pauling Institute, Micronutrient Information Center. https://lpi.oregonstate.edu/mic/vitamins/vitamin-E.

33 de Angelis, C., Galdiero, M., Pivonello, C., Garifalos, F. *et al.* (2017) 'The role of vitamin D in male fertility: A focus on the testis.' *Reviews in Endocrine and Metabolic Disorders 18*, 3, 285–305. doi:10.1007/s11154-017-9425-0.

34 Boxmeer, J., Smit, M., Utomo, E., Romjin, J. and Eijkemans, M. (2009) 'Low folate in seminal plasma is associated with increased sperm DNA damage.' *Fertility and Sterility 92*, 2, 548–556. doi:10.1016/j.fertnstert.2008.06.010.

35 Banihani, S.A. (2017) 'Vitamin B12 and semen quality.' *Biomolecules 7*, 2, 42. doi:10.3390%2Fbiom7020042.

36 Aksoy, Y., Aksoy, H., Altinkaynak, K., Aydin, H.R. and Ozkan, A. (2006) 'Sperm fatty acid composition in subfertile men.' *Prostaglandins, Leukotrienes and Essent Fatty Acids 75*, 2, 75–79. doi:10.1016/j.plefa.2006.06.002.

37 Safarinejad, M.R. and Safarinejad, S. (2012) 'The roles of omega-3 and omega-6 fatty acids in idiopathic male infertility.' *Asian Journal of Andrology 14*, 4, 514–515. doi:10.1038%2Faja.2012.46.

38 Safarinejad, M.R. and Safarinejad, S. (2012) 'The roles of omega-3 and omega-6 fatty acids in idiopathic male infertility.' *Asian Journal of Andrology 14*, 4, 514–515. doi:10.1038%2Faja.2012.46.

39 Micic, S., Lalic, N., Djordjevic, D., Bojanic, N. *et al.* (2019) 'Double-blind, randomised, placebo-controlled trial on the effect of L-carnitine and L-acetylcarnitine on sperm parameters in men with idiopathic oligoasthenozoospermia.' *Andrologia 51*, 6, e13267. doi:10.1111%2Fand.13267.

40 Menchini-Fabris, G.F., Canale, D., Izzo, P.L., Olivieri, L. and Bartelloni, M. (1984) 'Free L-carnitine in human semen: Its variability in different andrologic pathologies.' *Fertility and Sterility 42*, 2, 263–267. doi:10.1016/s0015-0282(16)48024-6.

41 Balercia, G., Regoli, F., Armeni, T., Koverech, A., Mantero, F. and Boscaro, M. (2005) 'Placebo-controlled double-blind randomized trial on the use of L-carnitine, L-acetylcarnitine, or combined L-carnitine and L-acetylcarnitine in men with idiopathic asthenozoospermia.' *Fertility and Sterility 84*, 3, 662–671.

42 Higdon, J. (2002) 'L-Carnitine.' Linus Pauling Institute, Micronutrient Information Center. https://lpi.oregonstate.edu/mic/dietary-factors/L-carnitine.

43 Schachter, A., Friedman, S., Goldman, J. and Eckerling, B. (1973) 'Treatment of oligospermia with the amino acid arginine.' *International Journal of Gynaecology and Obstetrics 11*, 5, 206–209. doi:10.1002/j.1879-3479.1973.tb00901.x.

44 Scibona, M., Meschini, P., Capparelli, S., Pecori, C., Rossi, P. and Menchini Fabris, G.F. (1994) '[L-arginine and male infertility].' *Minerva Urologcia e Nefrologica 46*, 4, 251–253.

45 Aydin, S., Inci, O. and Alagöl, B. (1995) 'The role of arginine, indomethacin and kallikrein in the treatment of oligoasthenospermia.' *International Urology and Nephrology 27*, 2, 199–202. doi:10.1007/bf02551320.

46 Tan, J. (2017) '7 arginine-rich foods to avoid if you're prone to cold sores.' A. Vogel. www.avogel.co.uk/health/immune-system/cold-sores/7-arginine-rich-foods-to-avoid-if-you-get-cold-sores.

47 Roseff, S.J. (2002) 'Improvement in sperm quality and function with French maritime pine tree bark extract.' *Journal of Reproductive Medicine 47*, 10, 821–824.

48 Stanislavov, R., Nikolova, V. and Rohdewald, P. (2009) 'Improvement of seminal parameters with Prelox: A randomized, double-blind, placebo-controlled, cross-over trial.' *Phytotherapy Research 23*, 3, 297–302. doi:10.1002/ptr.2592.

49 Colone, M., Marelli, G., Unfer, V., Bozzuto, G., Molinari, A. and Stringaro, A. (2010) 'Inositol activity in oligoasthenoteratospermia – an in vitro study.' *European Review for Medical and Pharmacological Sciences 14*, 10, 891–896.

50 Condorelli, R.A, La Vignera, S., Mongioi, L.M., Vitale, S.G. *et al.* (2017) 'Myo-inositol as a male fertility molecule: Speed them up!' *European Review for Medical and Pharmacological Sciences 21* (2 Suppl), 30–35.

51 Calogero, A.E., Gullo, G., La Vignera, S., Condorelli, R.A. and Vaiarelli, A. (2015) 'Myoinositol improves sperm parameters and serum reproductive hormones in patients with idiopathic infertility: A prospective double-blind randomized placebo-controlled study.' *Andrology 3*, 3, 491–495. doi:10.1016/j.fertnstert.2008.06.010.

52 Clements Jr, R.S. and Darnell, B. (1980) 'Myo-inositol content of common foods: Development of a high-myo-inositol diet.' *American Journal of Clinical Nutrition 33*, 9, 1954–1967. doi:10.1093/ajcn/33.9.1954.

53 Rowe, M., Veerus, L., Trosvik, P., Buckling, A. and Pizzari, T. (2020) 'The reproductive microbiome: An emerging driver of sexual selection, sexual conflict, mating systems, and reproductive isolation.' *Trends in Ecology and Evolution 35*, 3, 220–234. doi:10.1016/j.tree.2019.11.004.

54 Younes, J., Lievens, E., Hummelen, R., van der Westen, R., Reid, G. and Petrova, M. (2018) 'Women and their microbes: The unexpected friendship.' *Trends in Microbiology 26*, 1, 16–32. doi:10.1016/j.tim.2017.07.008.

55 Naz, R. (2011) 'Can curcumin provide an ideal contraceptive?' *Molecular Reproduction and Development 78*, 2, 116–123. doi:10.1002/mrd.21276.

56 Naz, R. (2011) 'Can curcumin provide an ideal contraceptive?' *Molecular Reproduction and Development 78*, 2, 116–123. doi:10.1002/mrd.21276.

57 Zhou, Q., Wu, X., Liu, Y., Wang, X. *et al.* (2020) 'Curcumin improves asthenozoospermia by inhibiting reactive oxygen species reproduction through nuclear factor erythroid 2-related factor 2 activation.' *Andrologia 52*, 2, e13491. doi:10.1111%2Fand.13491.

CHAPTER 5

1 Parekattil, S.J., Esteves, S.C. and Agarwal, A. (eds) (2020) *Male Infertility: Contemporary Clinical Approaches, Andrology, ART and Antioxidants.* Cham: Springer.

2 Laurentino, S. (2014) 'Epigenetic aspects of sperm: What could go wrong?' European Society of Human Reproduction and Embryology (ESHRE) Annual Meeting 2014.

3 Viville, S. (2015) 'Epigenetics of spermatogenesis.' ESHRE Annual Meeting 2015.

4 Agarwal, A., Schattman, G.L. and Esteves, S.C. (2015) *Unexplained Infertility: Pathophysiology, Evaluation and Treatment.* New York, NY: Springer.

5 McSwiggin, H.M. and O'Doherty, A.M. (2018) 'Epigentic reprogramming during spermatogenesis and male factor infertility.' *Reproduction 156*, 2, 9–21. doi:10.1530/REP-18-0009.

6 McSwiggin, H.M. and O'Doherty, A.M. (2018) 'Epigentic reprogramming during spermatogenesis and male factor infertility.' *Reproduction 156*, 2, 9–21. doi:10.1530/REP-18-0009.

7 Viville, S. (2015) 'Epigenetics of spermatogenesis.' ESHRE Annual Meeting 2015.

8 McSwiggin, H.M. and O'Doherty, A.M. (2018) 'Epigentic reprogramming during spermatogenesis and male factor infertility.' *Reproduction 156*, 2, 9–21. doi:10.1530/REP-18-0009.

9 Boissonnas, C.C., Jouannet, P. and Jammes, H. (2013) 'Epigenetic disorders and male subfertility.' *Fertility and Sterility 99*, 3, 624–631. doi:10.1016/j.fertnstert.2013.01.124.

10 Parekattil, S.J., Esteves, S.C. and Agarwal, A. (eds) (2020) *Male Infertility: Contemporary Clinical Approaches, Andrology, ART and Antioxidants.* Cham: Springer.

11 Boissonnas, C.C., Jouannet, P. and Jammes, H. (2013) 'Epigenetic disorders and male subfertility.' *Fertility and Sterility 99*, 3, 624–631. doi:10.1016/j.fertnstert.2013.01.124.

12 Parekattil, S.J., Esteves, S.C. and Agarwal, A. (eds) (2020) *Male Infertility: Contemporary Clinical Approaches, Andrology, ART and Antioxidants.* Cham: Springer.

13 Adiga, D., Eswaran, S., Sriharikrishnaa, S., Khan, G.N. and Kabekkodu, S.P. (2020) 'Role of epigenetic changes in reproductive inflammation and male infertility.' *Chemical Biology Letters 7*, 2, 140–155.

14 Adiga, D., Eswaran, S., Sriharikrishnaa, S., Khan, G.N. and Kabekkodu, S.P. (2020) 'Role of epigenetic changes in reproductive inflammation and male infertility.' *Chemical Biology Letters 7*, 2, 140–155.

15 McSwiggin, H.M. and O'Doherty, A.M. (2018) 'Epigentic reprogramming during spermatogenesis and male factor infertility.' *Reproduction 156*, 2, 9–21. doi:10.1530/REP-18-0009.

16 McSwiggin, H.M. and O'Doherty, A.M. (2018) 'Epigentic reprogramming during spermatogenesis and male factor infertility.' *Reproduction 156*, 2, 9–21. doi:10.1530/REP-18-0009.

17 Cui, X., Jing, X., Wu, X., Yan, M. *et al.* (2016) 'DNA methylation in spermatogenesis and male infertility (Review).' *Experimental and Therapeutic Medicine 12*, 1973–1979. doi:10.3892/etm.2016.3569.

18 Eroglu, A. and Layman, L.C. (2012) 'Role of ART in imprinting disorders.' *Seminars in Reproductive Medicine 30*, 2, 92–104. doi:10.1055/s-0032-1307417

CHAPTER 6

1 Parekattil, S.J., Esteves, S.C. and Agarwal, A. (eds) (2020) *Male Infertility: Contemporary Clinical Approaches, Andrology, ART and Antioxidants.* Cham: Springer.

2 Parekattil, S.J., Esteves, S.C. and Agarwal, A. (eds) (2020) *Male Infertility: Contemporary Clinical Approaches, Andrology, ART and Antioxidants.* Cham: Springer.

3 Parekattil, S.J., Esteves, S.C. and Agarwal, A. (eds) (2020) *Male Infertility: Contemporary Clinical Approaches, Andrology, ART and Antioxidants.* Cham: Springer.

4   Parekattil, S.J., Esteves, S.C. and Agarwal, A. (eds) (2020) *Male Infertility: Contemporary Clinical Approaches, Andrology, ART and Antioxidants*. Cham: Springer.

5   Parekattil, S.J., Esteves, S.C. and Agarwal, A. (eds) (2020) *Male Infertility: Contemporary Clinical Approaches, Andrology, ART and Antioxidants*. Cham: Springer.

6   Parekattil, S.J., Esteves, S.C. and Agarwal, A. (eds) (2020) *Male Infertility: Contemporary Clinical Approaches, Andrology, ART and Antioxidants*. Cham: Springer.

7   Parekattil, S.J., Esteves, S.C. and Agarwal, A. (eds) (2020) *Male Infertility: Contemporary Clinical Approaches, Andrology, ART and Antioxidants*. Cham: Springer.

8   Parekattil, S.J., Esteves, S.C. and Agarwal, A. (eds) (2020) *Male Infertility: Contemporary Clinical Approaches, Andrology, ART and Antioxidants*. Cham: Springer.

9   Salonia, A., Rastrelli, G., Hackett, G., Seminara, S.B. *et al.* (2019) 'Paediatric and adult-onset male hypogonadism.' *Nature Reviews: Disease Primers 5*, 1, 38. doi:10.1038/s41572-019-0087-y.

10   Dohle, G.R., Arver, S., Bertocchi, C., Jones, T.H. and Kliesch, S. (2012) 'Guidelines: Male hypogonadism.' European Association of Urology. https://d56bochluxqnz.cloudfront.net/media/2012-Male-Hypogonadism_LR.pdf.

11   Nieschlag, E. and Behre, H.M. (eds) (2001) *Andrology, Male Reproductive Health and Dysfunction, 2nd Edition*. Heidelberg: Springer; Nieschlag, E., Behre, H.M., Bouchard, P., Corrales, J.J. *et al.* (2004) 'Testosterone replacement therapy: Current trends and future directions.' *Human Reproduction Update 10*, 5, 409–419.

12   Paraiso, B., Salvador, Z. and Packan, R. (2019) 'Kallmann Syndrome (KS) – Symptoms, causes and treatment.' InviTRA. www.invitra.com/en/kallmann-syndrome.

13   Arafa, M.M., Majzoub, A., AlSaid, S.S., El Ansari, W. *et al.* (2017) 'Chromosomal abnormalities in infertile men with azoospermia and severe oligozoospermia in Qatar and their association with sperm retrieval intracytoplasmic sperm injection outcomes.' *Arab Journal of Urology 16*, 1, 132–139. doi:10.1016/j.aju.2017.11.009.

14   NHS (2019) 'Klinefelter syndrome.' www.nhs.uk/conditions/klinefelters-syndrome.

15   Mayo Clinic (n.d.) 'Klinefelter syndrome.' www.mayoclinic.org/diseases-conditions/klinefelter-syndrome/symptoms-causes/syc-20353949.

16   Paduch, D.A., Fine, R.G., Bolyakov, A. and Kiper, J. (2008) 'New concepts in Klinefelter syndrome.' *Current Opinion in Urology 18*, 6, 621–627.

17   Parekattil, S.J., Esteves, S.C. and Agarwal, A. (eds) (2020) *Male Infertility: Contemporary Clinical Approaches, Andrology, ART and Antioxidants*. Cham: Springer.

18   Bhambhani, V. and Muenke, M. (2014) 'Noonan syndrome.' *American Family Physician 89*, 1, 37–43.

19   Parekattil, S.J., Esteves, S.C. and Agarwal, A. (eds) (2020) *Male Infertility: Contemporary Clinical Approaches, Andrology, ART and Antioxidants*. Cham: Springer.

20   Parekattil, S.J., Esteves, S.C. and Agarwal, A. (eds) (2020) *Male Infertility: Contemporary Clinical Approaches, Andrology, ART and Antioxidants*. Cham: Springer.

21   Baker, K. and Sabanegh, Jr, E. (2013) 'Obstructive azoospermia: Reconstructive techniques and results.' *Clinics (Sao Paulo) 68*, Suppl 1, 61–73. doi:10.6061/clinics/2013(sup01)07.

22   Baker, K. and Sabanegh Jr, E. (2013) 'Obstructive azoospermia: Reconstructive techniques and results.' *Clinics (Sao Paulo) 68*, Suppl 1, 61–73. doi:10.6061/clinics/2013(sup01)07.

23   Parekattil, S.J., Esteves, S.C. and Agarwal, A. (eds) (2020) *Male Infertility: Contemporary Clinical Approaches, Andrology, ART and Antioxidants*. Cham: Springer.

24   Krause, W., Weidner, W., Sperling, H. and Diemer, T. (2011) *Andrologie: Krankheiten der männlichen Geschlechtsorgane*. Leipzig: Thieme, p.224.

25   Yurdakul, T., Gokce, G., Kilic, O. and Piskin, M.M. (2008) 'Transurethral resection of ejaculatory ducts in the treatment of complete ejaculatory duct obstruction.' *International Urology and Nephrology 40*, 2, 369–372. doi:10.1007/s11255-007-9273-z.

26   Rahban, R. and Nef, S. (2020) 'Regional difference in semen quality of young men: A review on the implication of environmental and lifestyle factors during fetal life and adulthood.' *Basic and Clinical Andrology 30*, 16. doi:10.1186/s12610-020-00114-4.

27   Coward, R.M., Rajanahally, S., Kovac, J.R., Smith, R.P., Pastuszak, A.W. and Lipshultz, L.I. (2013) 'Anabolic steroid induced hypogonadism in young men.' *Journal of Urology 190*, 6, 2200–2205. doi:10.1016/j.juro.2013.06.010.

28   Turek, P.J., Williams, R.H., Gilbaugh, J.H. and Lipshultz, L.I. (1995) 'The reversibility of anabolic steroid-induced azoospermia.' *Journal of Urology 153*, 5, 1628–1630.

29 Parekattil, S.J., Esteves, S.C. and Agarwal, A. (eds) (2020) *Male Infertility: Contemporary Clinical Approaches, Andrology, ART and Antioxidants*. Cham: Springer; Patel, A.S., Leong, J.Y., Ramos, L. and Ramasamy, R. (2019) 'Testosterone is a contraceptive and should not be used in men who desire fertility.' *World Journal of Men's Health 37*, 1, 45–54. doi:10.5534/wjmh.180036.

30 Parekattil, S.J., Esteves, S.C. and Agarwal, A. (eds) (2020) *Male Infertility: Contemporary Clinical Approaches, Andrology, ART and Antioxidants*. Cham: Springer.

31 Rahban, R. and Nef, S. (2020) 'Regional difference in semen quality of young men: A review on the implication of environmental and lifestyle factors during fetal life and adulthood.' *Basic and Clinical Andrology 30*, 16. doi:10.1186/s12610-020-00114-4.

32 Agarwal, A., Schattman, G.L. and Esteves, S.C. (2015) *Unexplained Infertility: Pathophysiology, Evaluation and Treatment*. New York, NY: Springer.

33 Agarwal, A., Schattman, G.L. and Esteves, S.C. (2015) *Unexplained Infertility: Pathophysiology, Evaluation and Treatment*. New York, NY: Springer.

34 Parekattil, S.J., Esteves, S.C. and Agarwal, A. (eds) (2020) *Male Infertility: Contemporary Clinical Approaches, Andrology, ART and Antioxidants*. Cham: Springer.

35 Rozati, R., Reddy, P.P., Reddanna, P. and Mujtaba, R. (2002) 'Role of environmental estrogens in the deterioration of male factor infertility.' *Fertility and Sterility 78*, 6, 1187–1194. doi:10.1016/s0015-0282(02)04389-3.

36 Vested, A., Giwercman, A., Bonde, J. and Toft, G. (2014) 'Persistent organic pollutants and male reproductive health.' *Asian Journal of Andrology 16*, 1, 71–80. doi:10.4103%2F1008-682X.122345.

37 Fisher, B.G., Thankamony, A., Mendiola, J., Petry, C.J. *et al.* (2020) 'Maternal serum concentrations of bisphenol A and propyl paraben in early pregnancy are associated with male infant genital development.' *Human Reproduction 35*, 4, 913–928.

38 Chavarro, J.E., Toth, T.L., Sadio, S.M. and Hauser, R. (2008) 'Soy food and isoflavone intake in relation to semen quality parameters among men from an infertility clinic.' *Human Reproduction 23*, 11, 2584–2590.

39 Swan, S.H., Main, K.M., Liu, F. and Stewart, S.L. et al. (2005) 'Decrease in anogenital distance among male infants with prenatal phthalate exposure.' *Environmental Health Perspectives 113*, 8; Mendiola, J., Stahlhut, R.W., Jørgensen, N., Liu, F. and Swan, S.H. (2011) 'Shorter anogenital distance predicts poorer semen quality in young men in Rochester, New York.' *Environmental Health Perspectives 119*, 7, 958–963. doi:10.1289/ehp.1103421.

40 Bonde, J.P., Flachs, E.M., Rimborg, S., Glazer, C.H. *et al.* (2016) 'The epidemiologic evidence linking prenatal and postnatal exposure to endocrine disrupting chemicals with male reproductive disorders: A systematic review and meta-analysis.' *Human Reproduction Update 23*, 1, 104–125. doi:10.1093%2Fhumupd%2Fdmw036.

41 Anway, M.D., Cupp, A.S., Uzumcu, M. and Skinner, M.K. (2005) 'Epigenetic transgenerational actions of endocrine disruptors and male fertility.' *Science 308*, 5727, 1466–1469.

42 Ramasamy, R., Chiba, K., Butler, P. and Lamb, D.L. (2015) 'Male biological clock: A critical analysis of advanced paternal age.' *Fertility and Sterility 103*, 6, 1402–1406. doi:10.1016/j.fertnstert.2015.03.011.

43 Hellstrom, W.J.G., Overstreet, J.W., Sikka, S.C., Denne, J. *et al.* (2006) 'Semen and sperm reference ranges for men 45 years of age and older.' *Journal of Andrology 27*, 3, 421–428. doi:10.2164/jandrol.05156.

44 McQueen, D.B., Zhang, J. and Robins, J.C. (2019) 'Sperm DNA fragmentation and recurrent pregnancy loss: A systematic review and meta-analysis.' *Fertility and Sterility 112*, 1, 54–60. doi:10.1016/j.fertnstert.2019.03.003.

45 Ramasamy, R., Chiba, K., Butler, P. and Lamb, D.L. (2015) 'Male biological clock: A critical analysis of advanced paternal age.' *Fertility and Sterility 103*, 6, 1402–1406. doi:10.1016/j.fertnstert.2015.03.011.

46 Khandwala, Y.S., Baker, V.L., Shaw, G.M., Stevenson, D.K. *et al.* (2018) 'Association of paternal age with perinatal outcomes between 2007 and 2016 in the United States: Population based cohort study.' *BMJ 2018*, 363, k4372. doi:10.1136/bmj.k4372.

47 Ford, W.C., North, K., Taylor, H., Farrow, A., Hull, M.G. and Golding, J. (2000) 'Increasing paternal age is associated with delayed conception in a large population of fertile couples: Evidence for declining fecundity in older men. The ALSPAC Study Team (Avon Longitudinal Study of Pregnancy and Childhood).' *Human Reproduction 15*, 8, 1703–1708.

48 Wiener-Megnazi, Z., Auslender, R. and Dirnfeld, M. (2012) 'Advanced paternal age and reproductive outcome.' *Asian Journal of Andrology 14*, 1, 69–76. doi:10.1038/aja.2011.69; Ramasamy, R., Chiba, K., Butler, P. and Lamb, D.L. (2015) 'Male biological clock: A critical analysis of advanced paternal age.' *Fertility and Sterility 103*, 6, 1402–1406. doi:10.1016/j.fertnstert.2015.03.011.

49 Khandwala, Y.S., Baker, V.L., Shaw, G.M., Stevenson, D.K. *et al.* (2018) 'Association of paternal age with perinatal outcomes between 2007 and 2016 in the United States: Population based cohort study.' *BMJ 2018*, 363, k4372. doi:10.1136/bmj.k4372.

50 Sermondade, N., Faure, C., Fezeu, L., Shayeb, A.G. *et al.* (2013) 'BMI in relation to sperm count: An updated systematic review and collaborative meta-analysis.' *Human Reproduction Update 19*, 3, 221–223. doi:10.1093%2Fhumupd%2Fdms050.

51 Bieniek, J.M., Kashian, J.A., Deibert, C.M., Grober, E.D. *et al.* (2016) 'Influence of increasing body mass index on semen and reproductive hormonal parameters in a multi-institutional cohort of subfertile men.' *Fertility and Sterility 106*, 5, 1070–1075. doi: 10.1016/j.fertnstert.2016.06.041.

52 Sallmén, M., Sandler, D.P., Hoppin, J.A., Blair, A. and Baird, D.D. (2006) 'Reduced fertility among over-weight and obese men.' *Epidemiology 17*, 5, 520–523. doi:10.1097/01.ede.0000229953.76862.e5.

53 McPherson, N.O. and Lane, M. (2015) 'Male obesity and subfertility, is it really about increased adiposity?' *Asian Journal of Andrology 17*, 3, 450–458. doi:10.4103/1008-682X.148076.

54 Bakos, H.W., Henshaw, R.C., Mitchell, M. and Lane, M. (2011) 'Paternal body mass index is associated with decreased blastocyst development and reduced live birth rates following assisted reproductive technology.' *Fertility and Sterility 95*, 5, 1700–1704. doi:10.1016/j.fertnstert.2010.11.044.

55 Keltz, J., Zapantis, A., Jindal, S.K., Lieman, H.J., Santoro, N. and Polotsky, A.J. (2010) 'Overweight men: Clinical pregnancy after ART is decreased in IVF but not in ICSI cycles.' *Journal of Assisted Reproduction and Genetics 27*, 9–10, 539–544.

56 Haddock, L., Gordon, S., Lewis, S.E.M., Larsen, P., Shehata, A. and Shehata, H. (2021) 'Sperm DNA fragmentation is a novel biomarker for early pregnancy loss.' *Reproductive BioMedicine Online 42*, 1, 175–184.

57 Jensen, T.K., Andersson, A.M., Jørgensen, N., Andersen, A.G. *et al.* (2004) 'Body mass index in relation to semen quality and reproductive hormones among 1,558 Danish men.' *Fertility and Sterility 82*, 4, 863–870.

58 Ma, J., Wu, L., Zhou, Y., Zhang, H. *et al.* (2019) 'Association between BMI and semen quality: An obser-vational study of 3966 sperm donors.' *Human Reproduction 34*, 1, 155–162. doi:10.1093/humrep/dey328.

59 Parekattil, S.J., Esteves, S.C. and Agarwal, A. (eds) (2020) *Male Infertility: Contemporary Clinical Approaches, Andrology, ART and Antioxidants*. Cham: Springer.

60 Parekattil, S.J., Esteves, S.C. and Agarwal, A. (eds) (2020) *Male Infertility: Contemporary Clinical Approaches, Andrology, ART and Antioxidants*. Cham: Springer.

61 Gallegos, G., Ramos, B., Santiso, R., Goyanes, V., Gosálvez, J. and Fernández, J.L. (2008) 'Sperm DNA fragmentation in infertile men with genitourinary infection by Chlamydia trachomatis and Myco-plasma.' *Fertility and Sterility 90*, 2, 328–334.

62 AWMF Online (2019) 'Diagnostik und Therapie der Gonorrhe.' www.awmf.org/leitlinien/detail/ll/059-004.html.

63 Weidner, W., Colpi, G.M., Hargreave, T.B., Papp, G.K., Pomerol, J.M., Ghosh, C., EAU Working Group on Male Infertility (2002) 'EAU guidelines on male infertility.' *European Urology 42*, 4, 313–322. doi:10.1016/s0302-2838(02)00367-6.

64 Lyu, Z., Feng, X., Li, N., Zhao, W. *et al.* (2017) 'Human papillomavirus in semen and the risk for male infertility: A systematic review and meta-analysis.' *BMC Infectious Diseases 17*, 1, 714. doi:10.1186/s12879-017-2812-z.

65 Dutta, S. and Sengupta, P. (2021) 'SARS-CoV-2 and male infertility: Possible multifaceted pathology.' Reproductive Sciences 28, 23–36. doi:10.1007/s43032-020-00261-z.

66 Roychoudhury, S., Das, A., Jha, N.K., Kesari, K.K. *et al.* (2021) 'Viral pathogenesis of SARS-CoV-2 infection and male reproductive health.' *Open Biology 11*, 1, 200347. doi:10.1098/rsob.200347.

67 Hu, B., Liu, K., Ruan, Y., Wei, X. et al. (2022) 'Evaluation of mid- and long-term impact of COVID-19 on male fertility through evaluating semen parameters.' *Translational Andrology and Urology 11*, 2, 159–167. doi:10.21037/tau-21-922.

68 World Health Organization (2016) 'Diabetes.' www.who.int/health-topics/diabetes#tab=tab_1.

69 Chemlal, H., Bensalem, S., Bendiab, K., Azzar, M. *et al.* (2021) 'High HbA1c levels affect motility parame-ters and overexpress oxidative stress of human mature spermatozoa.' *Andrologia 53*, 1, e13902. doi:10.1111/and.13902.

70 Parekattil, S.J., Esteves, S.C. and Agarwal, A. (eds) (2020) *Male Infertility: Contemporary Clinical Approaches, Andrology, ART and Antioxidants*. Cham: Springer.

71 Shindel, A. and Lue, T.F. (2021) 'Sexual Dysfunction in Diabetes.' In K.R. Feingold, B. Anawalt, A. Boyce *et al.* (eds) *Endotext* [Internet]. www.endotext.org.

72 Ivell, R. (2007) 'Lifestyle impact and the biology of the human scrotum.' *Reproductive Biology and Endocrinology 5*, 15. doi:10.1186/1477-7827-5-15.

73 Kompanje, E. (2013) '"Real men wear kilts." The anecdotal evidence that wearing a Scottish kilt has influence on reproductive potential: How much is true?' *Scottish Medical Journal 58*, 1, e1–e5. doi:10.1177/0036933012474600.

74 Ivell, R. (2007) 'Lifestyle impact and the biology of the human scrotum.' *Reproductive Biology and Endocrinology 5*, 15. doi:10.1186/1477-7827-5-15.

75 Bujan, L. (2000) 'Increase in scrotal temperature in car drivers.' *Human Reproduction 15*, 6, 1355–1357.

76 Nakata, K. (2019) 'Mounting evidence of harmful effects of WiFi router electromagnetic waves on sperm.' ASPIRE. http://aspire-reproduction.org/mounting-evidence-of-harmful-effects-of-wifi-router-electromagnetic-waves-on-sperm.

77 Partsch, C.J., Aukamp, M. and Sippell, W.G. (2000) 'Scrotal temperature is increased in disposable plastic lined nappies.' *Archives of Disease in Childhood 83*, 4, 364–368.

78 Mostafa, R.M., Nasrallah, Y.S., Hassan, M.M., Farrag, A.F., Majzoub, A. and Agarwal, A. (2018) 'The effect of cigarette smoking on human seminal parameters, sperm chromatin structure and condensation.' *Andrologia 50*, 3. doi:10.1111/and.12910.

79 Zitzmann, M., Rolf, C., Nordhoff, V., Schräder, G. *et al.* (2003) 'Male smokers have a decreased success rate for in vitro fertilization and intracytoplasmic sperm injection.' *Fertility and Sterility 79*, Suppl 3, 1550–1554.

80 Fowler, P.A., Cassie, S., Rhind, S.M., Brewer, M.J. *et al.* (2008) 'Maternal smoking during pregnancy specifically reduces human fetal desert hedgehog gene expression during testis development.' *Journal of Clinical Endocrinology and Metabolism 93*, 2, 619–626. doi:10.1210/jc.2007-1860.

81 Sobinoff, A.P., Sutherland, J.M., Beckett, E.L., Stanger, S.J. *et al.* (2014) 'Damaging legacy: Maternal cigarette smoking has long-term consequences for male offspring fertility.' *Human Reproduction 29*, 12, 2719–2735. doi:10.1093/humrep/deu235.

82 Ricci, E., Noli, S., Ferrari, S., La Vecchia, I. *et al.* (2018) 'Alcohol intake and semen variables: Cross-sectional analysis of a prospective cohort study of men referring to an Italian fertility clinic.' *Andrology 6*, 5, 690–696. doi:10.1111/andr.12521.9.

83 Jensen, T.K., Gottschau, M., Madsen, J.O.B., Andersson, A.M. *et al.* (2014) 'Habitual alcohol consumption associated with reduced semen quality and changes in reproductive hormones: A cross-sectional study among 1221 young Danish men.' *BMJ Open 4*, 9, e005462. doi:10.1136/bmjopen-2014-005462.

84 Yao, D.F. and Mills, J.N. (2016) 'Male infertility: Lifestyle factors and holistic, complementary, and alternative therapy.' *Asian Journal of Andrology 18*, 3, 410–418. doi:10.4103%2F1008-682X.175779.

85 Ricci, E., Al Beitawi, S., Cipriani, S., Candiani, M. *et al.* (2017) 'Semen quality and alcohol intake: A systematic review and meta-analysis.' *Reproductive Biomedicine Online 34*, 1, 38–47. doi:10.1016/j.rbmo.2016.09.012.

86 Ricci, E., Noli, S., Ferrari, S., La Vecchia, I. *et al.* (2018) 'Alcohol intake and semen variables: Cross-sectional analysis of a prospective cohort study of men referring to an Italian fertility clinic.' *Andrology 6*, 5, 690–696. doi:10.1111/andr.12521.9.

87 Ricci, E., Viganò, P., Cipriani, S., Somigliana, E. *et al.* (2017) 'Coffee and caffeine intake and male infertility: A systematic review.' *Nutrition Journal 16*, 37. doi:10.1186/s12937-017-0257-2.

88 Bu, F.L., Feng, X., Yang, X.Y., Ren, J. and Cao, H.J. (2020) 'Relationship between caffeine intake and infertility: A systematic review of controlled clinical studies.' *BMC Women's Health 20*, 1, 125. doi:10.1186/s12905-020-00973-z.

89 Krzastek, S.C., Farhim, J., Gray, M. and Smith, R.P. (2020) 'Impact of environmental toxin exposure on male fertility potential.' *Translational Andrology and Urology 9*, 6, 2797–2813. doi:10.21037/tau-20-685.

90 Pariz, J.R., Ranéa, C., Monteiro, R.A.C., Evenson, D.P., Drevet, J.R. and Hallak, J. (2019) 'Melatonin and caffeine supplementation used, respectively, as protective and stimulating agents in the cryopreservation of human sperm improves survival, viability, and motility after thawing compared to traditional TEST-yolk buffer.' *Oxidative Medicine and Cellular Longevity 2019*, 6472945. doi:10.1155/2019/6472945.

91 Schrott, R., Acharya, K., Itchon-Ramos, N. et al. (2020) 'Cannabis use is associated with potentially heritable widespread changes in autism candidate gene DLGAP2 DNA methylation in sperm.' *Epigenetics 15*, 1–2, 161–173. doi:10.1080/15592294.2019.1656158.

92 Schrott, R. and Murphy, S.K. (2020) 'Cannabis use and the sperm epigenome: A budding concern?.' *Environ Epigenet 6*, 1. doi:10.1093/eep/dvaa002)

93 Nasaan, F.L., Arvizu, M., Minguez-Alarcón, L., Williams, P.L. *et al.* (2019) 'Marijuana smoking and markers of testicular function among men from a fertility centre.' *Human Reproduction 34*, 4, 715–723.

94 Payne, K.S., Mazur, D.J., Hotaling, J.M. and Pastuszak, A.W. (2019) 'Cannabis and male fertility: A systematic review.' *Journal of Urology 202*, 4, 674–681. doi:10.1097/JU.0000000000000248.

95 Semet, M., Paci, M., Saïas-Magnan, J., Metzler-Guillemain, C. *et al.* (2017) 'The impact of drugs on male fertility: A review.' *Andrology 5*, 4, 640–663. doi:10.1111/andr.12366.

96 Parekattil, S.J., Esteves, S.C. and Agarwal, A. (eds) (2020) *Male Infertility: Contemporary Clinical Approaches, Andrology, ART and Antioxidants.* Cham: Springer.

97 Kristensen, D.M., Desdoits-Lethimonier, C., Mackey, A.L., Dalgaard, M.D. *et al.* (2018) 'Ibuprofen alters human testicular physiology to produce a state of compensated hypogonadism.' *PNAS 115*, 4, E715–E724. doi:10.1073/pnas.1715035115.

98 Meistrich, M.L. (2013) 'Effects of chemotherapy and radiotherapy on spermatogenesis in humans.' *Fertility and Sterility 100*, 5, 1180–1186. doi: 10.1016/j.fertnstert.2013.08.010.

99 Vaamonde, D., Da Silva, M.E., Poblador, M.S. and Lancho, J.L. (2006) 'Reproductive profile of physically active men after exhaustive endurance exercise.' *International Journal of Sports Medicine 27*, 9, 680–689. doi:10.1055/s-2005-872906.

100 Gaskins, A.J., Mendiola, J., Afeiche, M., Jørgensen, N., Swan, S.H. and Chavarro, J.E. (2015) 'Physical activity and television watching in relation to semen quality in young men.' *British Journal of Sports Medicine 49*, 4, 265–270. doi:10.1136/bjsports-2012-091644.

101 Jóźków, P. and Rossato, M. (2017) 'The impact of intense exercise on semen quality.' *American Journal of Men's Health 11*, 3, 654–662. doi:10.1177/1557988316669045.

102 Gaskins, A.J., Mendiola, J., Afeiche, M., Jørgensen, N., Swan, S.H. and Chavarro, J.E. (2015) 'Physical activity and television watching in relation to semen quality in young men.' *British Journal of Sports Medicine 49*, 4, 265–270. doi:10.1136/bjsports-2012-091644; Kipandula, W. and Lampiao, F. (2015) 'Semen profiles of young men involved as bicycle taxi cyclists in Mangochi District, Malawi: A case-control study.' *Malawi Medical Journal 27*, 4, 151–153.

103 Jóźków, P. and Rossato, M. (2017) 'The impact of intense exercise on semen quality.' *American Journal of Men's Health 11*, 3, 654–662. doi:10.1177/1557988316669045.

104 Safarinejad, M.R., Azma, K. and Kolahi, A.A. (2009) 'The effects of intensive, long-term treadmill running on reproductive hormones, hypothalamus-pituitary-testis axis, and semen quality: A randomized controlled study.' *Journal of Endocrinology 200*, 3, 259–271.

105 Chen, H.-G., Sun, B., Chen, Y.-J., Chavarro, J.E. *et al.* (2020) 'Sleep duration and quality in relation to semen quality in healthy men screened as potential sperm donors.' *Environment International 135*, 105368. doi:10.1016/j.envint.2019.105368.

106 Bonmati-Carrion, M.A., Arguelles-Prieto, R., Martinez-Madrid, M.J., Reiter, R. *et al.* (2014) 'Protecting the melatonin rhythm through circadian healthy light exposure.' *International Journal of Molecular Sciences 15*, 12, 23448–23500. doi:10.3390/ijms151223448.

107 Janevic, T., Kahn, L.G., Landsbergis, P., Cirillo, P.M. *et al.* (2014) 'Effects of work and life stress on semen quality.' *Fertility and Sterility 102*, 2, 530–553.

108 Pound, N., Javed, M.H., Ruberto, M., Shaikh, M.A., Del Valle, A.P. (2002) 'Duration of sexual arousal predicts semen parameters for masturbatory ejaculates.' *Physiology and Behavior 76*, 4–5, 685–689. doi:10.1016/s0031-9384(02)00803-x.

109 Elzanaty, S. and Malm, J. (2008) 'Comparison of semen parameters in samples collected by masturbation at a clinic and at home.' *Fertility and Sterility 89*, 6, 1718–1722. doi:10.1016/j.fertnstert.2007.05.044.

110 Joseph, P.N., Sharma, R.K., Agarwal, A. and Sirot, L. (2015) 'Men ejaculate larger volumes of semen, more motile sperm, and more quickly when exposed to images of novel women.' *Evolutionary Psychological Science 1*, 195–200. doi:10.1007/s40806-015-0022-8.

111 Pound, N., Javed, M.H., Ruberto, M., Shaikh, M.A. and Del Valle, A.P. (2002) 'Duration of sexual arousal predicts semen parameters for masturbatory ejaculates.' *Physiology and Behavior 76*, 4–5, 685–689. doi:10.1016/s0031-9384(02)00803-x.

112 Pham, M.N., Jeffery, A.J., Sela, Y. and Lynn, J.T. (2016) 'Duration of cunnilingus predicts estimated ejaculate volume in humans: A content analysis of pornography.' *Evolutionary Psychological Science 2*, 220–227. doi:10.1007/s40806-016-0057-5.

113 Chidambar, C.K., Shankar, S.M., Agarwal, R.K., Bhushan, K.S. and Gururaj. S.B. (2019) 'Evaluation of periodontal status among men undergoing infertility treatment.' *Journal of Human Reproductive Sciences 12*, 2, 130–135.

114 Salas-Hueto, A., Bulló, M. and Salas-Salvadó, J. (2017) 'Dietary patterns, foods and nutrients in male fertility parameters and fecundability: A systematic review of observational studies.' *Human Reproduction Update 23*, 4, 371–389; Karayiannis, D., Kontogianni, M.D., Mendorou, C.G., Douka, L., Mastrominas, M. and Yiannakouris, N. (2017) 'Association between adherence to the Mediterranean diet and semen quality parameters in male partners of couples attempting fertility.' *Human Reproduction 32*, 1, 215–222.

CHAPTER 7

1 Schlegel, P.N., Sigman, M., Collura, B., De Jonge, C.J. *et al.* (2021) 'Diagnosis and Treatment of Infertility in Men: AUA/ASRM Guideline PART II.' *Journal of Urology 205*, 1, 44–51. doi:10.1097/ju.0000000000001520.

2 Schlegel, P.N., Sigman, M., Collura, B., De Jonge, C.J. *et al.* (2021) 'Diagnosis and Treatment of Infertility in Men: AUA/ASRM Guideline PART II.' *Journal of Urology 205*, 1, 44–51. doi:10.1097/ju.0000000000001520.

3 Kasman, A.M., Del Giudice, F. and Eisenberg, M.L. (2020) 'New insights to guide patient care: The bidirectional relationship between male infertility and male health.' *Fertility and Sterility 113*, 3, 469–477. doi:10.1016/j.fertnstert.2020.01.002.

4 Stentz, N.C., Koelper, N., Barnhart, K.T., Sammel, M.D. and Senapati, S. (2020) 'Infertility and mortality.' *American Journal of Obstetrics and Gynecology 222*, 3, 251.e1–251.e10. doi:10.1016/j.ajog.2019.09.007.

5 Barratt, C.L.R., De Jonge, C.J., Anderson, R.A., Eisenberg, M.L. *et al.* (2021) 'A global approach to addressing the policy, research and social challenges of male reproductive health.' *Human Reproduction Open 2021*, 1, hoab009. doi:10.1093/hropen/hoab009.

6 Pozzi, E., Boeri, L., Capogrosso, P., Candela, L. *et al.* (2021) 'Infertility as a proxy of men's health: Still a long way to go.' *Turkish Journal of Urology.* doi:10.5152/tud.2021.20561.

7 Jacobsen, R., Bostofte, E., Engholm, G., Hansen, J. *et al.* (2000) 'Risk of testicular cancer in men with abnormal semen characteristics: Cohort study.' *BMJ 321*, 7264, 789-792. doi: 10.1136/bmj.321.7264.789.

8 Choy, J.T. and Eisenberg, M.L. (2018) 'Male infertility as a window to health.' *Fertility and Sterility 110*, 5, 810–814. doi:10.1016/j.fertnstert.2018.08.015.

9 Walsh, T.J., Schembri, M., Turek, P.J., Chan, J.M. *et al.* (2010) 'Increased risk of high-grade prostate cancer among infertile men.' *Cancer 116*, 9, 2140–2147. doi:10.1002/cncr.25075.

10 Kasman, A.M., Del Giudice, F. and Eisenberg, M.L. (2020) 'New insights to guide patient care: The bidirectional relationship between male infertility and male health.' *Fertility and Sterility 113*, 3, 469–477. doi:10.1016/j.fertnstert.2020.01.002.

11 Boeri, L., Capogrosso, P., Cazzaniga, W., Ventimiglia, E.A. *et al.* (2020) 'Infertile men have higher prostate-specific antigen values than fertile individuals of comparable age.' *European Journal of Urology 79*, 2, 234–240. doi:10.1016/j.eururo.2020.08.001.

12 Eisenberg, M.L., Li, S., Behr, B., Cullen, M.R. *et al.* (2014) 'Semen quality, infertility and mortality in the USA.' *Human Reproduction 29*, 7, 1567-1574. doi:10.1093/humrep/deu106.

13 Eisenberg, M.L., Betts, P., Herder, D., Lamb, D.J. and Lipshultz, L.I. (2013) 'Increased risk of cancer among azoospermic men.' *Fertility and Sterility 100*, 3, 681–685. doi:10.1016/j.fertnstert.2013.05.022.

14 Sermondade, N., Faure, C. Fezeu, L., Shayeb, A.G. *et al.* (2013) 'BMI in relation to sperm count: An updated systematic review and collaborative meta-analysis.' *Human Reproduction Update 19*, 3, 221–231. doi:10.1093/humupd/dms050.

15 Camacho, E.M., Huhtaniemi, I.T., O'Neill, T.W., Finn, J.D. *et al.* (2013) 'Age-associated changes in hypothalamic-pituitary-testicular function in middle-aged and older men are modified by weight change and lifestyle factors: Longitudinal results from the European Male Ageing Study.' *European Journal of Endocrinology 168*, 3, 445–455. doi:10.1530/EJE-12-0890.

16 Corona, G., Rastrelli, G., Monami, M., Saad, F. *et al.* (2013) 'Body weight loss reverts obesity-associated hypogonadotropic hypogonadism: A systematic review and meta-analysis.' *European Journal of Endocrinology 168*, 6, 829–843. doi:10.1530/EJE-12-095.

17 Ferlin, A., Garolla, A., Ghezzi, M., Selice, R. *et al.* (2019) 'Sperm count and hypogonadism as markers of general male health.' *European Urology Focus 7*, 1, 205–213. doi:10.1016/j.euf.2019.08.001.

18 Eisenberg, M.L., Li, S., Behr, B., Cullen, M.R. *et al.* (2014) 'Semen quality, infertility and mortality in the USA.' *Human Reproduction 29*, 7, 1567-1574. doi:10.1093/humrep/deu106.

19 Latif, T., Jensen, T.K., Mehlsen, J., Holmboe, S.A. *et al.* (2017) 'Semen quality as a predictor of subsequent morbidity: A Danish cohort study of 4,712 men with long-term follow-up.' *American Journal of Epidemiology 186*, 8, 910–917.

20 Eisenberg, M.L., Li, S., Cullen, M.R. and Baker, L.C. (2016) 'Increased risk of incident chronic medical conditions in infertile men: Analysis of United States claims data.' *Fertility and Sterility 105*, 3, 629–636. doi:10.1016/j.fertnstert.2015.11.011.

21 Boeri, L., Capogrosso, P., Cazzaniga, W., Ventimiglia, E.A. *et al.* (2020) 'Infertile men have higher prostate-specific antigen values than fertile individuals of comparable age.' *European Journal of Urology 79*, 2, 234–240. doi:10.1016/j.eururo.2020.08.001; Glazer, C.H., Bonde, J.P., Giwercman, A., Vassard, D. *et al.* (2017) 'Risk of diabetes according to male factor infertility: A register-based cohort study.' *Human Reproduction 32*, 7, 1474–1481. doi:10.1093/humrep/dex097.

22 Boeri, L., Capogrosso, P., Cazzaniga, W., Ventimiglia, E.A. *et al.* (2020) 'Infertile men have higher prostate-specific antigen values than fertile individuals of comparable age.' *European Journal of Urology 79*, 2, 234–240. doi:10.1016/j.eururo.2020.08.001.

23 Eisenberg, M.L., Li, S., Behr, B., Cullen, M.R. *et al.* (2014) 'Semen quality, infertility and mortality in the USA.' *Human Reproduction 29*, 7, 1567–1574. doi:10.1093/humrep/deu106.

24 Kasman, A.M., Del Giudice, F. and Eisenberg, M.L. (2020) 'New insights to guide patient care: The bidirectional relationship between male infertility and male health.' *Fertility and Sterility 113*, 3, 469–477. doi:10.1016/j.fertnstert.2020.01.002.

25 Glazer, C.H., Tøttenborg, S.S., Giwercman, A., Bräuner, E.V. *et al.* (2018) 'Male factor infertility and risk of multiple sclerosis: A register-based cohort study.' *Multiple Sclerosis Journal 24*, 14, 1835–1842. doi:10.1177/1352458517734069.

26 Brubaker, W.D., Li, S., Baker, L.C. and Eisenberg, M.L. (2018) 'Increased risk of autoimmune disorders in infertile men: Analysis of US claims data.' *Andrology 6*, 1, 94–98. doi:10.1111/andr.12436.

27 Choy, J.T. and Eisenberg, M.L. (2018) 'Male infertility as a window to health.' *Fertility and Sterility 110*, 5, 810–814. doi:10.1016/j.fertnstert.2018.08.015.

28 Schlegel, P.N., Sigman, M., Collura, B., De Jonge, C.J. *et al.* (2021) 'Diagnosis and Treatment of Infertility in Men: AUA/ASRM Guideline PART II.' *Journal of Urology 205*, 1, 44–51. doi:10.1097/ju.0000000000001520.

29 Schlegel, P.N., Sigman, M., Collura, B., De Jonge, C.J. *et al.* (2021) 'Diagnosis and Treatment of Infertility in Men: AUA/ASRM Guideline PART II.' *Journal of Urology 205*, 1, 44–51. doi:10.1097/ju.0000000000001520.

30 Schlegel, P.N., Sigman, M., Collura, B., De Jonge, C.J. *et al.* (2021) 'Diagnosis and Treatment of Infertility in Men: AUA/ASRM Guideline PART II.' *Journal of Urology 205*, 1, 44–51. doi:10.1097/ju.0000000000001520.

31 Snodgrass, W. (2012) 'Hypospadias.' In A. Wein, M.F. Campbell and P.C. Walsh (eds) *Campbell-Walsh Urology, 10th Edition*. Philadelphia, PA: Elsevier.

32 Chang, J., Wang, S. and Zheng, Z. (2020) 'Etiology of hypospadias: A comparative review of genetic factors and developmental processes between human and animal models.' *Research and Reports in Urology 12*, 673–686. doi:10.2147/RRU.S276141.

33 Boeri, L., Capogrosso, P., Ventimiglia, E., Cazzaniga, W. *et al.* (2021) 'Testicular volume in infertile versus fertile white-European men: A case-control investigation in the real-life setting.' *Asian Journal of Andrology 23*, 5, 501–509. doi:10.4103/aja.aja_93_20.

34 Parekattil, S.J., Esteves, S.C. and Agarwal, A. (eds) (2020) *Male Infertility: Contemporary Clinical Approaches, Andrology, ART and Antioxidants*. Cham: Springer.

35 Parekattil, S.J., Esteves, S.C. and Agarwal, A. (eds) (2020) *Male Infertility: Contemporary Clinical Approaches, Andrology, ART and Antioxidants*. Cham: Springer.

36 Parekattil, S.J., Esteves, S.C. and Agarwal, A. (eds) (2020) *Male Infertility: Contemporary Clinical Approaches, Andrology, ART and Antioxidants*. Cham: Springer.

37 Parekattil, S.J., Esteves, S.C. and Agarwal, A. (eds) (2020) *Male Infertility: Contemporary Clinical Approaches, Andrology, ART and Antioxidants*. Cham: Springer.

38 Nudell, D.M. (n.d.) 'Male infertility evaluation and treatment options.' https://www.drnudell.com/male-infertility-evaluation.

39 Schlegel, P.N., Sigman, M., Collura, B., De Jonge, C.J. *et al.* (2021) 'Diagnosis and Treatment of Infertility in Men: AUA/ASRM Guideline PART II.' *Journal of Urology 205*, 1, 44–51. doi:10.1097/ju.0000000000001520.

40 Russell, S. (n.d.) 'Elevated prolactin/hyperprolactinemia and male infertility.' www.maleinfertilityguide.com/elevated-prolactin.

41 La Vignera, S. and Vita, R. (2018) 'Thyroid dysfunction and semen quality.' *International Journal of Immunopathology and Pharmacology 32*, 2058738418775241. doi:10.1177/2058738418775241.

42 Cooper, T.G., Noonan, E., von Eckardstein, S., Auger, J. et al. (2010) 'World Health Organization reference values for human semen characteristics.' *Human Reproduction Update 16*, 3, 231–245. doi:10.1093/humupd/dmp048.

43 Andrade-Rocha, F.T. (2017) 'On the origins of the semen analysis: A close relationship with the history of the reproductive medicine.' *Journal of Human Reproductive Sciences 10*, 4, 242–255. doi:10.4103/jhrs. JHRS_97_17.

44 Andrade-Rocha, F.T. (2017) 'On the origins of the semen analysis: A close relationship with the history of the reproductive medicine.' *Journal of Human Reproductive Sciences 10*, 4, 242–255. doi:10.4103/jhrs. JHRS_97_17.

45 Andrade-Rocha, F.T. (2017) 'On the origins of the semen analysis: A close relationship with the history of the reproductive medicine.' *Journal of Human Reproductive Sciences 10*, 4, 242–255. doi:10.4103/jhrs. JHRS_97_17

46 Reproduced from World Health Organization (2021) *WHO Laboratory Manual for the Examination and Processing of Human Semen, 6th Edition*. Geneva: WHO, pp.1–2, Copyright 2021.

47 Reproduced from World Health Organization (2021) *WHO Laboratory Manual for the Examination and Processing of Human Semen, 6th Edition*. Geneva: WHO, p.14, Copyright 2021.

48 Reproduced from World Health Organization (2021) *WHO Laboratory Manual for the Examination and Processing of Human Semen, 6th Edition*. Geneva: WHO, Copyright 2021.

49 Reproduced from World Health Organization (2021) *WHO Laboratory Manual for the Examination and Processing of Human Semen, 6th Edition*. Geneva: WHO, p.14, Copyright 2021.

50 Du Plessis, S.S., Gokul, S. and Agarwal, A. (2013) 'Semen hyperviscosity: Causes, consequences, and cures.' *Frontiers in Bioscience-Elite 5*, 1, 224–231. doi:10.2741/e610.

51 Reproduced from World Health Organization (2021) *WHO Laboratory Manual for the Examination and Processing of Human Semen, 6th Edition*. Geneva: WHO, Copyright 2021.

52 Reproduced from World Health Organization (2021) *WHO Laboratory Manual for the Examination and Processing of Human Semen, 6th Edition*. Geneva: WHO, p.28, Copyright 2021.

53 Reproduced from World Health Organization (2021) *WHO Laboratory Manual for the Examination and Processing of Human Semen, 6th Edition*. Geneva: WHO, p.10, Copyright 2021.

54 Reproduced from World Health Organization (2021) *WHO Laboratory Manual for the Examination and Processing of Human Semen, 6th Edition*. Geneva: WHO, p.23, Copyright 2021.

55 Reproduced from World Health Organization (2021) *WHO Laboratory Manual for the Examination and Processing of Human Semen, 6th Edition*. Geneva: WHO, p.24, Copyright 2021.

56 Reproduced from World Health Organization (2021) *WHO Laboratory Manual for the Examination and Processing of Human Semen, 6th Edition*. Geneva: WHO, Copyright 2021.

57 Dearing, C., Jayasena, C. and Lindsay, K. (2019) 'Can the Sperm Class Analyser (SCA) CASA-Mot system for human sperm motility analysis reduce imprecision and operator subjectivity and improve semen analysis?' *Human Fertility 24*, 3, 208–218. doi:10.1080/14647273.2019.1610581.

58 Barratt, C.L.R., Björndahl, L., Menkveld, R. and Mortimer, D. (2011) 'ESHRE special interest group for andrology basic semen analysis course: A continued focus on accuracy, quality, efficiency and clinical relevance.' *Human Reproduction 26*, 12, 3207–3212. doi:10.1093/humrep/der312.

59 Van der Horst, G. (2020) 'Sperm motility across the species and how does it relate to humans.' ESHRE 2020.

60 Kirkman-Brown, J. (2015) 'Current and future relevance of sperm motility assessment in ART.' ESHRE 2015.

61 Reproduced from World Health Organization (2021) *WHO Laboratory Manual for the Examination and Processing of Human Semen, 6th Edition*. Geneva: WHO, Copyright 2021.

62 Pozzi, E., Boeri, L., Capogrosso, P., Candela, L. *et al.* (2021) 'Infertility as a proxy of men's health: Still a long way to go.' *Turkish Journal of Urology*. doi:10.5152/tud.2021.20561.

63 Reproduced from World Health Organization (2021) *WHO Laboratory Manual for the Examination and Processing of Human Semen, 6th Edition*. Geneva: WHO, p.42, Copyright 2021.

64 Reproduced from World Health Organization (2021) *WHO Laboratory Manual for the Examination and Processing of Human Semen, 6th Edition*. Geneva: WHO, p.49, Copyright 2021.

65 Reproduced from World Health Organization (2021) *WHO Laboratory Manual for the Examination and Processing of Human Semen, 6th Edition*. Geneva: WHO, p.51, Copyright 2021.

66 Kruger, T.F., Menkveld, R., Stander, F.S., Lombard, C.J. *et al.* (1986) 'Sperm morphologic features as a prognostic factor in in vitro fertilization.' *Fertility and Sterility 46*, 6, 1118–1123; Kruger, T.F., Acosta, A.A., Simmons, K.F., Swanson, R.J., Matta, J.F. and Oehninger, S. (1988) 'Predictive value of abnormal sperm morphology in in vitro fertilization.' *Fertility and Sterility 49*, 1, 112–117. Cited in World Health Organization (2021) *WHO Laboratory Manual for the Examination and Processing of Human Semen, 6th Edition*. Geneva: WHO.

67 Kruger, T.F., Menkveld, R., Stander, F.S., Lombard, C.J. *et al.* (1986) 'Sperm morphologic features as a prognostic factor in in vitro fertilization.' *Fertility and Sterility 46*, 6, 1118–1123; Kruger, T.F., Acosta, A.A., Simmons, K.F., Swanson, R.J., Matta, J.F. and Oehninger, S. (1988) 'Predictive value of abnormal sperm morphology in in vitro fertilization.' *Fertility and Sterility 49*, 1, 112–117; Menkveld, R., Stander, F.S., Kotze, T.J., Kruger, T.F. and van Zyl, J.A. (1990) 'The evaluation of morphological characteristics of human spermatozoa according to stricter criteria.' *Human Reproduction 5*, 5, 586–592. Cited in World Health Organization (2021) *WHO Laboratory Manual for the Examination and Processing of Human Semen, 6th Edition*. Geneva: WHO.

68 Reproduced from World Health Organization (2021) *WHO Laboratory Manual for the Examination and Processing of Human Semen, 6th Edition*. Geneva: WHO, Copyright 2021.

69 Grow, D.R., Oehninger, S., Seltman, H.J. et al. (1994) 'Sperm morphology as diagnosed by strict criteria: probing the impact of teratozoospermia on fertilization rate and pregnancy outcome in a large in vitro fertilization population.' *Fertility and Sterility 62*, 3, 559–567; Sukcharoen, N., Stewart Irvine, J.K.D. and Aitken, J.R. (1995) 'Predicting the fertilizing potential of human sperm suspensions in vitro: importance of sperm morphology and leukocyte contamination.' *Fertility and Sterility 63*, 6, 1293–1300.

70 Baker, R.R. and Bellis, M.A. (1989) 'Elaboration of the Kamikaze Sperm Hypothesis: A reply to Harcourt.' *Animal Behaviour 37*, 5, 865–867. doi:10.1016/0003-3472(89)90074-2.

71 Reproduced from World Health Organization (2021) *WHO Laboratory Manual for the Examination and Processing of Human Semen, 6th Edition*. Geneva: WHO, p.11, Copyright 2021.

72 Sobreiro, B.P., Lucon, A.M., Pasqualotto, F.F., Hallak, J., Athayde, K.S. and Arap. S. (2005) 'Semen analysis in fertile patients undergoing vasectomy: Reference values and variations according to age, length of sexual abstinence, seasonality, smoking habits and caffeine intake.' *Sao Paulo Medical Journal 123*, 4, 161–166.

73 Levitas, E., Lunenfeld, E., Weiss, N., Friger, M. *et al.* (2005) 'Relationship between the duration of sexual abstinence and semen quality: Analysis of 9,489 semen samples.' *Fertility and Sterility 83*, 6, 1680–1686. doi:10.1016/j.fertnstert.2004.12.045.

74 Levitas, E., Lunenfeld, E., Weiss, N., Friger, M. *et al.* (2005) 'Relationship between the duration of sexual abstinence and semen quality: Analysis of 9,489 semen samples.' *Fertility and Sterility 83*, 6, 1680–1686. doi:10.1016/j.fertnstert.2004.12.045.

75 Makkar, G., Ng, E.H., Yeung, W.S. and Ho, P.C. (2001) 'A comparative study of raw and prepared semen samples from two consecutive days.' *Journal of Reproductive Medicine 46*, 6, 565–572.

76 Levitas, E., Lunenfeld, E., Weisz, N., Friger, M., Har-Vardi, I. and Potashnik, G. (2006) 'Relationship between sexual abstinence duration and the acrosome index in teratozoospermic semen: Analysis of 1800 semen samples.' *Andrologia 38*, 3, 110–112. doi:10.1111/j.1439-0272.2006.00715.x.

77 Patil, P.S. (2013) 'Immature germ cells in semen – correlation with total sperm count and sperm motility.' *Journal of Cytology 30*, 3, 185–189. doi:10.4103/0970-9371.117682.

78 Reproduced from World Health Organization (2021) *WHO Laboratory Manual for the Examination and Processing of Human Semen, 6th Edition*. Geneva: WHO, Copyright 2021.

79 Cui, D., Han, G., Shang, Y., Liu, C. *et al.* (2015) 'Antisperm antibodies in infertile men and their effect on semen parameters: A systematic review and meta-analysis.' *Clinica Chimica Acta 444*, 29–36. doi:10.1016/j.cca.2015.01.033.

80 Pozzi, E., Boeri, L., Capogrosso, P., Candela, L. *et al.* (2021) 'Infertility as a proxy of men's health: Still a long way to go.' *Turkish Journal of Urology*. doi:10.5152/tud.2021.20561.

81 Reproduced from World Health Organization (2021) *WHO Laboratory Manual for the Examination and Processing of Human Semen, 6th Edition*. Geneva: WHO, Copyright 2021.

82 Kandil, H., Agarwal, A., Saleh, R., Boitrelle, F. *et al.* (2021) 'Editorial commentary on draft of World Health Organization Sixth Edition Laboratory Manual for the Examination and Processing of Human Semen.' *World Journal of Men's Health 39*, 4, 577–580. doi:10.5534/wjmh.210074.

CHAPTER 8

1 Jayasena, C.N., Radia, U.K., Figueiredo, M., Revill, L.F. *et al.* (2019) 'Reduced testicular steroidogenesis and increased semen oxidative stress in male partners as novel markers of recurrent miscarriage.' *Clinical Chemistry 65*, 1, 161–169.

2 Lewis, S.H. (2019) 'Sperm DNA damage, test everyone?' debate, ESHRE 2019.

3 Lewis, S.H. (2019) 'Sperm DNA damage, test everyone?' debate, ESHRE 2019.

4   Esteves, S.C. and Agarwal, A. (2011) 'Novel concepts in male infertility.' *International Brazilian Journal of Urology 37*, 1, 5–15. doi:10.1590/s1677-55382011000100002.

5   Sharma, R., Agarwal, A., Mohanty, G., Du Plessis, S.S. *et al.* (2013) 'Proteomic analysis of seminal fluid from men exhibiting oxidative stress.' *Reproductive Biology and Endocrinology 11*, 85. doi:10.1186/1477-7827-11-85.

6   Lewis, S.H. (2019) 'Sperm DNA damage, test everyone?' debate, ESHRE 2019.

7   Javed, A., Talkad, M.S. and Ramaiah, M.K. (2019) 'Evaluation of sperm DNA fragmentation using multiple methods: A comparison of their predictive power for male infertility.' *Clinical and Experimental Reproductive Medicine 46*, 1, 14–21. doi:10.5653/cerm.2019.46.1.14.

8   J. Kirkman-Brown (2021) 'The significance of male factor and sperm damage to the offspring.' talk, ESHRE 2021.

9   González-Marín, C., Gosálvez, J. and Roy, R. (2012) 'Types, causes, detection and repair of DNA fragmentation in animal and human sperm cells.' *International Journal of Molecular Sciences 13*, 11, 14026–14052. doi:10.3390/ijms131114026.

10 Ahmadi, A. and Ng, S.C. (1999) 'Fertilizing ability of DNA-damaged spermatozoa.' *Journal of Experimental Zoology 284*, 6, 696–704. doi:10.1002/(sici)1097-010x(19991101)284:6<696::aid-jez11>3.0.co;2-e.

11 González-Marín, C., Gosálvez, J. and Roy, R. (2012) 'Types, causes, detection and repair of DNA fragmentation in animal and human sperm cells.' *International Journal of Molecular Sciences 13*, 11, 14026–14052. doi:10.3390/ijms131114026.

12 Agarwal, A., Majzoub, A., Esteves, S.C., Ko, E., Ramasamy, R. and Zini, A. (2016) 'Clinical utility of sperm DNA fragmentation testing: Practice recommendations based on clinical scenarios.' *Translational Andrology and Urology 5*, 6, 935–950. doi:10.21037/tau.2016.10.03.

13 Gallegos, G., Ramos, B., Santiso, R., Goyanes, V., Gosálvez, J. and Fernández, J.L. (2008) 'Sperm DNA fragmentation in infertile men with genitourinary infection by Chlamydia trachomatis and Mycoplasma.' *Fertility and Sterility 90*, 2, 328–334. doi:10.1016/j.fertnstert.2007.06.035; Bibancos, M., Rocha, A.M., Hassun, P.A., Smith, G.D., Motta, E.L.A. and Serafini, P.C. (2008) 'Sperm DNA fragmentation decreases after oral anti-inflammatory and antibiotic treatment.' *Fertility and Sterility 90*, s467–468. doi:10.1016/j.fertnstert.2008.07.326.

14 Agarwal, A., Majzoub, A., Baskaran, S., Selvam, M.K.P. *et al.* (2020) 'Sperm DNA fragmentation: A new guideline for clinicians.' *World Journal of Men's Health 38*, 4, 412–471. doi:10.5534/wjmh.200128.

15 Lipovac, M., Nairz, V., Aschauer, J. and Riedl, C. (2021) 'The effect of micronutrient supplementation on spermatozoa DNA integrity in subfertile men and subsequent pregnancy rate.' *Gynecological Endocrinology 37*, 8, 1–5. doi:10.1080/09513590.2021.1923688.

16 Roque, M. and Esteves, S.C. (2018) 'Effect of varicocele repair on sperm DNA fragmentation: A review.' *International Urology and Nephrology 50*, 4, 583–603. doi:10.1007/s11255-018-1839-4.

17 Agarwal, A., Majzoub, A., Baskaran, S., Selvam, M.K.P. *et al.* (2020) 'Sperm DNA fragmentation: A new guideline for clinicians.' *World Journal of Men's Health 38*, 4, 412–471. doi:10.5534/wjmh.200128.

18 Gosálvez, J., González-Martínez, M., López-Fernández, C., Fernández, J.L. and Sánchez-Martín, P. (2011) 'Shorter abstinence decreases sperm deoxyribonucleic acid fragmentation in ejaculate.' *Fertility and Sterility 96*, 5, 1083–1086. doi:10.1016/j.fertnstert.2011.08.027.

19 Uppangala, S., Mathai, S.E., Salian, S.R., Kumar, D. *et al.* (2016) 'Sperm chromatin immaturity observed in short abstinence ejaculates affects DNA integrity and longevity in vitro.' *PLOS ONE 11*, 4, e0152942. doi:10.1371/journal.pone.0152942.

20 Pons, I., Cercas, R., Villas, C., Braña, C. and Fernández-Shaw, S. (2013) 'One abstinence day decreases sperm DNA fragmentation in 90% of selected patients.' *Journal of Assisted Reproduction and Genetics 30*, 9, 1211–1218. doi:10.1007/s10815-013-0089-8.

21 Esteves, S.C., Sánchez-Martín, F., Sánchez-Martín, P., Schneider, D.T. and Gosálvez, J. (2015) 'Comparison of reproductive outcome in oligozoospermic men with high sperm DNA fragmentation undergoing intracytoplasmic sperm injection with ejaculated and testicular sperm.' *Fertility and Sterility 104*, 6, 1398–1405. doi:10.1016/j.fertnstert.2015.08.028.

22 Robinson, L., Gallos, I.D., Conner, S.J., Rajkhowa, M. *et al.* (2012) 'The effect of sperm DNA fragmentation on miscarriage rates: A systematic review and meta-analysis.' *Human Reproduction 27*, 10, 2908–2917. doi:10.1093/humrep/des261.

23 Bungum, M., Humaidan, P., Axmon, A., Spano, M. *et al.* (2007) 'Sperm DNA integrity assessment in prediction of assisted reproduction technology outcome.' *Human Reproduction 22*, 1, 174–179. doi:10.1093/humrep/del326.

24 Lewis, S.E.M., Aitken, R.J., Conner, S.J., Iuliis, G.D. *et al.* (2013) 'The impact of sperm DNA damage in assisted conception and beyond: Recent advances in diagnosis and treatment.' *Reproductive Biomedicine Online 27*, 4, 325–337. doi:10.1016/j.rbmo.2013.06.014.

25 Johns Hopkins Medicine (n.d.) 'Sperm retrieval procedures.' www.hopkinsmedicine.org/health/treatment-tests-and-therapies/sperm-retrieval-procedures.

26 Henkel, R.R. and Schill, W.-B. (2003) 'Sperm preparation for ART.' *Reproductive Biology and Endocrinology 1*, 108. doi:10.1186/1477-7827-1-108.

27 Muratori, M., Tarozzi, N., Carpentiero, F., Danti, S. *et al.* (2019) 'Sperm selection with density gradient centrifugation and swim up: Effect on DNA fragmentation in viable spermatozoa.' *Scientific Reports 9*, 7492. doi:10.1038/s41598-019-43981-2.

28 Parekattil, S.J., Esteves, S.C. and Agarwal, A. (eds) (2020) *Male Infertility: Contemporary Clinical Approaches, Andrology, ART and Antioxidants.* Cham: Springer.

29 Muratori, M., Tarozzi, N., Carpentiero, F., Danti, S. *et al.* (2019) 'Sperm selection with density gradient centrifugation and swim up: Effect on DNA fragmentation in viable spermatozoa.' *Scientific Reports 9*, 1, 7492. doi:10.1038/s41598-019-43981-2.

30 Cassuto, N.G., Bouret, D., Hatem. G., Larue, L. *et al.* (2020) 'Using high magnification to select sperm: A large prospective cohort study comparing ICSI and IMSI.' *Clinical Obstetrics, Gynecology and Reproductive Medicine 6*, 1–5. doi:10.15761/COGRM.1000276.

31 Avalos-Durán, G., Cañedo-Del Ángel, A.M.E., Rivero-Murillo, J., Zambrano-Guerrero, J.E., Carballo-Mondragón, E. and Checa-Vizcaíno, M.Á. (2018) 'Physiological ICSI (PICSI) vs. conventional ICSI in couples with male factor: A systematic review.' *JBRA Assisted Reproduction 22*, 2, 139–147. doi:10.5935/1518-0557.20180027.

32 Miller, D., Pavitt, S., Sharma, V., Forbes, G. *et al.* (2019) 'Physiological, hyaluronan-selected intracytoplasmic sperm injection for infertility treatment (HABSelect): A parallel, two-group, randomised trial.' *Lancet 393*, 10170, 416–422. doi:10.1016/S0140-6736(18)32989-1.

33 J. Kirkman-Brown (2021) 'The significance of male factor and sperm damage to the offspring.' talk, ESHRE 2021.

34 Nova IVF Fertility (n.d.) 'Effects of MACS.' www.novaivffertility.com/fertility-help/what-is-magnetic-activated-cell-sorting-macs.

35 Parekattil, S.J., Esteves, S.C. and Agarwal, A. (eds) (2020) *Male Infertility: Contemporary Clinical Approaches, Andrology, ART and Antioxidants.* Cham: Springer.

36 Parekattil, S.J., Esteves, S.C. and Agarwal, A. (eds) (2020) *Male Infertility: Contemporary Clinical Approaches, Andrology, ART and Antioxidants.* Cham: Springer.

37 Samuel, R., Feng, H., Jafek, A., Despain, D., Jenkins, T. and Gale, B. (2018) 'Microfluidic-based sperm sorting and analysis for treatment of male infertility.' *Translational Andrology and Urology 7*, Suppl 3, S336–S347. doi:10.21037/tau.2018.05.08.

38 Hasanen, E., Elqusi, K., ElTanbouly, S., Hussin, A.E. *et al.* (2020) 'PICSI vs. MACS for abnormal sperm DNA fragmentation ICSI cases: A prospective randomized trial.' *Journal of Assisted Reproduction and Genetics 37*, 10, 2605–2613. doi:10.1007/s10815-020-01913-4.

CHAPTER 9

1 Loukas, M., Ferrauiola, J., Shoja, M.M., Tubbs, R.S. and Cohen-Gadol, A. (2010) 'Anatomy in Ancient China: The Yellow Emperor's Inner Canon of Medicine and Wang Qingren's Correcting the Errors in the Forest of Medicine.' *Clinical Anatomy 23*, 4, 364–369.

2 Schnorrenberger, C.C. (2013) 'Anatomical roots of acupuncture and Chinese Medicine.' *Swiss Journal of Integrative Medicine 25*, 2. doi:10.1159/000349905.

3 Loukas, M., Ferrauiola, J., Shoja, M.M., Tubbs, R.S. and Cohen-Gadol, A. (2010) 'Anatomy in Ancient China: The Yellow Emperor's Inner Canon of Medicine and Wang Qingren's Correcting the Errors in the Forest of Medicine.' *Clinical Anatomy 23*, 4, 364–369.

4 Damone, B. (2008) *Principles of Chinese Medical Andrology.* Fletcher, NC: Blue Poppy Press; Damone, B. (n.d.) 'Improving Men's Sexual Health and Reproductive Function.' Online seminar at https://bluepoppy.myabsorb.com/#/online-courses/ae1af4d9-ffac-4b82-850b-1e9ad0ae535d.

5 Maciocia, G. (n.d.) 'Male disorders.' Online seminar, www.maciociaonline.com.

6 Franconi, G. (2018) *Male Infertility: An Integrative Manual of Western and Chinese Medicine.* Sharjah, UAE: Bentham Sciences Publishers.

7   Damone, B. (n.d.) 'Improving Men's Sexual Health and Reproductive Function.' Online seminar at https://bluepoppy.myabsorb.com/#/online-courses/ae1af4d9-ffac-4b82-850b-1e9ad0ae535d.

8   Wisemen, N. (1998) *A Practical Dictionary of Traditional Chinese Medicine*. Boulder, CO: Paradigm Press, p.15.

9   Franconi, G. (2018) *Male Infertility: An Integrative Manual of Western and Chinese Medicine*. Sharjah, UAE: Bentham Sciences Publishers.

CHAPTER 10

1   Damone, B. (2008) *Principles of Chinese Medical Andrology*. Fletcher, NC: Blue Poppy Press.

2   Lin, A. (1992) *A Handbook of TCM Urology and Male Sexual Dysfunction*. Fletcher, NC: Blue Poppy Press.

3   Maciocia, G. (n.d.) 'Male disorders.' Online seminar, www.maciociaonline.com.

4   Maciocia, G. (n.d.) 'Men's Sexual and Prostate Problems in Chinese Medicine', blog 'The Three Treasures'. https://giovanni-maciocia.com/the-treatment-of-male-problems-in.

5   Noll, A.A. and Wilms, S. (2009) *Chinese Medicine in Fertility Disorders*. Stuttgart and New York, NY: Thieme.

6   Damone, B. (2008) *Principles of Chinese Medical Andrology*. Fletcher, NC: Blue Poppy Press.

7   Chen, Z. and Li, L. (2008) *The Clinical Practice of Chinese Medicine: Male and Female Infertility* (Bilingual, Translation Edition). Beijing: People's Medical Publishing House.

8   Damone, B. (2008) *Principles of Chinese Medical Andrology*. Fletcher, NC: Blue Poppy Press.

CHAPTER 11

1   Damone, B. (n.d.) 'Improving Men's Sexual Health and Reproductive Function.' Online seminar at https://bluepoppy.myabsorb.com/#/online-courses/ae1af4d9-ffac-4b82-850b-1e9ad0ae535d.

2   Damone, B. (n.d.) 'Improving Men's Sexual Health and Reproductive Function.' Online seminar at https://bluepoppy.myabsorb.com/#/online-courses/ae1af4d9-ffac-4b82-850b-1e9ad0ae535d.

3   Damone, B. (2008) *Principles of Chinese Medical Andrology*. Fletcher, NC: Blue Poppy Press, p.62.

4   Damone, B. (2008) *Principles of Chinese Medical Andrology*. Fletcher, NC: Blue Poppy Press, p.62.

5   Damone, B. (2008) *Principles of Chinese Medical Andrology*. Fletcher, NC: Blue Poppy Press.

6   Damone, B. (n.d.) 'Improving Men's Sexual Health and Reproductive Function.' Online seminar at https://bluepoppy.myabsorb.com/#/online-courses/ae1af4d9-ffac-4b82-850b-1e9ad0ae535d.

7   Damone, B. (2008) *Principles of Chinese Medical Andrology*. Fletcher, NC: Blue Poppy Press, p.58.

8   Damone, B. (2008) *Principles of Chinese Medical Andrology*. Fletcher, NC: Blue Poppy Press, p.67.

9   Damone, B. (2008) *Principles of Chinese Medical Andrology*. Fletcher, NC: Blue Poppy Press, p.67.

10 Damone, B. (2008) *Principles of Chinese Medical Andrology*. Fletcher, NC: Blue Poppy Press.

CHAPTER 12

1   Cakmak, Y.O., Akpinar, I.N., Ekinci, G. and Bekiroglu, N. (2008) 'Point- and frequency-specific response of the testicular artery to abdominal electroacupuncture in humans.' *Fertility and Sterility 90*, 5, 1732–1738. doi:10.1016/j.fertnstert.2007.08.013.

2   Lyttleton, J. (2013) *Treatment of Infertility with Chinese Medicine, 2nd Edition*. Edinburgh: Churchill Livingstone.

3   Rampa, G. 'Grundlagen Akupunktur. 'TCM Schweizerische Ärztegesellschaft für Akupunktur (Sacam).' (lecture handout).

4   Damone, B. (2008) *Principles of Chinese Medical Andrology*. Fletcher, NC: Blue Poppy Press, p.64.

5   Deadman, P., Al-Khafaji, M. and Baker, K. (1999) *A Manual of Acupuncture*. Hove: Journal of Chinese Medicine Publications.

6   Franconi, G. (2018) *Male Infertility: An Integrative Manual of Western and Chinese Medicine*. Sharjah, UAE: Bentham Sciences Publishers.

7   Deadman, P., Al-Khafaji, M. and Baker, K. (1999) *A Manual of Acupuncture*. Hove: Journal of Chinese Medicine Publications.

8   Bahr, F.R., Dorfer, L., Jost, F., Litscher, G., Suwanda, S. and Zeitler, H. (2006) *Das große Buch der klassischen Akupunktur*. Urban & Fischer Verlag/Elsevier.

9   Deadman, P., Al-Khafaji, M. and Baker, K. (1999) *A Manual of Acupuncture*. Hove: Journal of Chinese Medicine Publications.

10 Deadman, P., Al-Khafaji, M. and Baker, K. (1999) *A Manual of Acupuncture*. Hove: Journal of Chinese Medicine Publications.

11 Franconi, G. (2018) *Male Infertility: An Integrative Manual of Western and Chinese Medicine*. Sharjah, UAE: Bentham Sciences Publishers.

12 Rampa, G. 'Grundlagen Akupunktur. 'TCM Schweizerische Ärztegesellschaft für Akupunktur (Sacam).' (lecture handout).

13 Kirschbaum, B. (2012) *Die 8 außerordentlichen Gefäße in der traditionellen chinesischen Medizin*. Bamberg: Mediengruppe Oberfranken.

14 Kirschbaum, B. (2012) *Die 8 außerordentlichen Gefäße in der traditionellen chinesischen Medizin*. Bamberg: Mediengruppe Oberfranken.

15 Deadman, P., Al-Khafaji, M. and Baker, K. (1999) *A Manual of Acupuncture*. Hove: Journal of Chinese Medicine Publications.

16 Franconi, G. (2018) *Male Infertility: An Integrative Manual of Western and Chinese Medicine*. Sharjah, UAE: Bentham Sciences Publishers.

17 Kirschbaum, B. (2012) *Die 8 außerordentlichen Gefäße in der traditionellen chinesischen Medizin*. Bamberg: Mediengruppe Oberfranken.

18 Maciocia, G. (2007) *The Practice of Chinese Medicine, 2nd Edition*. Edinburgh: Churchill Livingston.

19 Deadman, P., Al-Khafaji, M. and Baker, K. (1999) *A Manual of Acupuncture*. Hove: Journal of Chinese Medicine Publications.

20 Kirschbaum, B. (2012) *Die 8 außerordentlichen Gefäße in der traditionellen chinesischen Medizin*. Bamberg: Mediengruppe Oberfranken.

21 Kirschbaum, B. (2012) *Die 8 außerordentlichen Gefäße in der traditionellen chinesischen Medizin*. Bamberg: Mediengruppe Oberfranken.

22 Bahr, F.R., Dorfer, L., Jost, F., Litscher, G., Suwanda, S. and Zeitler, H. (2006) *Das große Buch der klassischen Akupunktur*. Urban & Fischer Verlag/Elsevier.

23 Kirschbaum, B. (2012) *Die 8 außerordentlichen Gefäße in der traditionellen chinesischen Medizin*. Bamberg: Mediengruppe Oberfranken.

24 Deadman, P., Al-Khafaji, M. and Baker, K. (1999) *A Manual of Acupuncture*. Hove: Journal of Chinese Medicine Publications.

25 Maciocia, G. (2007) *The Practice of Chinese Medicine, 2nd Edition*. Edinburgh: Churchill Livingston.

CHAPTER 13

1   Lyttleton, J. (2013) *Treatment of Infertility with Chinese Medicine, 2nd Edition*. Edinburgh: Churchill Livingstone.

CHAPTER 14

1   Damone, B. (2008) *Principles of Chinese Medical Andrology*. Fletcher, NC: Blue Poppy Press.

2   Franconi, G. (2018) *Male Infertility: An Integrative Manual of Western and Chinese Medicine*. Sharjah, UAE: Bentham Sciences Publishers.

3   Franconi, G. (2018) *Male Infertility: An Integrative Manual of Western and Chinese Medicine*. Sharjah, UAE: Bentham Sciences Publishers.

CHAPTER 15

1   Deadman, P., Al-Khafaji, M. and Baker, K. (2007) *A Manual of Acupuncture, 2nd Edition*. Hove: Journal of Chinese Medicine Publications.

2   Lin, A. (1992) *A Handbook of TCM Urology and Male Sexual Dysfunction*. Fletcher, NC: Blue Poppy Press.

3   Dharmananda, S. (n.d.) 'Hua Tuo.' www.itmonline.org/arts/huatuo.htm; Amaro, J. (2009) 'Spinal Hua Tuo points.' *Acupuncture Today 10*, 12.

4   Dharmananda, S. (n.d.) 'Hua Tuo.' www.itmonline.org/arts/huatuo.htm; Amaro, J. (2009) 'Spinal Hua Tuo points.' *Acupuncture Today 10*, 12.

5   Damone, B. (2008) *Principles of Chinese Medical Andrology*. Fletcher, NC: Blue Poppy Press.

6   Maciocia, G. (n.d.) 'Men's Sexual and Prostate Problems in Chinese Medicine', blog 'The Three Treasures', https://giovanni-maciocia.com/the-treatment-of-male-problems-in.

7   Franconi, G. (2018) *Male Infertility: An Integrative Manual of Western and Chinese Medicine*. Sharjah, UAE: Bentham Sciences Publishers.

8   Glover, J. (2018) 'Treating male infertility with acupuncture and Chinese herbal medicine.' www.healthy-seminars.com/product/treating-male-infertility-acupuncture-and-chinese-herbal-medicine.

9   Lyttleton, J. (2013) *Treatment of Infertility with Chinese Medicine, 2nd Edition*. Edinburgh: Churchill Livingstone.

10 Maciocia, G. (n.d.) 'Men's Sexual and Prostate Problems in Chinese Medicine', blog 'The Three Treasures', https://giovanni-maciocia.com/the-treatment-of-male-problems-in.

11 Glover, J. (2018) 'Treating male infertility with acupuncture and Chinese herbal medicine.' www.healthy-seminars.com/product/treating-male-infertility-acupuncture-and-chinese-herbal-medicine.

12 Lyttleton, J. (2013) *Treatment of Infertility with Chinese Medicine, 2nd Edition*. Edinburgh: Churchill Livingstone.

13 Lyttleton, J. (2013) *Treatment of Infertility with Chinese Medicine, 2nd Edition*. Edinburgh: Churchill Livingstone.

14 Lyttleton, J. (2013) *Treatment of Infertility with Chinese Medicine, 2nd Edition*. Edinburgh: Churchill Livingstone.

15 Lyttleton, J. (2013) *Treatment of Infertility with Chinese Medicine, 2nd Edition*. Edinburgh: Churchill Livingstone.

16 Chen, Z. and Li, L. (2008) *The Clinical Practice of Chinese Medicine: Male and Female Infertility* (Bilingual, Translation Edition). Beijing: People's Medical Publishing House.

17 Weixin, J. (1999) *Diagnosis of Sterility and Its Traditional Chinese Medical Treatment*. Shandong: Shandong Science and Technology Press.

18 Szmelskyj, I. and Aquilina, L. (2015) *Acupuncture for IVF and Assisted Reproduction: An Integrated Approach to Treatment and Management*. Edinburgh: Churchill Livingstone.

19 Glover, J. (2018) 'Treating male infertility with acupuncture and Chinese herbal medicine.' www.healthy-seminars.com/product/treating-male-infertility-acupuncture-and-chinese-herbal-medicine.

20 Lyttleton, J. (2013) *Treatment of Infertility with Chinese Medicine, 2nd Edition*. Edinburgh: Churchill Livingstone.

21 Franconi, G. (2018) *Male Infertility: An Integrative Manual of Western and Chinese Medicine*. Sharjah, UAE: Bentham Sciences Publishers.

22 Weixin, J. (1999) *Diagnosis of Sterility and Its Traditional Chinese Medical Treatment*. Shandong: Shandong Science and Technology Press.

23 Franconi, G. (2018) *Male Infertility: An Integrative Manual of Western and Chinese Medicine*. Sharjah, UAE: Bentham Sciences Publishers.

24 Franconi, G. (2018) *Male Infertility: An Integrative Manual of Western and Chinese Medicine*. Sharjah, UAE: Bentham Sciences Publishers.

25 Szmelskyj, I. and Aquilina, L. (2015) *Acupuncture for IVF and Assisted Reproduction: An Integrated Approach to Treatment and Management*. Edinburgh: Churchill Livingstone.

26 Lyttleton, J. (2013) *Treatment of Infertility with Chinese Medicine, 2nd Edition*. Edinburgh: Churchill Livingstone.

27 Glover, J. (2018) 'Treating male infertility with acupuncture and Chinese herbal medicine.' www.healthy-seminars.com/product/treating-male-infertility-acupuncture-and-chinese-herbal-medicine.

28 Lyttleton, J. (2013) *Treatment of Infertility with Chinese Medicine, 2nd Edition*. Edinburgh: Churchill Livingstone.

29 Szmelskyj, I. and Aquilina, L. (2015) *Acupuncture for IVF and Assisted Reproduction: An Integrated Approach to Treatment and Management*. Edinburgh: Churchill Livingstone.

30 Szmelskyj, I. and Aquilina, L. (2015) *Acupuncture for IVF and Assisted Reproduction: An Integrated Approach to Treatment and Management*. Edinburgh: Churchill Livingstone.

31 Lyttleton, J. (2013) *Treatment of Infertility with Chinese Medicine, 2nd Edition*. Edinburgh: Churchill Livingstone.

CHAPTER 16

1   Xu, J.X. (2003) '[Treatment of hyperprolactinemic impotence by Jiawei Shaoyao Gancao Tang: A clinical observation of 58 cases]' (Chinese). *Xin Zhongyi 35*, 21–22.

2   'Formula Shao Fu Zhu Yu Tang – Decoction for Treating Infertility.' https://musculoskeletalkey.com/formula-shao-fu-zhu-yu-tang-decoction-for-treating-infertility

3   Huo Jingiun (1995) *Acupuncture and Moxibustion Therapy in Gynecology and Obstretics*. Beijing: Science and Technology Press.

4   Clavey, S. (2003) 'Notes on the treatment of male infertility.' *Journal of Chinese Medicine 73*, 45–52.

5   Noll, A.A. and Wilms, S. (2009) *Chinese Medicine in Fertility Disorders*. Stuttgart and New York, NY: Thieme.

6   Becker, S. (2008) 'Fertilitätsstörungen des Mannes.' *Extrakt Zeitschrift*, 2008.

7   Tiandong Lin and Xianxun Huang (2007) 'Treatment of male infertility.' *Journal of Traditional Chinese Medicine 27*, 2, 119–123.

8   Weixin, J. (1999) *Diagnosis of Sterility and Its Traditional Chinese Medicine Treatment*. Shandong: Shandong Science and Technology Press.

CHAPTER 17

1   Zhou, S.H., Deng, Y.F., Weng, Z.W., Weng, H.W. and Liu, Z.D. (2019) 'Traditional Chinese Medicine as a remedy for male infertility: A review.' *World Journal of Men's Health 37*, 2, 175–185. doi:10.5534/wjmh.180069.

2   Zhou, S.H., Deng, Y.F., Weng, Z.W., Weng, H.W. and Liu, Z.D. (2019) 'Traditional Chinese Medicine as a remedy for male infertility: A review.' *World Journal of Men's Health 37*, 2, 175–185. doi:10.5534/wjmh.180069.

3   Zhou, S.H., Deng, Y.F., Weng, Z.W., Weng, H.W. and Liu, Z.D. (2019) 'Traditional Chinese Medicine as a remedy for male infertility: A review.' *World Journal of Men's Health 37*, 2, 175–185. doi:10.5534/wjmh.180069.

4   Zhou, S.H., Deng, Y.F., Weng, Z.W., Weng, H.W. and Liu, Z.D. (2019) 'Traditional Chinese Medicine as a remedy for male infertility: A review.' *World Journal of Men's Health 37*, 2, 175–185. doi:10.5534/wjmh.180069.

5   Zhou, S.H., Deng, Y.F., Weng, Z.W., Weng, H.W. and Liu, Z.D. (2019) 'Traditional Chinese Medicine as a remedy for male infertility: A review.' *World Journal of Men's Health 37*, 2, 175–185. doi:10.5534/wjmh.180069.

6   Zhou, S.H., Deng, Y.F., Weng, Z.W., Weng, H.W. and Liu, Z.D. (2019) 'Traditional Chinese Medicine as a remedy for male infertility: A review.' *World Journal of Men's Health 37*, 2, 175–185. doi:10.5534/wjmh.180069.

7   Zhou, S.H., Deng, Y.F., Weng, Z.W., Weng, H.W. and Liu, Z.D. (2019) 'Traditional Chinese Medicine as a remedy for male infertility: A review.' *World Journal of Men's Health 37*, 2, 175–185. doi:10.5534/wjmh.180069.

8   Zhou, S.H., Deng, Y.F., Weng, Z.W., Weng, H.W. and Liu, Z.D. (2019) 'Traditional Chinese Medicine as a remedy for male infertility: A review.' *World Journal of Men's Health 37*, 2, 175–185. doi:10.5534/wjmh.180069.

9   Zhou, S.H., Deng, Y.F., Weng, Z.W., Weng, H.W. and Liu, Z.D. (2019) 'Traditional Chinese Medicine as a remedy for male infertility: A review.' *World Journal of Men's Health 37*, 2, 175–185. doi:10.5534/wjmh.180069.

10 Zhou, S.H., Deng, Y.F., Weng, Z.W., Weng, H.W. and Liu, Z.D. (2019) 'Traditional Chinese Medicine as a remedy for male infertility: A review.' *World Journal of Men's Health 37*, 2, 175–185. doi:10.5534/wjmh.180069.

11 Lian, F., Sun, J., Guo, L., Sun, Z. and Wu, H. (2014) 'Effects of Shengjing Formula on the expression of H19 imprinted gene in infertile patients caused by oligoasthenospermia with kidney deficiency syndrome.' *Journal of Traditional Chinese Medicine 55*, 1113–1116.

CHAPTER 18

1   Jerng, U.M., Jo, J.-Y., Lee, S., Lee, J.-M., Kwon, O. *et al.* (2014) 'The effectiveness and safety of acupuncture for poor semen quality in infertile males: A systematic review and meta-analysis.' *Asian Journal of Andrology 16*, 884–891.

2   Tafuri, S., Ciani, F., Iorio, E.L., Esposito, L. and Cocchia, N. (2015) 'Reactive Oxygen Species (ROS) and Male Fertility.' In B. Wu (ed.) *New Discoveries in Embryology.* IntechOpen.

3   Gröber, U. (2011) *Mikronährstoffe, Metabolic Tuning Prävention Therapie*, 3. Auflage. Stuttgart: Wissenschaftliche Verlagsgesellschaft, p.54.

4   Espinoza, J.A., Schulz, M.A., Sánchez, R. and Villegas, J.V. (2009) 'Integrity of mitochondrial membrane potential reflects human sperm quality.' *Andrologia 41*, 1, 51–54.

5   Goldstein, S.F. (1969) 'Irradiation of sperm tails by laser microbeam.' *Journal of Experimental Biology 51*, 2, 431–441.

6   Sato, H., Landthaler, M., Haina, D. and Schill, W.B. (1984) 'The effects of laser light on sperm motility and velocity in vitro.' *Andrologia 16*, 1, 23–25.

7   Salman Yazdi, R., Bakhshi, S., Jannat Alipoor, F., Akhoond, M.R. *et al.* (2014) 'Effect of 830-nm diode laser irradiation on human sperm motility.' *Lasers in Medical Science 29*, 1, 97–104.

8   Shkuratov, D.Y., Chudnovskiy, V.M. and Drozdov, A.L. (1997) 'The influence of low-intensity laser radiation and superhigh-frequency electromagnetic fields on gametes of marine invertebrates.' *Tsitologiya 39*, 1, 25–28.

9   Huang, Y.Y., Chen, A.C.H., Carroll, J.D. and Hamblin, M.R. (2009) 'Biphasic dose response in low-level light therapy.' *Dose-Response 7*, 4, 358–383.

10   Firestone, R.S., Esfandiari, N., Moskovtsev, S.I., Burstein, E. *et al.* (2012) 'The effects of low-level laser light exposure on sperm motion characteristics and DNA damage.' *Journal of Andrology 33*, 3, 469–473.

11   Fernandes, G.H.C., de Carvalho, P. de T.C., Serra, A.J., Crespilho, A.M. *et al.* (2015) 'The effect of low-level laser irradiation on sperm motility, and integrity of the plasma membrane and acrosome in cryopreserved bovine sperm.' *PLOS ONE 10*, 3, e0121487. doi:10.1371/journal.pone.0121487.

12   Behtaj, S. and Weber. M. (2019) 'Using laser acupuncture and low-level laser therapy (LLLT) to treat male infertility by improving semen quality: Case report.' *Archives of Clinical and Medical Case Reports 3*, 5, 349–352.

13   Moskvin, S.V. and Apolikhin, O.I. (2018) 'Review article: Effectiveness of low level laser therapy for treating male infertility.' *BioMedicine 8*, 2, 7.

14   Espey, B.T., Kielwein, K., van der Ven, H., Steger, K. *et al.* (2021) 'Effects of pulsed-wave photobiomodulation therapy on human spermatozoa.' *Lasers in Surgery and Medicine.* doi:10.1002/lsm.23399.

Further Reading

Acharya, N., Majumdar, S. and Ramayya, R. (2015) *Handbook of Male Infertility and Andrology*. New Delhi: Jaypee Brothers.

Agarwal, A., Schattman, G.L. and Esteves, S.C. (2015) *Unexplained Infertility: Pathophysiology, Evaluation and Treatment*. New York, NY: Springer.

Al-Harbi, M. (n.d.) 'Male hypogonadism.' (PowerPoint). https://pt.slideshare.net/33221144/male-hypogonadism.

Chen, Z. and Li, L. (2008) *The Clinical Practice of Chinese Medicine: Male and Female Infertility* (Bilingual, Translation Edition). Beijing: People's Medical Publishing House.

Clavey, S. (2003) 'Notes of the treatment of male infertility.' *Journal of Chinese Medicine* 73, 45–52.

Damone, B. (2008) *Principles of Chinese Medical Andrology*. Fletcher, NC: Blue Poppy Press.

Deadman, P. (2008) 'The treatment of male subfertility with acupuncture.' *Journal of Chinese Medicine* 88, 5–16.

Dias, T.R., Samanta, L., Agarwal, A., Pushparaj, P.N., Selvam, M.K.P. and Sharma, R. (2019) 'Proteomic signatures reveal differences in stress response, antioxidant defense and proteasomal activity in fertile men with high seminal ROS levels.' *International Journal of Molecular Sciences* 20, 1, 203.

Giacone, F., Cannarella, R., Mongioì, L.M., Alamo, A. *et al.* (2019) 'Epigenetics of male fertility: Effects on assisted reproductive techniques.' *World Journal of Men's Health* 37, 2, 148–156. doi:10.5534/wjmh.180071.

Gunasekaran, K. and Pandiyan, N. (2017) *Male Infertility: A Clinical Approach*. New Delhi: Springer India.

Krause, W., Weidner, W., Sperling, H. and Diemer, T. (2011) *Andrologie: Krankheiten der männlichen Geschlechtsorgane*. Leipzig: Thieme.

Lin, A. (1992) *A Handbook of TCM Urology and Male Sexual Dysfunction*. Fletcher, NC: Blue Poppy Press.

Lyttleton, J. (2013) *Treatment of Infertility with Chinese Medicine, 2nd Edition*. Edinburgh: Churchill Livingstone.

Maciocia, G. (n.d.) 'Male disorders.' Online seminar. www.maciociaonline.com.

Parekattil, S.J., Esteves, S.C. and Agarwal, A. (eds) (2020) *Male Infertility: Contemporary Clinical Approaches, Andrology, ART and Antioxidants*. Cham: Springer.

Smith, J. (n.d.) 'Hypogonadism and testosterone replacement' (PowerPoint). https://slideplayer.com/slide/1034883.

Steger, K. (2014) 'The sperm egigenome.' ESHRE Campus Symposium 2014. www.eshre.com.

Tvrda, E., Gosalvez, J. and Agarwal, A. (2015) 'Epigenetics and Its Role in Male Infertility.' In R. Watson (ed.) *Handbook of Fertility: Nutrition, Diet, Lifestyle and Reproductive Health*. Amsterdam: Elsevier.

Unschuld, P.U. (2003) *Huangdi Nei Jing Su Wen*. Oakland, CA: University of California Press.

Unschuld, P.U. (2016) *Huangdi Nei Jing Ling Shu*. Oakland, CA: University of California Press.

Unschuld, P.U. (2016) *Huangdi Nei Jing Nan Jing*. Oakland, CA: University of California Press.

Weixin, J. (1999) *Diagnosis of Sterility and Its Traditional Chinese Medical Treatment*. Shandong: Shandong Science and Technology Press.

Zhanjiang Dou (2008) 'Eight TCM treatment methods for male infertility caused by sperm disorders.' *Journal of the Association of Traditional Chinese Medicine* 15, 2.

Figure Sources

Acknowledgements

This book would have never been possible without the help of two of the world's most fantastic men: Sandro Graca and my father, Wolfgang Pojer. Thank you both from the bottom of my heart for all your support, the proof reading of every single chapter and for always cheering me up in difficult times! You are the secret heroes of this book!

Thanks to Sandra Lemp-Dorfer and Simon Becker for helping me with the very important herbal chapters. Special thanks to my brother-in-law Patrick Böcker for bringing Sam the Sperm and his friends to life, what a masterstroke! Thank you to Roland Geyer for creating brilliant charts and drawings and, of course, Kali MacIsaac and Michael Weber for their fantastic contributing chapters.

I am grateful to my 'work-wife' Ursula Ritz for being such an amazing friend and brave colleague in realizing our dream by founding our integrative fertility clinic Femme&Fertile. Special thanks to my favourite andrologist Markus Margreiter for being so open-minded and innovative and inviting me to collaborate and work in his Men's health clinic in Vienna.

Thank you to Claire Wilson from Singing Dragon for asking me to write this book and going on that journey with me.

My dearest thanks to Jane Lyttleton (my TCM fertility goddess) and Ashok Agarwar (my andrology hero) for writing the forewords, this meant the world to me.

Finally, thanks to that one special man for always having an open ear, grounding and calming me.

Subject Index

Sub-headings in *italics* indicate figures.

Author Index